T0201422

Polycystic Ovary Syndrome

Polycystic Ovary Syndrome

Edited by

Gabor T. Kovacs
Monash University, Melbourne, Australia

Bart C. J. M. Fauser
University Medical Center, Utrecht, Netherlands

Richard S. Legro
Penn State Medical Center, Hershey, PA, USA

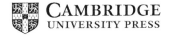

CAMBRIDGE
UNIVERSITY PRESS

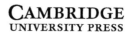

University Printing House, Cambridge CB2 8BS, United Kingdom

One Liberty Plaza, 20th Floor, New York, NY 10006, USA

477 Williamstown Road, Port Melbourne, VIC 3207, Australia

314–321, 3rd Floor, Plot 3, Splendor Forum, Jasola District Centre, New Delhi – 110025, India

103 Penang Road, #05–06/07, Visioncrest Commercial, Singapore 238467

Cambridge University Press is part of the University of Cambridge.

It furthers the University's mission by disseminating knowledge in the pursuit of education, learning, and research at the highest international levels of excellence.

www.cambridge.org
Information on this title: www.cambridge.org/9781108839334
DOI: 10.1017/9781108989831

© Cambridge University Press 2007, 2022

This publication is in copyright. Subject to statutory exception and to the provisions of relevant collective licensing agreements, no reproduction of any part may take place without the written permission of Cambridge University Press.

First published 2002
Second edition 2007
Third edition 2022

Printed in the United Kingdom by TJ Books Limited, Padstow Cornwall

A catalogue record for this publication is available from the British Library.

Library of Congress Cataloging-in-Publication Data
Names: Kovacs, Gabor, 1947 April 6– editor. | Fauser, B. C. J. M. (Bart C. J. M.), editor. | Legro, Richard S., 1957– editor.
Title: Polycystic ovary syndrome / edited by Gabor T. Kovacs, Bart Fauser, Richard S. Legro.
Other titles: Polycystic ovary syndrome (Kovacs)
Description: Third edition. | Cambridge ; New York, NY : Cambridge University Press, 2022. | Preceded by Polycystic ovary syndrome / edited by Gabor T. Kovacs, Robert Norman. 2nd ed. 2007. | Includes bibliographical references and index.
Identifiers: LCCN 2021024021 (print) | LCCN 2021024022 (ebook) | ISBN 9781108839334 (hardback) | ISBN 9781108989831 (ebook)
Subjects: MESH: Polycystic Ovary Syndrome
Classification: LCC RG480.S7 (print) | LCC RG480.S7 (ebook) | NLM WP 320 | DDC 618.1/1–dc23
LC record available at https://lccn.loc.gov/2021024021
LC ebook record available at https://lccn.loc.gov/2021024022

ISBN 978-1-108-83933-4 Hardback

Cambridge University Press has no responsibility for the persistence or accuracy of URLs for external or third-party internet websites referred to in this publication and does not guarantee that any content on such websites is, or will remain, accurate or appropriate.

Every effort has been made in preparing this book to provide accurate and up-to-date information that is in accord with accepted standards and practice at the time of publication. Although case histories are drawn from actual cases, every effort has been made to disguise the identities of the individuals involved. Nevertheless, the authors, editors, and publishers can make no warranties that the information contained herein is totally free from error, not least because clinical standards are constantly changing through research and regulation. The authors, editors, and publishers therefore disclaim all liability for direct or consequential damages resulting from the use of material contained in this book. Readers are strongly advised to pay careful attention to information provided by the manufacturer of any drugs or equipment that they plan to use.

Contents

Contributors

Adam Balen MBBS, MD, DSc, FRCOG, Professor of Reproductive Medicine and Surgery, Leeds Teaching Hospitals, Leeds, UK

Martina Capuzzo Department of Medical and Surgical Sciences for Mother, Child and Adult, University of Modena and Reggio Emilia, Modena, Italy Clinica EUGIN, Modena, Italy

Ozlem Celik Division of Endocrinology and Metabolism, Department of Internal Medicine, Acibadem University School of Medicine, Istanbul, Turkey

Anuja Dokras MD, PhD, Professor of Obstetrics and Gynecology Director, Penn Polycystic Ovary Syndrome Center; Medical Director, Hospital of the University of Pennsylvania Reproductive Surgical Facility; The Perelman School of Medicine of the University of Pennsylvania, Philadelphia, PA, USA

Bart C. J. M. Fauser MD, PhD, Emeritus Professor of Reproductive Medicine, University of Utrecht, Utrecht, the Netherlands

Stephen Franks FRCP, MD, FMedSci, Institute of Reproductive and Developmental Biology, Imperial College London, Hammersmith Hospital, London, UK

Harry Frydenberg AM, FRACS, Director, Surgeon, Epworth Centre for Bariatric Surgery Richmond, Victoria, Australia

Rhonda Garad PhD, Senior Lecturer and Research Fellow, Monash Centre for Health Research and Implementation, Monash University

Rhonda Garad PhD, MPH, RN Div.1 Monash Centre for Health Research and Implementation, Mona, Monash University, Victoria, Australia

Paul Hardiman MBBS MD FRCOG Associate Professor Institute for Women's Health, University College London Honorary Consultant in Obstetrics and Gynaecology, Royal Free and Whittington Hospitals London

Roger J. Hart MBBS, MD, FRANZCOG, FRCOG CREI, Division of Obstetrics and Gynaecology, University of Western Australia, Perth, Western Australia; Fertility Specialists of Western Australia, Bethesda Hospital, Claremont, Western Australia; King Edward Memorial Hospital

Roy Homburg FRCOG, Homerton University Hospital NHS Trust, London, UK

Susie Jacob MBBS, MD, MRCOG, Consultant in Reproductive Medicine, Calderdale and Huddersfield NHS Foundation Trust, UK

Femi Janse MD, PhD, Department of Reproductive Medicine and Gynecology, University Medical Center Utrecht, University of Utrecht, the Netherlands

Eleni A. Kandaraki MD, PhD, MRCPUK, European University Cyprus, Nicosia, Cyprus Hygeia Hospital, Athens, Greece

Gabor T. Kovacs AM, MD, FRANZCOG, FRCOG, CREI, Grad Dip Mgt, FAICD, Professor of Obstetrics and Gynaecology, Monash University, Melbourne, Australia

Antonio La Marca Professor, Obstetrics, Gynecology and Reproductive Medicine University of Modena and Reggio Emilia Policlinico di Modena, Italy

Sabra Lane BA, President, National Press Club of Australia, Canberra Presenter, AM program, Australian Broadcasting Commission

Joop S. E. Laven Division Reproductive Endocrinology and Infertility, Department of Obstetrics and Gynaecology, Erasmus University Medical Center, Rotterdam, the Netherlands

Siew Lim PhD, MND, BSc (Biomedical), Monash Centre for Health Research and Implementation, Monash Public Health and Preventive Medicine, Monash University, and Monash Health, Melbourne, Victoria, Australia

Yvonne V. Louwers Division Reproductive Endocrinology and Infertility, Department of Obstetrics and Gynaecology, Erasmus University Medical Center, Rotterdam, the Netherlands

Marla E. Lujan PhD, MS, Division of Nutritional Sciences, Cornell University, Ithaca, NY, USA

Lisa Moran PhD, BND, BSc (Hons), G Dip Pub Health, Monash Centre for Health Research and Implementation, Monash Public Health and Preventive Medicine, Monash University, and Monash Health, Melbourne, Victoria, Australia

Robert J. Norman AO, MD, FRANZCOG, FRCPA, CREI, FAHMS, GAICD, Professor of Reproductive and Periconceptual Medicine, Robinson Research Institute; Professor of Women's Health at the Monash Centre for Health Research and Implementation MCHRI, Monash University; Consultant and Subspecialist in Reproductive Endocrinology and Infertility, Fertility SA, Royal Adelaide Hospital, Adelaide, Australia

Lisa Owens MB, BCh, BAO, MRCPI, PhD, Consultant Physician & Endocrinologist St James's Hospital, Dublin, Ireland; Clinical Senior Lecturer in Medicine, Trinity College Dublin, Ireland and Honorary Senior Lecturer, Imperial College London, UK

Olga Papalou MD, PhD, Hygeia Hospital, Athens, Greece

Claudia Raperport MRCOG, PGCert (MedEd), BMBS, BMedSCi, Homerton University Hospital NHS Trust, London, UK

Larisa Suturina MD, PhD, Head of the Department of Reproductive Health Protection, Scientific Center for Family Health and Human Reproduction Problems, Irkutsk, Russian Federation

Helena Teede MBBS, FRACP, PhD, FAAHMS, Executive Director Monash Partners Academic Health Research Translation Centre, Director Monash Centre for Health Research and Implementation, Monash University, Endocrinologist Monash Health, Melbourne, Victoria, Australia

Evert J. P. van Santbrink MD, PhD, Department of Reproductive Medicine, Reinier de Graaf Group, the Netherlands

Heidi Vanden Brink PhD, MS, RDMS, Division of Nutritional Sciences, Cornell University, Ithaca, NY, USA

Melanie Walls BSc, BMedSci, PhD, Division of Obstetrics and Gynaecology, University of Western Australia, Perth, Western Australia; Fertility Specialists of Western Australia, Bethesda Hospital, Claremont, Western Australia; School of Medical and Health Sciences, Edith Cowan University, Joondalup, Western Australia

Bülent Okan Yildiz MD, Professor of Medicine and Endocrinology, Hacettepe University School of Medicine, Department of Internal Medicine Division of Endocrinology and Metabolism, Ankara, Turkey

Introduction to and History of Polycystic Ovary Syndrome

Gabor T. Kovacs

Although the modern history of polycystic ovary syndrome (PCOS) started with the pivotal paper by Stein and Leventhal in 1935,[1] there are suggestions that the "syndrome" was referred to as early as in the time of Hippocrates (ca. 460–377 BC). Medical notes at the time referred to women "whose menstruation is less than three days or is meager, are robust, with a healthy complexion and a masculine appearance; yet they are not concerned about bearing children nor do they become pregnant" and suggest that they may have been describing women with PCOS.[2]

It has also been recorded that Soranus of Ephesus (ca. AD 98–138) described some women "who did not menstruate at all, whose bodies are of a masculine type . . . we observe that the majority of those not menstruating are rather robust, like mannish and sterile women." More recent accounts of women who probably had PCOS are given by Maimonides (1135–1204): "there are women whose skin is dry and hard, and whose nature resembles the nature of a man. However, if any woman's nature tends to be transformed to the nature of a man, this does not arise from medications, but is caused by heavy menstrual activity"; and by the sixteenth-century obstetrician and surgeon Ambroise Paré (1510–1590), who observed: "Many women, when their flowers or tearmes be stopped, degenerate after a manner into a certaine manly nature, whence they are called Viragines, that is to say stout, or manly women; therefore their voice is loud and bigger, like unto a mans, and they become bearded."

All these observations fit the symptomatology of PCOS – menstrual irregularity, subfertility, masculine features and obesity. However, it was the 1934 presentation and subsequent publication by Irving Stein and Michael Leventhal that identified this condition as a reproductive disorder and proposed an effective treatment – bilateral ovarian wedge resection (BOWR) – for the associated subfertility.[1]

Irving Stein was born in Chicago on September 19, 1887, the seventh of ten children, to Adolf Stein and Emma Freiler. Stein initially completed a science degree at the University of Michigan and subsequently obtained a medical degree from Rush Medical College in Chicago in 1912. After a two-year internship at Michael Reese Hospital in Chicago, he joined the hospital's obstetrics and gynecology department as an assistant in surgery, focusing on women's reproductive health and obstetrics and reaching "attending physician" status by 1915. He married Lucile Oberfelder in 1921, and they had two children, a son, Irving F. Stein Junior, and a daughter, Eleanor H. Rusnak. Stein was also a professor at Northwestern University and established a private practice at Highland Park Hospital, Illinois.[3]

Stein was known as a warm and caring doctor as well as a dignified and respected teacher, often found with a large group of fellow doctors and nurses following him while he did his rounds. One of his colleagues, Melvin Cohen, stated that "Stein was meticulous in everything he did, including patient care, surgery, and even his appearance, as Stein often wore a boutonniere to the hospital."

Michael Leventhal joined Stein at the Michael Reese Hospital in 1926, where they collaborated on research into "sterility in women." Michael Leo Leventhal was also born in Chicago and graduated from Rush Medical College, but 12 years after Stein (1924). Apart from military service as a medical officer in the US Army, he spent his entire career working at the Michael Reese Hospital.

Before Leventhal, Stein was working with Robert Arens studying ovarian abnormalities and developed a method for imaging the reproductive organs by injecting carbon dioxide into the pelvis and iodized oil into the fallopian tubes, combined with X-ray examination. This enabled measuring the dimensions of the ovaries and the patency of the tubes. It was through using this technology

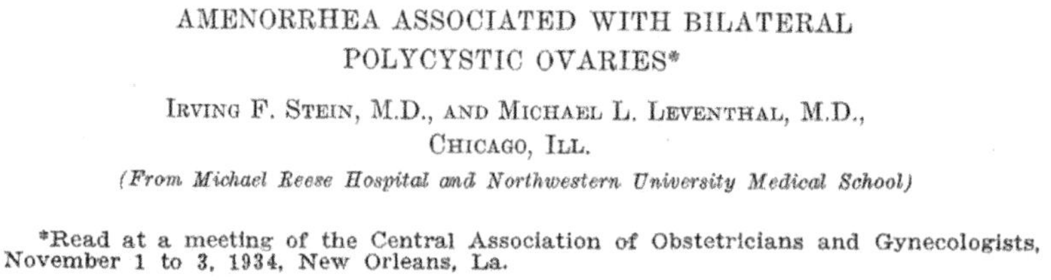

AMENORRHEA ASSOCIATED WITH BILATERAL
POLYCYSTIC OVARIES*

IRVING F. STEIN, M.D., AND MICHAEL L. LEVENTHAL, M.D.,
CHICAGO, ILL.

(From Michael Reese Hospital and Northwestern University Medical School)

*Read at a meeting of the Central Association of Obstetricians and Gynecologists,
November 1 to 3, 1934, New Orleans, La.

Figure 1.1 The Stein and Leventhal paper of 1935

that Stein was able to observe a group of women with abnormally large ovaries – two to four times the normal size – who became the subject of Stein and Leventhal's seminal 1935 paper.

In an article commemorating the 80th anniversary of Stein and Leventhal's original publication, Ricardo Azziz and Eli Adashi wrote that the research, "although not flawless, was both seminal and transformative."[4] They pointed out that not only was the Stein and Leventhal paper the first report of a case series but it also described a possible therapy, BOWR. Azziz and Adashi concluded that "we have much to celebrate, as we commemorate the 80th anniversary of the publication of the report by Stein and Leventhal in 1935, for a new disorder was described, one that we know today affects, in its various forms, 1 in every 7–17 women worldwide." We will therefore look at the 1935 paper in detail. The title and details of this paper are shown in Figure 1.1.

In their paper, they commence by commenting that bilateral polycystic ovaries are usually described in association with uterine bleeding and endometrial hyperplasia, but no mention is made of bilateral polycystic ovaries and amenorrhea. They then describe a series of patients with ovaries enlarged up to four times the normal size, associated with absent menses. They described the cortex as hypertrophied and the tunica as tough fibrotic and thickened. The cysts were follicular, contained clear fluid and were confined to the surface of the cortex, numbering from 20 to 100 in each ovary. On section, the ovary was "oyster grey" with corpora lutea rarely found, and if present they were small and deeply placed. They described the uteri as either normal sized or smaller and firmer than normal. They also reported masculinizing changes in some patients, with rhomboid escutcheon and hirsutism on the arms, legs and face. The external genitalia were

reported as normal in most, but some showed hypertrophied labia minora and clitoris.

They then described seven women with PCOS, all amenorrheic, who underwent bilateral wedge resection of the ovaries, all of whom reported a regular 28-day cycle postoperatively, with one woman (their first patient) conceiving two children. Stein and Leventhal recommended that diagnosis should include pneumo-roentgenography as pelvic examination of ovarian size was not reliable. Their reference for normal size of the ovary was "about one fourth the size of the uterine corpus." They also discussed the etiology of this condition and disputed the previous hypothesis that it was the result of an inflammatory process, as there was never any evidence of adhesions that one would expect if it was due to infection. They postulated an endocrine causal relationship.

In summary, they concluded that the treatment of PCOS by estrogenic hormone was unsatisfactory, whereas surgical wedge resection was successful in restoring physiologic function – menstruation – with pregnancies in two out of seven patients. A recurrence of polycystic change in the ovary was not found in the follow-up of any of these women. With respect to the pathophysiology of PCOS, they believed that mechanical overcrowding of the cortex by cysts interferes with the progress of normal Graafian follicle to the surface of the ovary.

By 1964, Stein had expanded his experience and reported on a successful series of 108 women treated by "wedge resection."[5] Consequently, BOWR became the standard treatment for anovulation associated with PCOS. An example of the efficacy and widespread acceptance of BOWR as a treatment for PCOS-associated anovulation came from Sweden, where Lunde and colleagues reported on 149 women with polycystic ovarian syndrome (PCOS), who were treated at a university teaching hospital 15–25 years after ovarian wedge resection (BOWR) and studied three times by means of a questionnaire.[6] Life-table analysis showed a cumulative rate of spontaneous pregnancies of 76%, increasing to 88% when induced pregnancies were included, with a cumulated live birth rate of 78% and with a regular menstrual pattern restored up to 25 years after BOWR.

When less invasive alternatives for the treatment of anovulation using oral clomiphene citrate and injectable follicle-stimulating hormone (FSH) preparations became available in the 1960s, the popularity of BOWR waned.[7, 8] Furthermore, evidence emerged that BWRO could be followed by periovarian/peritubal scarring, which had its own negative effect on fertility. Toaff and colleagues reported in 1976 that all seven patients who underwent laparoscopy subsequent to BOWR had extensive periovarian and peritubal adhesions.[9] They concluded that "our observations support the plea to relegate the surgical approach to a minor position in patients with Stein-Leventhal syndrome." The current status of surgical management of PCOS is discussed in detail in Chapter 12.

The Historical Development of Diagnostic Criteria for PCOS

Ovarian Enlargement/Appearance

In the time of Stein and Leventhal, PCOS was diagnosed on a history of irregular menses associated with some androgenization in the presence of enlarged ovaries. Ovarian enlargement was diagnosed by palpation, which is very subjective especially in obese women (as many PCOS patients are). Stein improved the diagnostic accuracy by introducing pneumo-roentgenography as in his 1935 report. As BOWR became popular, histological features of hypertrophied ovarian cortex with thickened fibrotic tunica became the criteria for diagnosis.[10]

Hormonal Assays

The next diagnostic criteria evolved with the availability of radioimmunoassay during the 1970s, and PCOS was diagnosed on the basis of elevated levels of luteinizing hormone (LH) and raised testosterone (T).[11] The limitations of using hormonal criteria include the imprecise nature of assays, the variability in hormone levels and the pulsatile

manner of gonadotropin secretions. To improve preciseness not only absolute levels but ratios of LH:FSH between 2:1 and 3:1 were suggested as a diagnostic criterion. Nevertheless, many women had clinical symptoms of PCOS who did not fulfill the endocrine criteria.

Ultrasound Appearance

With the development of noninvasive visualization of the ovaries using ultrasonic scanning, it was possible to easily and reliably count ovarian follicles as well as measure ovarian and follicular size. In addition, the sclerotic stroma could also be identified. The first description of polycystic ovaries visualized on ultrasound came from Swanson and colleagues.[12] Both laparoscopic and histologic comparisons showed excellent correlations with ultrasonic examination. Adams and colleagues defined an ovary as polycystic if "there were multiple cysts (10 or more) 2–8 mm in diameter arranged either peripherally around a dense core of stroma or scattered throughout an increased amount of stroma."[13] This became the basis of the diagnosis of polycystic ovaries (PCO) in what is known as the "Rotterdam criteria."[14]

It also became apparent that many more women had PCO, now called polycystic ovarian morphology (PCOM), than those who had the syndrome (PCOS). Women could be separated into those with PCO appearance on ultrasound and those who had associated symptoms of oligo/amenorrhea and/or hyperandrogenism (PCOS). In population studies, it appeared that about half of the women with PCO developed PCOS sometime during their lifetime.[15]

Anti-Müllerian Hormone (AMH) Levels

It has been recognized for nearly two decades that anti-Müllerian hormone (AMH) is produced by the granulosa cells of pre-antral and small antral ovarian follicles.[16] Consequently, there is a correlation between the antral follicle count (AFC) and AMH levels, and it is hoped that the measurement of AMH will be a diagnostic tool for the presence of PCOM. Unfortunately, owing to the heterogeneity of the AFC and AMH levels, it should not yet be used for the diagnosis of PCOM. It is hoped that with improved and better standardized assays, as well as large-scale validation studies, the threshold level of AMH to diagnose PCOM may be established.[17]

From Ovarian Pathology of Stein-Leventhal Syndrome to a Multisystem Endocrine Disease

Stein-Leventhal syndrome was a recognized disorder for more than five decades until the focus shifted to it being a "metabolic multisystem syndrome." In 1990, an expert conference was sponsored by the National Institute of Child Health and Human Development (NICHD) of the National Institutes of Health (NIH). The expert group concluded that diagnostic criteria should include (in order of importance):

> 1. hyperandrogenism and/or hyperandrogenemia,
> 2. menstrual dysfunction with the exclusion of other known disorders.[18]

The subsequent discovery that many women with PCOS are insulin-resistant with compensatory hyperinsulinemia designated this condition as a reproductive-metabolic disorder, with broader implications than those defined by the NIH in 1990.

To arrive at an international agreement on the diagnostic criteria, and to define the clinical implications of PCOS, a consensus conference chaired by Basil Tarlatzis (Greece) and Bart Fauser (Netherlands) was held on May 1–3, 2003, in Rotterdam, the Netherlands.[14] A scientific committee consisting of Jeff Chang (USA), Ricardo Azziz (USA), Rick Legro (USA), Didier Dewailly (France), Steve Franks (UK), Basil Tarlatzis (Greece) and Bart Fauser (Netherlands) was established. Also invited were a number of international experts as discussants: Adam Balen (UK), Phillipe Bouchard (France), Eva Dahlgren (Sweden), Luigi Devoto (Chile), Evita Diamanti (Greece), Andrea Dunaif (USA), Marco Filicori (Italy), Roy Homburg (Israel), Lourdes Ibanez (Spain), Joop Laven (Netherlands), Dennis Magoffin (USA), John Nestler (USA), Rob Norman (Australia), Renato Pasquali (Italy), Michel Pugeat (France), Jerome Strauss (USA), Seang Lin Tan (Canada), Anne Taylor (USA), Robert Wild (USA) and Sarah Wild (UK). This symposium was financially sponsored by an unconditional grant from NV Organon and by the European Society of Human Reproduction (ESHRE) and the American Society for Reproductive Medicine (ASRM). They concluded that PCOS is a syndrome of ovarian dysfunction along with the cardinal features of hyperandrogenism and PCO morphology. A finding of at least 12 follicles in one ovary, or an ovarian volume of 10 cc, was considered the ultrasonic diagnostic criterion for PCO. They agreed that clinical manifestations may include menstrual irregularities, signs of androgen excess and obesity. They noted that insulin resistance and elevated serum LH levels were also common features in PCOS, and PCOS was associated with an increased risk of type 2 diabetes and cardiovascular events.[14]

Although the Rotterdam Conference concentrated on a definition for diagnosis, there was a need for consensus on which treatments should be offered. To define appropriate therapeutic guidelines another consensus conference was organized on March 2–3, 2007, in Thessaloniki, Greece. The experts invited included Basil Tarlatzis (Greece), Bart Fauser (Netherlands), Rick Legro (USA), Rob Norman (Australia), Kathleen Hoeger (USA), Renato Pasquali (Italy), Steve Franks (UK), Ioannis Messinis (Greece), Robert Casper (Canada), Roy Homburg (Israel), Rick Lobo (USA), Robert Rebar (USA), Richard Fleming (UK), B. R. Carr (USA), Phillipe Bouchard (France), J. Chang (USA), J. N. Hugues (France), R. Azziz (USA), Efstratios Kolibianakis (Greece), George Griesinger (Germany), Klaus Diedrich (Germany), Adam Balen (UK), Cindy Farquhar (New Zealand), Paul Devroey (Belgium), Pak Chung Ho (Hong Kong), John Collins (Canada), Dimitrios Goulis (Greece), René Eijkemans (Netherlands), Piergiorgio Crosignani (Italy), Alan DeCherney (USA) and Andre van Steirteghem (Belgium). This symposium was also supported by an unconditional grant from NV Organon and by ESHRE and ASRM.

A number of interventions were reviewed and recommendations were made including lifestyle modifications (diet and exercise), administration of pharmaceutical agents such as clomiphene citrate (CC), insulin-sensitizing agents, gonadotropins and gonadotropin-releasing hormone (GnRH) analogues, the use of laparoscopic ovarian drilling and the application of assisted reproductive techniques (ART).[19]

A third consensus conference was held in 2011 in Amsterdam to summarize the then current knowledge and to identify knowledge gaps regarding various women's health aspects of PCOS.[20] Topics addressed included PCOS in adolescence, the symptoms of hirsutism and acne, contraceptive options, menstrual cycle abnormalities, quality of life, ethnicity, pregnancy complications, long-term metabolic and cardiovascular health and, finally, cancer risk. Participants included Bart Fauser (Netherlands), Basil Tarlatzis (Greece), Robert Rebar (USA), Rick Legro (USA), Adam Balen (UK), Rick Lobo (USA), E. Carmina (Sicily), Jeff Chang (USA), Bulent Yildiz (Turkey), Joop Laven (Netherlands), J. Boivin (UK), F. Petraglia (Italy), C. N. Wijeyeratne (Sri Lanka), Rob Norman (Australia), Andrea Dunaif (USA), Steve Franks (UK), Robert Wild (USA), Daniel Dumesic (USA) and Kurt Barnhart (USA). For each aspect, the consensus committee published concluding statements (where there was agreement), a summary of areas of disagreement (if any) and knowledge gaps with recommended directions for future research.

Simultaneously, in Australia, the Australian government's Department of Health and Ageing funded a Guideline Development Group, chaired by Helena Teede. The Department of Health recognized that PCOS has potential for major metabolic consequences, including obesity and type 2 diabetes mellitus (DM2) as well as cardiovascular disease (CVD), all of which were national health priority areas. The recommendations of the group were published as a supplement to the *Medical Journal of Australia* in 2011.[21]

A European approach to define the criteria required for the diagnosis of PCO emphasized the phenotypic heterogeneity of the syndrome. [22] The group focused on the impact of metabolic issues, specifically insulin resistance and obesity, and the susceptibility to develop earlier than expected glucose intolerance states, including type 2 diabetes. They concentrated on an endocrine and European perspective in the debate on the definition of PCOS listed as etiological factors, such as early life events, potentially involved in the development of the disorder. They placed an emphasis on the laboratory evaluation of androgens and other potential biomarkers of ovarian and metabolic dysfunctions. They considered the role of obesity, sleep disorders and neuropsychological aspects of PCOS as well as the relevant pathogenetic aspects of cardiovascular risk factors. They also discussed how to target

treatment choices according to the phenotype and individual patient's needs.

In November 2015, the American Association of Clinical Endocrinologists (AACE), the American College of Endocrinology (ACE), and the Androgen Excess and PCOS Society (AE-PCOS) released new guidelines in the evaluation and treatment of PCOS. They recommended that diagnosis be based on the presence of at least two of the following three criteria: chronic anovulation, hyperandrogenism (clinical or biological) and PCO. They stated that free T levels are more sensitive than the measurement of total T and that the value of measuring levels of androgens other than T in patients with PCOS is relatively low. With respect to imaging, new ultrasound machines allow a threshold for diagnosis of PCOM in patients having at least 25 small follicles (2–9 mm) in the whole ovary, and ovarian size greater than 10 mL should be considered increased ovarian size. They felt that AMH was useful for diagnosis of PCOS.

They recommended that management of women with PCOS should include reproductive function, as well as the care of hirsutism, alopecia and acne. They also recognized the increased prevalence of endometrial hyperplasia and endometrial cancer. They highlighted that, in PCOS, hirsutism develops gradually and intensifies with weight gain and that girls with severe acne may have a 40% likelihood of developing PCOS. It was also pointed out that oral contraceptives can effectively lower androgens. They further warned against diagnosis in the first few years after menarche, as many features of PCOS, including acne, menstrual irregularities and hyperinsulinemia, are common in normal puberty.[23]

The Australian group was important, as it was the catalyst for the formation of the International PCOS Network driven by Helena Teede and Rob Norman, who then undertook the development of international evidence-based guidelines on the assessment and management of polycystic ovary syndrome. Funding for the group came principally from the Australian National Health and Medical Research Council (NHMRC) through the funded Centre for Research Excellence in Polycystic Ovary Syndrome (CREPCOS) as well as from ESHRE and ASRM.

The International Advisory Panel (representatives from six continents) was chaired by Bart Fauser (Netherlands), the deputy chair Rob

Norman (Australia) and included JuhaTapanainen (Finland), Zephne van der Spuy (South Africa), Duru Shah (Inida), Rick Legro (USA), Frank Broekmans (Germany), Anuja Dokras (USA), Marie Misso (Austalia), Chir Ruey Tzeng (Taiwan), Jie Qiao (China) and Poli Mara Spritzer (Brazil).

The International PCOS Network was able to collaborate and engage with 37 organizations (including consumers) across 71 countries and organized 23 face-to-face international meetings over 15 months. The various groups involved more than 3000 health professionals and consumers internationally.[17] These international evidence-based guidelines included the assessment and management of PCOS and were designed to provide clear information to assist clinical decision-making and support optimal patient care. Addressing psychological, metabolic and reproductive features of PCOS, there were 60 prioritized clinical questions involving 40 systematic and 20 narrative reviews, generating 166 recommendations and practice points. This is discussed in detail in Chapter 5.

How Has PCOS Survived Natural Selection?

The inheritance of PCO/PCOS is still poorly understood and is discussed in detail in Chapter 2. However, there is consensus that there is some genetic hereditary factor. One may then ask, how did these series of symptoms, which have a reproductive handicap (subfertility, cardiac disease, diabetes), survive natural selection?

If we go back to the hunter-gatherer existence, while the phenotype of PCOS had a reproductive disadvantage, being a female with the greatest capacity for the energy storage necessary to endure prolonged episodes of starvation, the so-called thrifty genotype, was an advantage, as women with PCOS were able to survive during periods of food deprivation. Furthermore, insulin resistance that diminishes energy expenditure in times of famine was an additional evolutionary advantage. Also, despite a community belief that women with PCOS are sterile, they are certainly not but they do have lower fertility. Consequently, in the absence of contraception, they will have lower fecundity and therefore have longer spacing between pregnancies, which would have resulted in better maternal health. Birth-associated

mortality was also high, so that having fewer pregnancies and births was also an advantage. For women who were nomadic hunters, having fewer children made it easier for them to be transported and, additionally, there were fewer mouths to feed. With delayed fecundity and aging parturition, PCOS women may have attained significant nurturing skills, given their wisdom and strength in surviving a physically demanding environment. They also created an environment suitable for child-rearing as it was not focused on or threatened by pregnancy.

At the individual level, the greater lean muscle mass and bone mineral density of women with PCOS would have been advantageous to their own survival and that of their progeny. It could therefore be argued that PCOS favored the survival of those family units containing women with PCOS.

With a change to human settlement in communities that underwent a shift to agricultural farming and animal husbandry, with sufficient food becoming available, there was a need to have several children in order to provide a rural workforce, therefore PCOS should have become a teleological disadvantage. However, for PCOS women, even in sedentary agricultural societies, they could still conceive, albeit at a rate lower than normal, and they may have had lower maternal mortality and would have been sturdier than average. Even for agricultural societies during the eighteenth and nineteenth centuries, significant periodic famines remained a fact of life for which women with PCOS were better suited to survive.

Considering the male genetically related relatives of PCOS women, they may have symptoms and signs of androgen excess and insulin resistance but neither their ability to attract partners nor their fertility has been shown to be impaired, and, as discussed, they also carry the metabolic advantage of being able to survive famine. All these factors seem to have potentially counterbalanced any disadvantages arising from the overall lower number of children conceived by PCOS women and explain why the condition has not been teleologically genetically eliminated.

We still have a lot to learn about PCO(M)/PCOS, especially about its etiology and pathogenesis. Long-term studies, or "big data" analysis, may answer some of these questions. Certainly, this introductory chapter on the history of PCOS will need to be updated for the fourth edition of *Polycystic Ovary Syndrome*.

References

1 Stein, I. F. and Leventhal, M. L. Amenorrhoea associated with bilateral polycystic ovaries. *Am J Obstet Gynecol* 1935; 29(2): 181–191.

2 Azziz, R. Dumesic, D. A. and Goodarzi, M. O. Polycystic ovary syndrome: An ancient disorder? *Fertil Steril* 2011; 95(5): 1544–1548.

3 Darby, A. Irving Freiler Stein Sr. (1887–1976). *Embryo Project Encyclopedia*, July 20, 2017. http://embryo.asu.edu/handle/10776/12956

4 Azziz, R. and Adashi, E. Y. Stein and Leventhal: 80 years on. *Am J Obstet Gynecol* 2016; (214) 2: 247.

5 Stein, I. F. Duration of fertility following ovarian wedge resection: Stein-Leventhal syndrome. *West J Surg Obstet Gynecol* 1964; 72: 237–242.

6 Lunde, O., Djoseland, O. and Grottum, P. Polycystic ovarian syndrome: A follow-up study on fertility and menstrual pattern in 149 patients 15–25 years after ovarian wedge resection. *Hum Reprod* 2001; 16(7): 1479–1485.

7 Greenblatt, R. B., Barfield, W. E. and Jungck, E. C. Induction of ovulation with MRL/41: Preliminary report. *JAMA* 1961; 178: 101–104.

8 Gemzell, C. A., Diczfalusy, E. and Tillinger, G. Clinical effect of human pituitary follicle-stimulating hormone (FSH). *J Clin Endocrinol Metab* 1958; 18(12): 1333–1348.

9 Toaff, R., Toaff, M. E., Peyser and M. R. Infertility following wedge resection of the ovaries. *Am J Obstet Gynecol* 1976; 124(1): 92–96.

10 Goldzieher, J. W. and Green, J. A. The polycystic ovary: I. Clinical and histological features. *J Clin Endocrinol Metab* 1962; 22: 325–328.

11 Yen, S. S. C., Vela, P. and Rankin, J. Inappropriate secretion of follicle-stimulating hormone and luteinizing hormone in polycystic ovarian disease. *J Clin Endocrinol Metab* 1970; 30: 442.

12 Swanson, M., Sauerbrei, E. E. and Cooperberg, P. L. Medical implications of ultrasonically detected polycystic ovaries. *J Clin Ultrasound* 1981; 9(5): 219–222.

13 Adams, J., Polson, D. W. and Franks, S. Prevalence of polycystic ovaries in women with anovulation and idiopathic hirsutism. *Br Med J* 1986; 293 (6543): 355–359.

14 The Rotterdam ESHRE/ASRM-Sponsored PCOS Consensus Workshop Group. Revised 2003 consensus on diagnostic criteria and long-term health risks related to polycystic ovary syndrome (PCOS). *Hum Reprod* 2004; 19(1): 41–47.

15 Lowe, P., Kovacs, G. and Howlett, D. Incidence of polycystic ovaries and polycystic ovary syndrome amongst women in Melbourne, Australia. *Aust N Z J Obstet Gynaecol* 45(1): 17–19.

16 Cook, C. L. et al. Relationship between serum müllerian-inhibiting substance and other reproductive hormones in untreated women with polycystic ovary syndrome and normal women. *Fertil Steril* 2002; 77(1): 141–146.

17 Teede, H., Misso, M. , Costello, M. et al. *International Evidence-Based Guideline for the Assessment and Management of Polycystic Ovary Syndrome.* Melbourne: Monash University and NHMRC, Centre for Research Excellence in PCOS and the Australian PCOS Alliance, 2018.

18 Zawadski, J. K. and Dunaif, A. Diagnostic criteria for polycystic ovary syndrome: Towards a rational approach. In A. Dunaif, J. R. Givens, F. P. Haseltine and G. R. Merriam, eds. *Polycystic Ovary Syndrome.* Boston, MA: Blackwell Scientific Publications, 1992: 377–384.

19 The Thessaloniki ESHRE/ASRM-Sponsored PCOS Consensus Workshop Group. Consensus on infertility treatment related to polycystic ovary syndrome. Fertil Steril 2008; 89(3): 505–522.

20 The Amsterdam ESHRE/ASRM-Sponsored 3rd PCOS Consensus Workshop Group. Consensus on women's health aspects of polycystic ovary syndrome (PCOS). *Hum Reprod* 2011; 27(1): 14–24.

21 Teede, H., Misso, M. L., Deeks, A. A. et al. Assessment and management of polycystic ovary syndrome: summary of an evidence-based guideline. *Med J Aust* 2011; 195(6): S65.

22 Conway, G., Dewailly, D., Diamanti-Kandarakis, E. et al. The polycystic ovary syndrome: A position statement from the European Society of Endocrinology. *Eur J Endocrinol* 2014; 171: P1–29.

23 Goodman, N. F., Cobin, R. H., Futterweit, W. et al. American Association of Clinical Endocrinologists, American College of Endocrinology, and Androgen Excess and PCOS Society disease state clinical review: Guide to the best practices in the evaluation and treatment of polycystic ovary syndrome–part 1. *Endocr Pract* 1915; 21(11): 1291–1300.

Polycystic Ovary Syndrome: From Phenotype to Genotype

Joop S. E. Laven and Yvonne V. Louwers

Introduction

Polycystic ovary syndrome (PCOS) is the most common endocrine disorder in women and is characterized by ovulatory dysfunction, hyperandrogenism and polycystic ovaries. Ovulatory dysfunction is generally associated with anovulation, leading to irregular menstrual bleeding. Hyperandrogenism could manifest itself either clinically, through hirsutism, or biochemically, through elevated serum levels of (free) androgens. Finally, polycystic ovaries are defined according to their typical morphology on ultrasound. Polycystic ovarian morphology (PCOM) is defined as an excessive number of preantral follicles in one or both ovaries. The clinical presentation is highly heterogeneous and can be categorized into several phenotypes, depending on the presence or absence of the three characteristic features. PCOS is therefore a diagnosis of exclusion, based primarily on the presence of hyperandrogenism, ovulatory dysfunction and PCOM.[1]

PCOS is also associated with metabolic disturbances such as obesity and insulin resistance, giving rise to a perturbed carbohydrate metabolism and an increased risk for developing type 2 diabetes mellitus. Moreover, women with PCOS are more often suffering from dyslipidemia with relatively low levels of high-density lipoprotein (HDL) and high low-density lipoprotein (LDL) and triglyceride levels. The incidence of so-called metabolic syndrome is also increased among women with PCOS. Taking the latter three factors together, they might also be at risk for developing cardiovascular disease in later life.[2] More recently, it was found that PCOS is also associated with psychological complaints such as an increased risk of depression and anxiety symptoms as well as low self-esteem.[3]

Genetics of PCOS

Familial clustering and the results from twin studies strongly support an underlying genetic basis for PCOS. For example, having a mother or sister with PCOS conveys a 50% risk of developing PCOS. The correlation for PCOS between monozygotic twin sisters was twice as high as the dizygotic twin correlation. Genetic factors were suggested to explain around 70% of the variance according to the several genetic models.[4] Moreover, there is evidence of clustering of metabolic syndrome, hypertension and dyslipidemia in mothers, fathers, sisters and brothers of women with PCOS.[5] Finally, recent research indicates that the genetic architecture seems to be polygenic with a rather complex genetic inheritance pattern. Despite its clinical importance and high heritability, the underlying genetic etiology of PCOS remains incompletely understood.[6]

There are basically two different approaches available to identify genes or genetic variants involved in complex genetic traits such as PCOS. The first approach is the so-called candidate gene approach, which looks at the effect of single nucleotide polymorphisms (SNPs) in genes that are thought to play a role in the pathophysiology of the disease under study. This approach makes use of an a priori hypothesis about the role of that particular SNP as a causative variant of the disease. The second approach, the so-called genome-wide association study (GWAS), looks for associations between common SNPs and the disease without a predefined hypothesis about the possible role of genetic variants in the pathophysiology.[7]

Candidate gene studies are particularly useful for validating and deciphering the functional impact of gene loci identified by a GWAS to contextualize clinical relevance. A multitude of candidate gene studies have been conducted in PCOS, identifying SNPs that may contribute to the genetic basis of PCOS. These studies provide an effective approach for detecting genetic variants that either are causative or belong to a shared haplotype that is causative. However, candidate gene studies have many common limitations, such as small sample size and selection bias from confounding variables including ancestry, diagnostic criteria, body mass index (BMI), source and the ethnicity of participants, which can limit statistical power and result in different findings among different studies. The lack of consistency between studies might also be attributable to the fact that most studies assessed only one or two variants genotyped in the gene of interest instead of the whole gene. Although GWAS studies are, by definition, hypothesis-free, a common misunderstanding about GWAS is that they identify specific causal genes. They merely provide information about a genetic region (gene loci) that is significantly associated with the trait. The identified gene loci might be directly involved in gene function if located in or near a gene but they might also have a regulatory function for genes located further up- or downstream in the genome. Hence, genetic loci detected by GWAS provide ideal a priori candidate genes that are located within these loci to investigate (Table 2.1).[7]

Candidate Gene Studies in PCOS

A recent meta-analysis looking at candidate genes for PCOS identified 934 unique publications. Of these, after screening for a priori selection criteria, title and/or abstract, 340 studies remained for assessment of full text. Of these, 143 articles were excluded due to quality issues and hence 197 studies remained for full text review. After this review, only 21 papers remained that were used in that meta-analysis. The authors categorized the identified SNPs into five major categories, namely gonadotropins and their receptors; anti-Müllerian hormone (AMH) and its receptors; sex steroid metabolism and the androgen receptor; metabolism; and inflammation.[7]

Gonadotropins

The follicle-stimulating hormone receptor (FSHR) is a G-protein-coupled receptor comprising transmembrane, intracellular and extracellular domains. The FSHR gene, which is located on chromosome 2p21, has 10 exons and 9 introns. Only two FSHR polymorphisms are known (p.Thr307Ala and p.Asn680Ser); both are located in exon 10. The p.Asn680Ser variant allele is associated with a higher basal FSH level, longer menstrual cycles and higher ovarian threshold to ovulation induction, reflecting the difference of receptor sensitivity between the two different phenotypes. Although there is some inconsistency between different studies, most studies confirm that FSHR polymorphisms do alter the phenotype of PCOS in that they either alter the response to exogenous FSH or increase the risk of having PCOS. Although most research has focused on the role of FSHR polymorphisms, there seems to also be some evidence showing that SNPs in the luteinizing hormone/choriogonadotropin receptor (LHCGR) as well as those in the FSH-beta gene might also alter the phenotype of PCOS.[8]

Anti-Müllerian Hormone (AMH) and the AMH Type 2 Receptor (AMHR2)

One of the first candidate gene studies to look at the role of genetic variants in AMH revealed that the frequency of AMH Ile(49)Ser and AMH type 2 receptor -482 A>G polymorphisms were similar in PCOS women and controls. However, within the group of PCOS women, carriers of the AMH (49)Ser allele less often had polycystic ovaries and had lower androgen levels compared to noncarriers. In addition, in vitro studies demonstrated that the bioactivity of the AMH (49)Ser protein is diminished, compared with the AMH (49)Ile protein. Hence genetic variants in the AMH and AMH type 2 receptor gene do not influence PCOS susceptibility per se but they might contribute to the severity of the PCOS phenotype.[9] However, subsequent studies generated contradictory results and the recent meta-analysis could not detect a clear-cut relationship between the studied SNPs in AMH and the AMHR2 and PCOS.[7] Recently, 24 rare AMH variants in patients with PCOS and control subjects were described. Eighteen of those were specific to women with PCOS, whereas the others were also found in controls. All but one of the PCOS-specific variants had significantly reduced AMH signaling, whereas none of the six variants observed in control subjects showed significant defects in signaling. It was suggested that AMH therefore might play a significant role in regulating androgen synthesis through interference with Cyp17 activity.[10] The same group identified 20 additional variants in/near AMH and AMHR2 with significantly reduced signaling activity. In total, there were 37 variants with impaired activity in/near AMH and AMHR2 in women with PCOS that were not identified in controls.[11]

Sex Steroid Metabolism and the Androgen Receptor

Both CYP17 and HSD11B1 genes have been previously studied for their possible relationship with PCOS, yielding inconsistent results in numerous studies. Most of the studies as well as a meta-analysis indicate that SNPs in these two genes are associated neither with PCOS nor with the quantitative traits characteristic of PCOS, suggesting that these genes are not major risk factors for the syndrome.[12]

Many studies have reported the associations of polymorphic CAG repeats in the androgen receptor (AR) gene with PCOS risk but with inconsistent results. A meta-analysis could not detect an evident association between the CAG length variations in the AR gene and PCOS risk. However, the CAG length in the AR appears to be positively associated with testosterone serum concentrations in women suffering from PCOS.[13]

Sex hormone binding globulin (SHBG) specifically transports testosterone, dihydrotestosterone (DHT) and estradiol. The motif (TAAAA)n is present in the upstream region of the SHBG promoter, and it has been shown to influence transcriptional activity in vitro. In addition, (TAAAA)n polymorphism affects SHBG mRNA and further affects SHBG levels. Longer repeat sequences of (TAAAA)n are associated with lower SHBG expression. The correlation between SHBG gene polymorphisms and serum SHBG levels is attracting increasing attention. Indeed, recent research indicated that long SHBG (TAAAA)n alleles (> 8 repeats) exhibit a positive correlation with PCOS. Hence, SHBG polymorphisms have been regarded as important predictors of hyperandrogenism in women with PCOS. However, the results of association between SHBG and PCOS are controversial. Indeed, some studies suggested a significant association between SHBG and PCOS, whereas others (mostly in European and Asian populations) could not confirm such a relationship.[14]

Metabolism

Numerous genes involved in metabolic function have been studied in similarly numerous studies. The most frequently investigated genes were Insulin Receptor (INSR), Adiponectin, Transcription factor 7-like 2 (TCF7L2), Insulin Receptor Substrate-1 (IRS-1), Insulin Receptor Substrate-2 (IRS-2), Calpain-10, Cytochrome P450 1A1 (CYP1A1), Cytochrome P450 11A1 (CYP11A1), Paraoxonase-1 (PON1), DENN domain-containing protein 1A (DENND1A), and the Insulin gene-variable number of tandem repeats (INS-VNTR).

In two systematic reviews, the SNP rs1801278 in IRS-1 was associated with an increased susceptibility for PCOS in those carrying the A allele, in a combined cohort of women from different ancestries. Similarly, the III allele in INS-VNTR was associated with an increased risk of PCOS compared to I allele in a combined cohort of multiple ancestries.[15]

Carriers of the rs4646903 SNP in the CYP1A1 gene and those having the CYP11A1 microsatellite [TTTA] n repeat polymorphism were more susceptible to developing PCOS, although not across all ancestries. In contrast, the T allele of the rs1501299 SNP in the adiponectin gene was protective against PCOS. Again, ancestry modulated that risk considerably with a significant association found only among a mixed population of East Asians.[16]

Three SNPs in Calpain-10 were associated with an increased risk of PCOS, with ancestry again playing a major role and a significant association only found in a mixed population of "Asian" ancestry. The two SNPs in PON1 were associated with an increased risk of PCOS overall but, again, this was restricted to specific ancestries and diagnostic criteria.[17]

Two SNPs in DENND1A (rs10818854 and rs10986105) were associated with an increased risk of PCOS, while the SNP (rs2479106) in DENND1A was only associated in the women of mixed "Asian" ancestry.[18]

In summary, the genes IRS-1, INS-VNTR, Calpain-10, PON1, CYP1A1, CYP11A1, DENND1A and Adiponectin were found to be associated with risk of PCOS. Some of the SNPs in these genes were not consistent across ancestries, indicating that future genetic studies should include larger samples sizes and investigation of other SNPs within these genes to uncover the causal SNP variant associated with PCOS in different ancestries (Figure 2.1 and Table 2.2).[7]

Table 2.1 SNPs identified by GWAS in PCOS

Study	Diagnostic Criteria	Gene Locus	SNPs	Nearest Gene
Chen et al. (2011)[19]	Rotterdam 2004	2p16.3	rs 13405728	LHCGR,STON1-GTF2A1L
		2p21	rs 12468394	THADA
			rs 13429458	
			rs 12478601	
		9q33.3	rs 10818854	DENND1A
			rs 2479106	
			rs 10986105	
Shi et al. (2012)[20]	Rotterdam 2004	2p16.3	rs 13405728	LHCGR,STON1-GTF2A1L
		2p16.3	rs 2268361	FSHR
			rs 2349415	
		2p21	rs 12468394	THADA
			rs 13429458	
			rs 12478601	
		9q33.3	rs 10818854	DENND1A
			rs 2479106	
			rs 10986105	
		9q22.32	rs 4385527	C9orf3
			rs 3802457	
		11q22.1	rs 18974116	YAP1
		12q13.2	rs 705702	RAB5B, SUOX
		12q14.3	rs 2272046	HMGA2
		16q12.1	rs 4784165	TOX3
		19p13.3	rs 2059807	INSR
		20q13.2	rs 6022786	SUMO1P1
Hwang et al. (2012)[21]	Rotterdam 2004	12p12.2	rs 10841843	GYS2
			rs 6487237	
			rs 7485509	
Lee et al. (2015)[22]	Rotterdam 2004	8q24.2	rs 10505648	KHDRBS3, LINC02055
Hayes et al. (2015)[23]	National Institute of Health (NIH)	8p32.1	rs 804279	GATA4,NEIL2
		9q22.32	rs 10993397	C9orf3
		11p14.1	rs 11031006	ARL14EP, FSHB
Day et al. (2015)[24]	National Institute of Health (NIH) / Rotterdam 2003	2q34	rs 1351592	ERBB4
		2q21	rs 7563201	THADA
		5q31.1	rs 13164856	RAD50
		11p14.1	rs 11031006	FSHB
		11q22.1	rs 11225154	YAP1
		12q21.2	rs 1275468	KRR!

Inflammation

Inflammation potentially acts as a link between insulin resistance and hyperandrogenism in PCOS and is associated with both. Two candidate gene systematic reviews focused on SNPs in the TNF-alpha gene, which is a pro-inflammatory cytokine that has been associated with PCOS, ovarian function and ovulation and is a known mediator of insulin resistance. Neither reported significant associations between the rs1800629 SNP and PCOS.[25, 26] However, the SNP rs1799964 was positively associated with PCOS, suggesting this may be the causal polymorphism in the TNF-alpha gene for susceptibility to PCOS.[27]

Four systematic reviews examined the SNP rs1800795 in the IL-6 gene and found a decreased risk of PCOS when carrying the C allele. Caution is warranted as when only primary studies with control groups in Hardy–Weinberg equilibrium (HWE) were included, this association was no longer significant based on three of the candidate gene systematic reviews.[7] However, the most recent systematic review with the largest sample size found that this association remained when controls were in HWE, indicating that rs1800795 in IL-6 may be associated with PCOS.[28] However, regarding the possible controversies, further studies are needed before definitive

Table 2.2 The 14 genome-wide significant SNPs associated with PCOS in a meta-analysis

Chr. Position[1]	rs ID	EA[2]	OA[3]	EAF[4]	Beta	OR[5]	95%CI[6]	Std Error	Nearest Gene	P-value	Effective N[7]
2:43561780	rs7563201	A	G	0.451	−0.108	0.90	(0.86±0.92)	0.0172	THADA	3.86 e 10	17192
2:21391766	rs2178575	A	G	0.151	0.166	1.18	(1.13±1.23)	0.0219	ERBB4	3.34 e 14	17192
5:131813204	rs13164856	T	C	0.729	0.124	1.13	(1.08±1.17)	0.0193	IRF1/RAD50	1.45 e 10	17192
8:11623889	rs804279	A	T	0.262	0.128	1.14	(1.09±1.17)	0.184	GATA4/NEIL2	3.76 e 12	16865
9:5440589	rs10739076	A	C	0.308	0.110	1.12	(1.07±1.15)	0.0197	PLGRKT	2.51 e 08	17192
9:97723266	rs7864171	A	G	0.428	−0.093	0.91	(0.88±0.94)	0.0168	FANCC	2.95 e 08	17192
9:126619233	rs969009	A	G	0.068	0.202	1.22	(1.15±1.30)	0.0311	DENND1A	7.96 e 11	17192
11:30226365	rs11031005	T	C	0.854	−0.159	0.85	(0.81±0.89)	0.0223	ARL14EP/FSHB	8.66 e 13	17192
11:102043240	rs11225154	A	G	0.094	0.179	1.20	(1.13±1.26)	0.0272	YAP1	5.44 e 11	17192
11:113949232	rs1784692	T	C	0.824	0.144	1.15	(1.10±1.20)	0.0226	ZBTB16	1.88 e 10	17192
12:56477694	rs2271194	A	T	0.416	0.097	1.10	(1.06±1.13)	0.0166	ERBB3/RAB5B	4.57 e 09	17192
12:75941042	rs1795379	T	C	0.240	−0.117	0.89	(0.85±0.92)	0.0195	KRR1	1.81 e 09	17192
16:52373777	rs8043701	A	T	0.815	−0.127	0.88	(0.84±0.91)	0.0208	TOX3	9.61 e 10	17192
20:31420757	rs853854	A	T	0.499	−0.098	0.91	(0.87±0.93)	0.0163	MAPRE1	2.36 e 09	17192

[1] Chromosome number and position on that chromosome in hg19; 2 EA: Effect Allele; 3 OA: Other Allele; 4 EAF: Effect Allele Frequency; 5 OR: Odds Ratio; 6 95% CI: 95% Confidence Interval; 7 Effective N: Effective sample size

Source. Modified after Day, F., Karaderi, T., Jones, M. R. et al., Large-scale genome-wide meta-analysis of polycystic ovary syndrome suggests shared genetic architecture for different diagnosis criteria. PLOS Genetics 14 (12): e1008517.

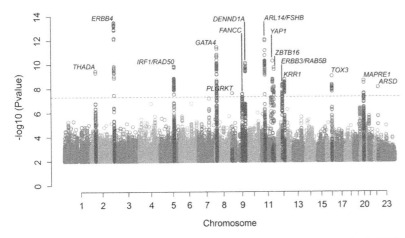

Figure 2.1 Manhattan plot showing results of meta-analysis for SNPs associated with PCOS
Source. With permission from Day, F., Karaderi, T., Jones, M. R. et al., Large-scale genome-wide meta-analysis of polycystic ovary syndrome suggests shared genetic architecture for different diagnosis criteria, *PLOS Genetics* 2018; 14 (12): 1–20. Manhattan plot showing results of meta-analysis for PCOS status, adjusting for age. The inverse $\log^{10}$ of the p-value $(-\log^{10}(p))$ is plotted on the y-axis. The green dashed line designates the minimum p-value for genome-wide significance $(< 5.0 \times 10^{-8})$. Genome-wide significant loci are denoted with a label showing the nearest gene to the index SNP at each locus. SNPs with p-values $< 1.0 \times 10^{-2}$ are not depicted.

conclusions can be made. SNPs in the genes IL-β, IL-10 and IL-18 were not associated with PCOS.[7]

In summary, evidence suggests that TNF-α (rs1800795) and IL-6 (rs1800795) may be associated with PCOS, but larger sample sizes and further studies with appropriate control groups are required to confirm these findings.[7]

GWAS in PCOS

To date, seven GWAS have been conducted to identify gene loci that are associated with PCOS. Four GWAS were conducted in women with Han Chinese ancestry (both North and South)[19–20, 22, 29] and two in women with Korean ancestry. [21–22] Two further GWAS have been performed in women from European ancestry determined by genetic analysis of local ancestry.[23–24] Presently, there has only been one large-scale meta-analysis of GWAS conducted in women with European ancestry.[30] In total, 19 genetic loci associated with risk of PCOS have been identified in three biogeographical ancestries, Korean, Han Chinese, and European. Eleven of the nineteen loci are common to Han Chinese and European ancestry. This meta-analysis also identified three novel loci that were significantly associated with PCOS. Moreover, only one locus differed significantly in its association by

diagnostic criteria. Otherwise, the genetic architecture was similar between PCOS diagnosed by self-report and PCOS diagnosed by the National Institute of Health (NIH) or Rotterdam criteria across common identified variants. The identified common genetic variants were associated with hyperandrogenism, gonadotropin regulation and testosterone levels in affected women. Moreover, linkage disequilibrium score regression analysis revealed genetic correlations with obesity, fasting insulin, type 2 diabetes, lipid levels and coronary artery disease, indicating shared genetic architecture between metabolic traits and PCOS. Finally, Mendelian randomization analyses suggested variants associated with BMI, fasting insulin, menopause timing, depression and male-pattern balding play a causal role in PCOS.[30]

Gonadotropins

Follicular arrest, menstrual dysfunction and anovulation are commonly observed in PCOS and are linked to hyperandrogenism, elevated LH/FSH ratios as well as elevated AMH serum levels. In the recent meta-analysis, eight variants were associated with PCOM and nine variants were associated with ovulatory dysfunction. SNPs associated with PCOM were near genes ERBB4, THADA,GATA4/NEIL2, DENND1A, C9orf3, Yap1, YAP1, ZBTB16 and ERBB3/RAB5B, all genes that are expressed at the ovarian level and some of which are known to play a role in folliculogenesis. The ones that were associated with ovulatory dysfunction were near the genes ERBB4, THADA, GATAS/NEIL2, DENND1A, C9orf3, ARL14P/FSHB, Yap1, ZBTB16, KRR1 and ERBB3/RAB5B. Again, some play a role in folliculogenesis, whereas others are involved in the processing of large protein hormones.[30]

In the first and second GWAS in Han Chinese women a locus near the FSHR gene was significantly associated with PCOS.[19–20] Indeed, in phenotypic studies the FSHR locus has been associated with serum FSH and LH concentrations. However, that was only the case in the Chinese studies, which used the former NIH criteria and therefore included the more severe phenotypes in their studies. A meta-analysis as well as a recent review emphasized that this particular SNP could be much more related to the polycystic ovarian morphology characteristic rather than to PCOS per se.[31, 8] Very recently, another study by a Chinese group again revealed that the FSHR region on chromosome 2p16.3 had a genome-wide significant association with serum FSH levels. Moreover, in that particular study the two most commonly studied SNPs (rs1665, Thr307Ala and rs1666, Asn680Ser) in the FSHR were also replicated. The effect of the newly identified SNP was, however, independent and about seven times stronger compared to the rs1665 and rs1666. It could therefore be that rs2300441 has effects on FSHR expression or action, resulting in a need for altering FSH levels to stimulate the receptor for follicle growth.[29] Although most research has focused on the role of FSHR polymorphisms, there seems to also be some evidence that SNPs in the LHCGR as well as those in the FSH-beta gene might also alter the phenotype of PCOS.[8] Indeed, a recent study in women with PCOS showed that rs11031006, nearest to the FSHB gene, was significantly associated with free testosterone serum concentrations and LH levels. However, the number of menstrual cycles per year, the antral follicle number, the ovarian volume and insulin sensitivity were not associated with any particular SNP.[32] Two loci in the combined GWAS were associated with ovulatory dysfunction, one of which was the locus near FSHB. This locus was also associated with LH and FSH levels.[30] In the meta-analysis, an SNP (rs804279) near the GATA4/NEIL2 gene was significantly different across diagnostic PCOS criteria and most strongly associated in NIH compared to the Rotterdam phenotype and self-reported cases. Deletion of GATA4 results in abnormal responses to exogenous gonadotropins and impaired fertility in mice.[30] Finally, patients with the AA genotype of rs13429458 in the THADA gene were older and had higher serum LH and testosterone (T) levels compared to those with the AC and CC genotypes. Similarly, the LH/FSH ratio was also higher in those patients with the AA genotype. These differences were independent of age and BMI.[33]

Anti-Müllerian Hormone (AMH) and the AMH Type 2 Receptor (AMHR2)

Neither AMH nor the AMHR2 have yet been identified as being significantly associated with PCOS in GWAS. However, genetic susceptibility to later menopause was associated with a higher PCOS risk and PCOS-susceptibility alleles are associated with higher serum AMH concentrations in girls.[24] Indeed, recent candidate gene approaches have established a role for genetic variants in AMH that are solely found among women with PCOS and could modify the phenotype.[10]

Sex Steroid Metabolism and the Androgen Receptor

The locus also encompasses the promoter region of FDFT1, the first enzyme in the cholesterol biosynthesis pathway, which is the substrate for testosterone synthesis and is associated with non-alcoholic fatty liver disease, a risk factor for women with PCOS. Four variants at the C9orf3, DENND1A, TOX3 and ERBB3/RAB5B were associated with hyperandrogenism in Europeans as well as in Han Chinese women. Furthermore, the association between the IRF1/RAD50 variant and testosterone levels may indicate a regulatory role in testosterone production. Moreover, male-pattern balding–associated variants showed strong effects on PCOS, suggesting that this might be a male manifestation of PCOS pathways, as has been previously suggested.[34] This observation may reflect the biology of hair follicle sensitivity to androgens, seen in androgenetic alopecia, a well-recognized feature of hyperandrogenism in PCOS. Moreover, ZBTB16 (also known as PLZF) has been marked as an androgen-responsive gene with anti-proliferative activity in prostate cancer cells.[30] Genetic variants within the locus near the THADA gene seem to cause differences in testosterone serum levels in women with PCOS.[33] A functional analysis looking at candidate loci including LHCGR, FSHR, ZNF217, YAP1, INSR, RAB5B and C9orf3 proposes that these candidates comprise a hierarchical signaling network by which DENND1A, LHCGR, INSR, RAB5B, adapter proteins and associated downstream signaling cascades converge to regulate theca cell androgen biosynthesis.[35] Moreover, DENND1A produces two different proteins called variant 1 and 2 (DENND1A.V1 and DENND1A. V2). In particular, the DENND1A.V2 protein and mRNA levels are increased in PCOS theca cells. Further research indicated that exosomal DENND1A.V2 RNA was significantly elevated in urine from PCOS women compared to healthy control women. Forced overexpression of DENND1A.V2 in normal theca cells resulted in a PCOS phenotype of augmented CYP17A1 and CYP11A1 gene transcription, mRNA abundance and androgen biosynthesis. In contrast to these findings, knockdown of DENND1A.V2 in PCOS theca cells reduced androgen biosynthesis and CYP17A1 and CYP11A1 gene transcription. Moreover, an IgG specific to DENND1A.V2 also reduced androgen biosynthesis and CYP17 and CYP11A1 mRNA when added to the medium of cultured PCOS theca cells. Hence, it seems that DENND1A plays a key role in the hyperandrogenemia associated with PCOS.[36]

Metabolism

Using a recessive model for rs12478601 near the THADA gene, the subjects with PCOS with the CC genotype were significantly older and had elevated serum LDL levels. The LDL levels remained increased after correction for age and BMI.[33] PLGRKT, a plasminogen receptor and several genes in the insulin super family (INSL6, INSL4) as well as RLN1, RLN2, which are endocrine hormones secreted by the ovary and testis, are suspected to impact follicle growth and ovulation. Furthermore, PLZF activates GATA4 gene transcription and mediates cardiac hypertrophic signaling from the angiotensin II receptor 2. It is also upregulated during adipocyte differentiation. SNPs in the MAPRE1 gene, which interacts

with the LDL receptor related protein 1 (LRP1), is also important in the control of adipogenesis. MAPRE1 might additionally mediate ovarian angiogenesis and follicle development.[30]

Mendelian randomization also indicated a shared biology between PCOS and different metabolic traits such as BMI and obesity, fasting insulin levels and type 2 diabetes, HDL and triglyceride levels and coronary artery disease.[30, 23]

In a recent study, it was shown that cluster analysis was capable of identifying two reproducible but different PCOS phenotypes, a reproductive one and one with a more metabolic background. Furthermore, these subtypes were associated with novel susceptibility loci previously not discovered in GWAS (Figure 2.2).[37]

Phenome-Wide Association Studies (PheWAS)

Candidate gene and GWAS have identified genetic variants that modulate risk for PCOS. Many of these associations require further study to replicate the results. A way to do this is through the so-called phenome-wide association study (PheWAS). A PheWAS is a study design in which the association between genetic variants is tested across a large number of different phenotypes. Hence, it is an unbiased approach to replicate previously reported relationships and discover new ones between genotypical and phenotypical features of PCOS. Polygenic risk scores (PRSs) represent the cumulative effect of common genetic variation summed per individual into a single risk score, providing an intuitive way to translate GWAS findings into clinically relevant information such as a patient's risk of disease. From a precision medicine perspective, PRSs hold significant promise especially for a multifactorial condition with complicated clinical manifestations, such as PCOS.[6]

The first study attempting to develop a risk score for PCOS used a weighted genetic risk score. The odds for having PCOS defined by the former NIH criteria or using the Rotterdam consensus criteria were based on genetic risk score from across the identified genome-wide significant loci. That study showed that women in the highest quintiles had a four-times higher risk for having PCOS compared to those in the lowest quintile. [30] Another more recent study identified four independent predictors of PCOS, namely the

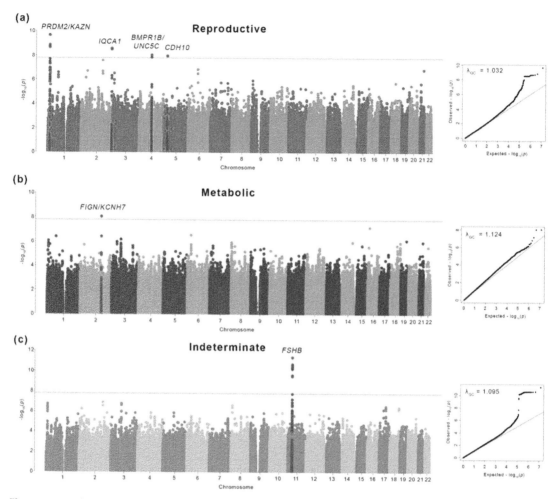

Figure 2.2 Manhattan plots for (a) reproductive, (b) metabolic and (c) indeterminate PCOS subtypes
Source. With permission taken from Dapas, M., Lin, F. T. J., Nadkarni, G. N. et al. Distinct subtypes of polycystic ovary syndrome with novel genetic associations: An unsupervised, phenotypic clustering analysis. *PLoS Medicine* 2020; 17: e1003132.
Genome-wide association results. Manhattan plots for (a) reproductive, (b) metabolic and (c) indeterminate PCOS subtypes. The horizontal line indicates genome-wide significance (P < 1.67 × 10⁻⁸). Genome-wide significant loci are colored in green and labeled according to nearby gene(s). Quantile–quantile plots with genomic inflation factor, λGC, are shown adjacent to corresponding Manhattan plots. PCOS, polycystic ovary syndrome.

free androgen index, 17-OHP, AMH and waist circumference. PCOS women with a high-risk score presented with a worse metabolic profile characterized by significantly higher two-hour glucose, insulin, triglycerides, C-reactive protein and lower HDL cholesterol compared to those with lower risk score for PCOS.[38]

The latest PheWAS enhanced the polygenic risk prediction by integrating additional disease component phenotypes retrieved from electronic health records into a polygenic and phenotypical risk score (PPRS). This integrated polygenic prediction improved the average performance for PCOS detection about 60-fold over the null model using the genuine diagnostic criteria. The subsequent PRS-powered PheWAS identified a high level of shared biology between PCOS and a range of metabolic and endocrine outcomes, especially with obesity and diabetes. Relevant PCOS-associated comorbidities were morbid obesity, type 2 diabetes, hypercholesterolemia, disorders of lipid metabolism, hypertension and sleep apnea reaching phenome-wide significance. This novel approach has provided a new methodological opportunity to stratify patients' genetic risk and to discover the phenomics network associated

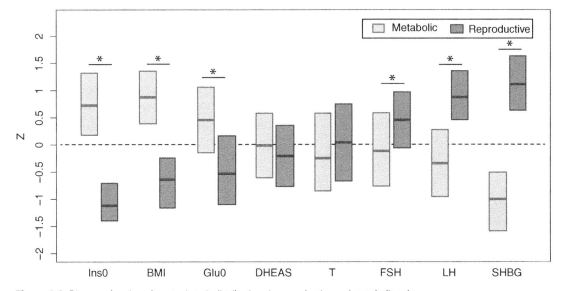

Figure 2.3 Diagram showing phenotypic trait distributions in reproductive and metabolic subtypes
Source. With permission taken from Dapas, M., Lin, F. T. J., Nadkarni, G. N. et al. Distinct subtypes of polycystic ovary syndrome with novel genetic associations: An unsupervised, phenotypic clustering analysis. *PLoS Medicine* 2020; 17: e1003132.
Phenotypic trait distributions in reproductive and metabolic subtypes. Median and IQRs are shown for normalized, adjusted quantitative trait distributions of genotyped PCOS cases with reproductive or metabolic subtype. The figure illustrates the traits for which the subtypes differ significantly with an asterisk (* Bonferroni adjusted Wilcoxon, P adjusted < 0.05): Ins0, BMI, Glu0, FSH, LH, and SHBG.
BMI, body mass index; DHEAS, dehydroepiandrosterone sulfate; FSH, follicle-stimulating hormone; Glu0, fasting glucose; Ins0, fasting insulin; IQR, interquartile range; LH, luteinizing hormone; PCOS, polycystic ovary syndrome; SHBG, sex hormone binding globulin; T, testosterone.

with PCOS pathogenesis. Moreover, it also permits detection of PCOS patients prior to diagnosis by a physician, allowing earlier interventions and thereby reducing costs from long-term complications (Figures 2.3 and 2.4).[6]

Other Genetic Approaches

A recent study looking at microRNAs (miRNAs) sequencing revealed 34 exosomal miRNAs that were differentially expressed in PCOS patients compared to controls. By using a quantitative reverse transcriptase polymerase chain reaction (qRT-PCR), 5 out of these 34 differentially expressed miRNAs (miR-126-3p, miR-146a-5p, miR-20b-5p, miR-106a-5p and miR-18a-3p) were identified. Further analyses predicted target functions of these miRNAs within pathways important for axon guidance, mitogen-activated protein kinase (MAPK) signaling, endocytosis, circadian rhythms and cancer pathways. Moreover, the expression of these miRNAs correlated with menstrual cycle, antral follicle count and hormone levels in women with PCOS. Finally, combined they yielded an area under the

receiver operating characteristic curve of 0.781, which was fairly good in discriminating PCOS patients from controls. Therefore, such plasma exosomal miRNAs may confer a risk of PCOS and may thereby be helpful in distinguishing PCOS patients from controls. Certain miRNA expression may be associated to the disease progression, which could help to elucidate the epigenetic components of the pathophysiology of PCOS.[39] MicroRNAs (miRNA) play a key role in the regulation of gene expression through the translational suppression and control of posttranscriptional modifications. Indeed, a recent review demonstrated that miRNAs conduct the pathways involved in human reproduction including maintenance of primordial germ cells, spermatogenesis, oocyte maturation, folliculogenesis and corpus luteum function. The association of differences in miRNA expression and infertility and more specifically PCOS, premature ovarian failure (POF) and repeated implantation failure has been reported. Furthermore, there is evidence that some miRNAs are involved in embryonic development and implantation.[40]

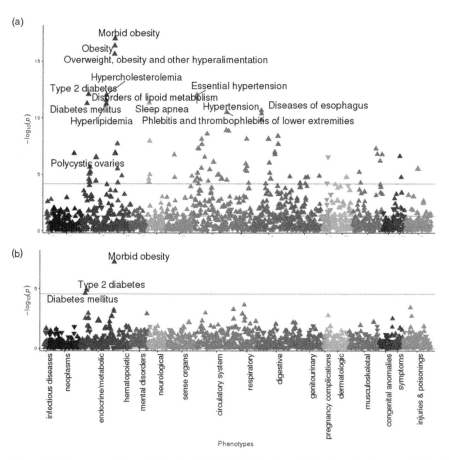

Figure 2.4 Phenome-wide association study (PheWAS) Manhattan plot of polygenic risk scores (PRSs) of SNPs in the phenomes of 49 343 female participants
Source. With permission taken from Joo, Y. Y., Actkins, K., Pacheco, J. A. et al. A polygenic and phenotypic risk prediction for polycystic ovary syndrome evaluated by phenome-wide association studies. *Clin Endocrinol Metab* 2020; 105(6): 1918–1936. https://doi.org/10 .1210/clinem/dgz326
PheWAS Manhattan plot of PRS (SNVs with P ≤ 1) in the phenomes of 49 343 female participants; In Manhattan plots (a) and (b), the x-axis represents the EHR phenotype categorical group and the y-axis represents the negative log(10) of the PheWAS P-value. Horizontal lines indicate the cutoff for phenome-wide significance. For readability, only the most significant associations are annotated.

Conclusions

GWAS have identified genetic loci that are significantly associated with PCOS. The identified common genetic variants were associated with hyperandrogenism, gonadotropin regulation and testosterone levels. Moreover, linkage disequilibrium score regression analysis revealed genetic correlations with obesity, fasting insulin, type 2 diabetes, lipid levels and coronary artery disease, indicating shared genetic architecture between metabolic traits and PCOS. Finally, Mendelian randomization analyses suggested variants associated with BMI, fasting insulin, menopause timing, depression and male-pattern balding play a causal role in PCOS. PheWAS have identified shared biology between PCOS and a range of metabolic and endocrine outcomes such as morbid obesity, type 2 diabetes, hypercholesterolemia, disorders of lipid metabolism, hypertension and sleep apnea.

References

1 Revised 2003 consensus on diagnostic criteria and long-term health risks related to polycystic ovary syndrome (PCOS). *Hum Reprod* 2004; 19(1): 41–47.

2 Fauser, B. C., Tarlatzis, B. C., Rebar, R. W. et al. Consensus on women's health aspects of polycystic ovary syndrome (PCOS): The Amsterdam ESHRE/ASRM-Sponsored 3rd PCOS Consensus Workshop Group. *Fertil Steril* 2012; 97(1): 28–38 e25.

3   Teede, H. J., Misso, M. L., Costello, M. F. et al. Recommendations from the international evidence-based guideline for the assessment and management of polycystic ovary syndrome. *Clin Endocrinol (Oxf)* 2018; 89(3): 251–268.

4   Vink, J. M., Sadrzadeh, S., Lambalk, C. B. and Boomsma, D. I. Heritability of polycystic ovary syndrome in a Dutch twin-family study. *J Clin Endocrinol Metab* 2006; 91(6): 2100–2104.

5   Yilmaz, B., Vellanki, P., Ata, B. and Yildiz, B. O. Metabolic syndrome, hypertension, and hyperlipidemia in mothers, fathers, sisters, and brothers of women with polycystic ovary syndrome: A systematic review and meta-analysis. *Fertil Steril* 2018; 109(2): 356–364 e332.

6   Joo, Y. Y., Actkins, K., Pacheco, J. A. et al. A polygenic and phenotypic risk prediction for polycystic ovary syndrome evaluated by phenome-wide association studies. *J Clin Endocrinol Metab* 2020; 105(6): 1918–1936. https://doi.org/10.1210/clinem/dgz326

7   Hiam, D., Moreno-Asso, A., Teede, H. J. et al. The genetics of polycystic ovary syndrome: An overview of candidate gene systematic reviews and genome-wide association studies. *J Clin Med* 2019; 8(10): 1606.

8   Laven, J. S. E. Follicle stimulating hormone receptor (FSHR) polymorphisms and polycystic ovary syndrome (PCOS). *Front Endocrinol (Lausanne)* 2019; 10: 23.

9   Kevenaar, M. E., Laven, J. S., Fong, S. L. et al. A functional anti-Müllerian hormone gene polymorphism is associated with follicle number and androgen levels in polycystic ovary syndrome patients. *J Clin Endocrinol Metab* 2008; 93(4): 1310–1316.

10   Gorsic, L. K., Kosova, G., Werstein, B. et al. Pathogenic anti-Müllerian hormone variants in polycystic ovary syndrome. *J Clin Endocrinol Metab* 2017; 102(8): 2862–2872.

11   Gorsic, L. K., Dapas, M., Legro, R. S., Hayes, M. G. and Urbanek M. Functional genetic variation in the anti-Müllerian hormone pathway in women with polycystic ovary syndrome. *J Clin Endocrinol Metab* 2019; 104(7): 2855–2874.

12   Zhao, H., Lv, Y., Li, L. and Chen, Z. J. Genetic studies on polycystic ovary syndrome. *Best Pract Res Clin Obstet Gynaecol* 2016; 37: 56–65.

13   Zhang, T., Liang, W., Fang, M., Yu, J., Ni, Y. and Li, Z. Association of the CAG repeat polymorphisms in androgen receptor gene with polycystic ovary syndrome: A systemic review and meta-analysis. *Gene* 2013; 524(2): 161–167.

14   Zhu, J. L., Chen, Z., Feng, W. J., Long, S. L. and Mo, Z. C. Sex hormone-binding globulin and polycystic ovary syndrome. *Clin Chim Acta* 2019; 499: 142–148.

15   Ruan, Y., Ma, J. and Xie, X. Association of IRS-1 and IRS-2 genes polymorphisms with polycystic ovary syndrome: A meta-analysis. *Endocr J* 2012; 59(7): 601–609.

16   Shen, W., Li, T., Hu, Y., Liu, H. and Song, M. Common polymorphisms in the CYP1A1 and CYP11A1 genes and polycystic ovary syndrome risk: A meta-analysis and meta-regression. *Arch Gynecol Obstet* 2014; 289(1): 107–118.

17   Shen, W., Li, T., Hu, Y., Liu, H. and Song, M. Calpain-10 genetic polymorphisms and polycystic ovary syndrome risk: A meta-analysis and meta-regression. *Gene* 2013; 531(2): 426–434.

18   Gao, J., Xue, J. D., Li, Z. C., Zhou, L. and Chen, C. The association of DENND1A gene polymorphisms and polycystic ovary syndrome risk: A systematic review and meta-analysis. *Arch Gynecol Obstet* 2016; 294(5): 1073–1080.

19   Chen, Z. J., Zhao, H., He, L. et al. Genome-wide association study identifies susceptibility loci for polycystic ovary syndrome on chromosome 2p16.3, 2p21 and 9q33.3. *Nat Genet* 2011; 43(1): 55–59.

20   Shi, Y., Zhao, H., Shi, Y. et al. Genome-wide association study identifies eight new risk loci for polycystic ovary syndrome. *Nat Genet* 2012; 44(9): 1020–1025.

21   Hwang, J. Y., Lee, E. J., Jin, G. M. et al. Genome-wide association study identifies GYS2 as a novel genetic factor for polycystic ovary syndrome through obesity-related condition. *J Hum Genet* 2012; 57(10): 660–664.

22   Lee, H., Oh, J. Y., Sung, Y. A. et al. Genome-wide association study identified new susceptibility loci for polycystic ovary syndrome. *Hum Reprod* 2015; 30(3): 723–731.

23   Hayes, M. G., Urbanek, M., Ehrmann, D. A. et al. Genome-wide association of polycystic ovary syndrome implicates alterations in gonadotropin secretion in European ancestry populations. *Nat Commun* 2015; 6: 7502.

24   Day, F. R., Hinds, D. A., Tung, J. Y. et al. Causal mechanisms and balancing selection inferred from genetic associations with polycystic ovary syndrome. *Nat Commun* 2015; 6: 8464.

25   Guo, R., Zheng, Y., Yang, J. and Zheng, N. Association of TNF-alpha, IL-6 and IL-1beta gene polymorphisms with polycystic ovary syndrome: a meta-analysis. *BMC Genet* 2015; 16(1): 5.

26   Jia, H., Yu, L., Guo, X., Gao, W. and Jiang, Z. Associations of adiponectin gene polymorphisms

with polycystic ovary syndrome: A meta-analysis. *Endocrine* 2012; 42(2): 299–306.

27 Wu, H., Yu, K. and Yang, Z. Associations between TNF-alpha and interleukin gene polymorphisms with polycystic ovary syndrome risk: A systematic review and meta-analysis. *J Assist Reprod Genet* 2015; 32(4): 625–634.

28 Chen, L., Zhang, Z., Huang, J. and Jin, M. Association between rs1800795 polymorphism in the interleukin-6 gene and the risk of polycystic ovary syndrome: A meta-analysis. *Medicine (Baltimore)* 2018; 97(29): e11558.

29 Yan, J., Tian, Y., Gao, X. et al. A genome-wide association study identifies FSHR rs2300441 associated with follicle-stimulating hormone levels. *Clin Genet* 2020; 97(6): 869–877.

30 Day, F., Karaderi, T., Jones, M. R. et al. Large-scale genome-wide meta-analysis of polycystic ovary syndrome suggests shared genetic architecture for different diagnosis criteria. *PLoS Genet* 2018; 14 (12): e1007813.

31 Qiu, L., Liu, J. and Hei, Q. M. Association between two polymorphisms of follicle stimulating hormone receptor gene and susceptibility to polycystic ovary syndrome: a meta-analysis. *Chin Med Sci J* 2015; 30(1): 44–50.

32 Hong, S. H., Hong, Y. S., Jeong, K., Chung, H., Lee, H. and Sung, Y. A. Relationship between the characteristic traits of polycystic ovary syndrome and susceptibility genes. *Sci Rep* 2020; 10(1): 10479.

33 Cui, L., Li, G., Zhong, W. et al. Polycystic ovary syndrome susceptibility single nucleotide polymorphisms in women with a single PCOS clinical feature. *Hum Reprod* 2015; 30(3): 732–736.

34 Carey, A. H., Chan, K. L., Short, F., White, D., Williamson R. and Franks, S. Evidence for a single gene effect causing polycystic ovaries and male pattern baldness. *Clin Endocrinol (Oxf)* 1993; 38(6): 653–658.

35 McAllister, J. M., Legro, R. S., Modi, B. P. and Strauss, J. F., 3rd. Functional genomics of PCOS: From GWAS to molecular mechanisms. *Trends Endocrinol Metab* 2015; 26(3): 118–124.

36 McAllister, J. M., Modi, B., Miller et al. Overexpression of a DENND1A isoform produces a polycystic ovary syndrome theca phenotype. *Proc Natl Acad Sci U S A* 2014; 111(15): E1519–1527.

37 Dapas, M., Lin, F. T. J., Nadkarni, G. N. et al. Distinct subtypes of polycystic ovary syndrome with novel genetic associations: An unsupervised, phenotypic clustering analysis. *PLoS Med* 2020; 17(6): e1003132.

38 Deshmukh, H., Papageorgiou, M., Kilpatrick, E. S., Atkin, S. L. and Sathyapalan, T. Development of a novel risk prediction and risk stratification score for polycystic ovary syndrome. *Clin Endocrinol (Oxf)* 2019; 90(1): 162–169.

39 Jiang, X., Li, J., Zhang, B. et al. Differential expression profile of plasma exosomal microRNAs in women with polycystic ovary syndrome. *Fertil Steril* 2021; 115(3): 782–792.

40 Kamalidehghan, B., Habibi, M., Afjeh, S. S. et al. The importance of small non-coding RNAs in human reproduction: A review article. *Appl Clin Genet* 2020; 13: 1–11.

Chapter 3

The Epidemiology of Polycystic Ovary Syndrome

Larisa Suturina

Epidemiology of PCOS

The prevalence of polycystic ovary syndrome (PCOS), considered one of the most common female endocrine disorders, depends on the diagnostic criteria used and the study population (referral or unselected). PCOS prevalence is also influenced by race and ethnicity.

PCOS Prevalence with the Different Diagnostic Criteria

The US National Institutes of Health (NIH) consensus, presented in 1990, has been historically used in epidemiological PCOS studies. It defined the diagnostic criteria for PCOS as the presence of ovarian dysfunction and hyperandrogenism with or without polycystic ovarian morphology (see Chapter 1). The average prevalence of PCOS, estimated under the NIH 1990 criteria, is 5.7–8.7%.[1, 2, 3, 4, 5, 6, 7, 8, 9, 10, 11] However, the prevalence reported based on the same criteria varies throughout the world: 4.8–7.1% in Iranians,[7, 8, 12] 13% in Mexican Americans and 15% among Australian Indigenous women.[13, 14] This heterogeneity may be related to the differences in study design and racial diversity in the population.

A higher prevalence of PCOS was demonstrated in studies that used the European Society of Human Reproduction (ESHRE) and American Society for Reproductive Medicine (ASRM) (Rotterdam 2003) criteria. This may be attributed to the inclusion of the additional "non-androgenic" and "ovulatory" phenotypes.[15] The estimates with the Androgen Excess and PCOS (AE-PCOS) Society 2006 (AES) criteria were also greater

than those obtained with the classic NIH 1990 diagnostic criteria, mainly due to the inclusion of PCOS patients without oligo-anovulation.[6–9, 11, 12, 14, 16] Currently, there are three published systematic reviews and meta-analysis summarizing the comparative prevalence studies conducted using different PCOS definitions (Table 3.1).

In a large meta-analysis with a total study population of 19226 Iranian females aged 10–45 years, the PCOS prevalence using NIH 1990 criteria was 6.8% vs. 19.5% when the Rotterdam 2003 criteria were used.[17] In 2016, the systematic review and meta-analysis of 24 eligible articles presented the overall prevalence of PCOS according to the diagnostic criteria of the NIH, Rotterdam and the AES.[18] The review demonstrated a significantly higher prevalence of PCOS patients when using Rotterdam and the AES diagnostic criteria vs. the "classic" NIH criteria. The prevalence of hirsutism, hyperandrogenemia, polycystic ovaries (PCO) and oligo-anovulation was reported in the article as follows: 13%, 11%, 28% and 15%, respectively. The authors highlighted the heterogeneity among studies and concluded that better standardization of the methods is required to increase the comparability of PCOS prevalence around the globe. The systematic review published by Skiba and colleagues in 2018 included 21 reports of PCOS prevalence studies performed between the years of 1990 and 2018.[19] In this review, the authors presented the pooled prevalence estimates of PCOS based on the NIH criteria as significantly lower than those identified in studies performed under the Rotterdam criteria (P < 0.0001). However, the pooled estimates for the Rotterdam and AES classification were not different (P = 0.201).

Table 3.1 PCOS prevalence depending on the different diagnostic criteria: systematic reviews and meta-analysis

Author(s), year	Study design*	NIH 1990	Rotterdam 2003	AE-PCOS Society 2006
		% [95% CI]		
Jalilian et al., 2015[17]	A meta-analysis	6.8 [4.1–8.5]	19.5 [2.24–8.14]	–
Bozdag et al., 2016[18]	A systematic review and meta-analysis	6 [5–8]	10 [8–13]	10 [7–13]
Skiba et al., 2018 [19]	A systematic review and meta-analysis	7 [6–7]	12 [10–15]	10 [6–13]

* as defined by the authors

The authors suggested that the higher prevalence of PCOS reported in the studies using the latest diagnostic approaches was due to the inclusion of ovarian morphology as the additional diagnostic criterion. In their opinion, the broad spectrum of clinical phenotypes, the lack of standardization of diagnostic cutoffs and the potential differences between the study populations may have led to the heterogeneity in the estimates of PCOS prevalence.

PCOS Prevalence in Referral Populations

It is well documented that PCOS prevalence and distribution of PCOS phenotypes significantly differ in selected (referred) vs. unselected (medically unbiased) populations. According to studies performed in the last decades, PCOS is a common finding in clients of medical clinics dealing with hirsutism, acne, oligo-anovulation, infertility and obesity. Farah and colleagues reported that 39 (12%) of the 315 hirsute women seeking treatment from community electrologists met the diagnostic criteria for PCOS, although they were not receiving appropriate treatment.[20] Among 873 patients with clinically evident androgen excess, PCOS was observed in 82% of all cases.[21] In 2006, Carmina and colleagues found PCOS in 72.1% of 950 women referred with clinical hyperandrogenism, 56.6% of whom had the classic anovulatory phenotype.[22]

Alen and colleagues demonstrated androgen excess and, consequently, PCOS in 38% of patients referred to the university-based outpatient clinic with a long history of oligo-ovulation.[23] In this study, in the cohort of women with short-lived episodes of ovulatory dysfunction, PCOS occurred in only 5%. Approximately 40%

of nonhirsute oligo-ovulatory women with 45-day menstrual cycles or longer were diagnosed with PCOS.[23]

According to the retrospective survey of the transvaginal ultrasound of 100 female partners of sterile males, the prevalence of polycystic ovaries reached 23%, with 12% of women achieving the full PCOS under the Rotterdam criteria.[24] Furthermore, in a cross-sectional observational study conducted at an infertility clinic in a university hospital, PCOS was found in 46% of infertile women and was considered one of the leading causes of infertility.[25] Another cross-sectional analysis of 104 patients reported that PCOS in infertile women depends on their race origin: 44.2% among South Asians vs. 11.5% in Caucasians, OR of 6.1 [95 % CI 2.2, 16.7].[26]

The association between obesity and PCOS is well established.[27] Yildiz and colleagues analyzed Turkish data from two population studies on PCOS prevalence and a hospital database of all untreated PCOS patients. In this study, the reported prevalence rates of PCOS in underweight, normal-weight, overweight and obese women in Turkey were as follows: 8.2%, 9.8%, 9.9% and 9.0% respectively. In this study, the highest rates of PCOS (12.4 and 11.5%) were found in women with a BMI of 35–40 kg/m^2 and greater than 40 kg/m^2.[28] The proportion of PCOS in 421 obese Chinese patients was also high (67%) and did not correlate with the presence of metabolic syndrome.[29]

Some studies of PCOS prevalence utilize public healthcare databases and resources of the medical insurance system. A cross-sectional study by Gabrielli and Aquino looked at 859 Brazilian women undergoing cervical cancer screening in the primary care setting.[30] They found a PCOS prevalence of 8.5% as defined by the Rotterdam criteria. Concurrently, the prevalence of PCOS among privately insured women in the USA was 1 585.1 per 100 000 or less than 1.6%.[31]

Limited epidemiological data have been derived from the secondary analysis of databases and registries from non-PCOS studies. In 2005, Goodarzi and colleagues recruited 156 unselected premenopausal women from the UCLA/Cedars-Sinai Mexican-American Coronary Artery Disease (MACAD) Project, a study of Mexican American families with a parent who has coronary artery disease.[13] In this project, 13% of participants met the NIH 1990 criteria for PCOS by self-reporting irregular menses and clinical signs of hyperandrogenism. A notable limitation of this study is that the authors used the self-reported data only, with no inclusion of objective examinations or laboratory data. A high prevalence of PCOS under the NIH 1990 definition in this study possibly resulted from the selection of participants based on a preexisting family history of coronary artery disease, which may account for this finding. Indeed, later, in 2010, Moran and colleagues reported a lower estimate of PCOS prevalence in Mexican female volunteers: 6% (NIH 1990) or 6.6% (Rotterdam 2003).[32] Among 827 female participants in a cross-sectional study of a nested cohort from the Dallas Heart Study (2000–2002), PCOS prevalence as defined by the classic NIH 1990 was 8%, and 19.6% as defined by Rotterdam 2003.[33]

PCOS Prevalence in Medically Unbiased Populations

Although the abovementioned studies are valuable, the results of the PCOS assessment at the referral settings are definitely at risk of bias due to the selection of participants.[34] Consequently, the unselected (medically unbiased) populations are more representative and thus preferable for epidemiological studies. These populations, as identified in the nonclinical settings, allow investigators to establish population-based "controls" and determine the prevalence of PCOS and the "naturally" occurring PCOS phenotype. The population-related differences were also significant when comparing the prevalence and distribution of the PCOS phenotype. A systematic

review and meta-analysis of 41 studies found the "classic" PCOS phenotype to be more prevalent in PCOS patients identified in referral vs. unselected populations under the Rotterdam 2003 diagnostic criteria.[35] The main characteristics and results of studies of PCOS performed in unselected populations are summarized in Table 3.2.

A population-based model is a "gold standard" for prevalence studies, although it is more challenging to perform and may suffer from incomplete data. When applying this model, different approaches to recruiting participants are used, examples include – though not exhaustive – random sampling from households, communities and birth cohorts. Kumarapeli and colleagues carried out a community-based, cross-sectional study to estimate PCOS prevalence and phenotype in a community setting in Sri Lanka in 2008.[36] The authors utilized an interviewer-administered questionnaire to screen for "probable cases" of PCOS and then referred selected "probable cases" for further assessment. With the previously diagnosed cases, the total prevalence under the Rotterdam 2003 diagnostic criteria was 6.3%.[36] Later, in a retrospective birth cohort study in 2010, March and colleagues demonstrated that the PCOS prevalence estimates under the Rotterdam and AES definitions were up to two times higher than those obtained with the NIH criteria. Interestingly, 68–69% of patients with PCOS identified in this study did not have a preexisting diagnosis.[6]

In the community-based sample of premenopausal women randomly selected from the different geographic regions of Iran, the prevalence of PCOS depending on diagnostic criteria was 7.1–14.6%.[8] These data were consistent with the previously reported estimated prevalence of PCOS in Iranian women referred to the mandatory pre-marriage screening clinic: 7%–15.2% under different diagnostic criteria.[7] In 2014, Rashidi and colleagues conducted a large community-based study in the southwest of Iran, with estimated PCOS prevalence as follows: 4.8% under the NIH definition, 14.1% using the Rotterdam approach and 12% by the AES criteria.[12]

As mentioned, 15.3% of Australian Indigenous women were diagnosed with PCOS as assessed using the NIH 1990 criteria.[14] A large-scale community-based study in China in 2013 demonstrated a much lower PCOS prevalence (5.6%)

according to the Rotterdam 2003 definition.[10] In 2014, Zhuang and colleagues found that the prevalence of PCOS in Chinese women aged 12–44 years varied from 7.1 to 11.2%, depending on the diagnostic criteria used.[11]

An institution-based model helps to determine the PCOS in unselected populations requiring medical assessment for nonmedical reasons: pre-employment, yearly employment and so on. A well-designed prospective study was performed at the pre-employment physical check of 277 reproductive-aged women in the southeastern USA. In this study, PCOS as defined under the NIH criteria was found in 4% of examined women.[37] In 2004, the cumulative PCOS prevalence of 6.6% was reported for a large representative unselected population of women seeking a pre-employment physical at the University of Alabama at Birmingham.[4] These data led the authors to conclude that PCOS is one of the most common reproductive endocrine disorders of women in the USA. The prevalence rates of PCOS among employees of a governmental institution in Turkey varied depending on the PCOS definitions, from 6.1% to 19.9%.[9]

Another model for unbiased epidemiological studies utilizes populations undergoing medical assessment for nonreproductive medical reasons. In 2008, Chen and colleagues evaluated 915 Chinese women of reproductive age undergoing their annual physical examination. This representative epidemiological study demonstrated a 2.4% prevalence of PCOS as defined by the Rotterdam 2003 criteria and 2.2% by the AES 2006 criteria.[38]

Table 3.2 PCOS prevalence in unselected, medically unbiased populations

Authors (year)	Country	Study design*	Population	Prevalence, % [95% CI], if presented, diagnostic criteria
Asunción et al. (2000)[3]	Spain	Prospective study	154 women, aged 18–45 years, blood donors from Madrid	6.5% NIH 1990
Azziz et al. (2004)[4]	USA	Prospective study	400 women, aged 18–45 years, pre-employment physical assessment, the University of Alabama at Birmingham	6.6% NIH 1990 (8.0% in black women, 4.8% in white women)
Boyle et al. (2012)[14]	Australia	Cross-sectional study	248 Indigenous women, aged 15–44 years, living in a defined area in and around Darwin, Northern Territory	15.3% [10.8–19.8] NIH 1990
Chen et al. (2008)[38]	China	Observational study	915 women, aged 20–45 years, living in Guangzhou, investigated at the time of their annual physical examination	2.4% Rott 2003 2.2% AES 2006
Diamanti-Kandarakis et al. (1999)[1]	Greece	Cross-sectional study	192 women, aged 17–45 years, living on the Greek island of Lesbos	6.77% NIH 1990
Knochenhauer et al. (1998)[37]	USA	Prospective study	277 women, aged 18–45 years, pre-employment physical assessment, the University of Alabama at Birmingham	4% NIH 1990 (3.4% in black women, 4.7% in white women)
Kumarapeli (2008)[36]	Sri Lanka	Community-based, cross-sectional study	A random sample of 2915 women, aged 15–39 years, permanent residents of the district of Gampaha	6.3% [5.9–6.8] Rott 2003

Table 3.2 (cont.)

Authors (year)	Country	Study design*	Population	Prevalence, % [95% CI], if presented, diagnostic criteria
Lauritsen et al. (2014)[16]	Denmark	Prospective, cross-sectional study	447 women, aged 20–40 years, employed at Copenhagen University Hospital, Rigshospitalet	16.6% Rott 2003
Li et al. (2013)[10]	China	Community-based study	15924 women, aged 19–45 years, residents of 152 cities and 112 villages of 10 provinces and municipalities in China	5.6% Rott 2003
March et al. (2010)[6]	Australia	Retrospective birth cohort study	728 women born during 1973–1975 in a single maternity hospital in Adelaide, interviewed in adulthood, aged 27–34 years	8.7% NIH 1990 11.9% Rott 2003 10.2% AES 2006
Mehrabian et al. (2011)[7]	Iran	Cross-sectional study	820 females, aged 17–34 years, recruited during the mandatory pre-marriage screening clinic in Isfahan	7% NIH 1990 15.2% Rott 2003 7.92% AES 2006
Michelmore et al. (1999)[2]	UK	Cross-sectional study	230 women, aged 18–25 years – volunteers from two universities and two general practice surgeries in Oxford	8% NIH 1990
Moran et al. (2010)[32]	Mexico	Prospective cross-sectional study	150 female Mexican volunteers, aged 20–45 years, employees of an Obstetrics and Gynecology Hospital of the Mexican Institute of Social Security, Mexico City	6% [1.9–10.1] NIH 1990 6.6% [2.3–10.9] Rott 2003
Rashidi et al. (2014)[12]	Iran	Community-based study	646 women, aged 18–45, living in urban areas of three randomly selected cities of Khouzestan province	4.8% NIH 1990 14.1% Rott 2003 12% AES 2006
Tehrani et al. (2011)[8]	Iran	Community-based study	1126 women, aged 18–45 years, randomly selected from the population of different geographic regions of Iran	7.1% [5.4–8.8] NIH 1990 14.6% [12.3–16.9] Rott 2003 11.7% [9.5–13.7] AES 2006
Yildiz et al. (2012)[9]	Turkey	Cross-sectional study	392 women, aged 18–45 years, employees of the government-based institute in Ankara	6.1 % NIH 1990 19.9 % Rott 2003 15.3% AES 2006
Zhuang et al. (2014)[11]	China	A community-based cross-sectional study	1645 female residents of Chengdu, aged 12–44 years	7.1 % NIH 1990 11.2% Rott 2003 7.4% AES 2006

* as defined by the authors

Studies of medical staff or healthy volunteers are also helpful but of lower quality due to selection bias. Michelmore and colleagues, in 1990, determined the prevalence of PCO and associated clinical and biochemical features in two universities and two general practice surgeries. The prevalence of PCOS in this group was estimated as 8% when using the NIH 1990 criteria and as high as 26% when UK criteria were applied.[2] Asunción and colleagues analyzed the prevalence of PCOS, as defined by the NIH 1990 criteria, in blood donors. In this minimally biased population, PCOS was found in 6.5% of participants.[3] Among premenopausal women employed at the Copenhagen University Hospital, the prevalence of PCOS was much higher (16.6% according to the Rotterdam 2003 criteria). Still, the prevalence significantly decreased with age: from 33.3% in women younger than 30 years to 10.2% in those over the age of 35 years ($P < 0.001$). The authors suggest that the study population (healthcare workers) and the exclusion of hormonal contraceptive users may have caused selection bias.[16]

PCOS Prevalence: Contribution of Race and Ethnicity

There is some evidence to date that race and ethnicity contribute to the heterogeneity of prevalence and clinical manifestation of PCOS. In general, East Asians are likely to have a lower rate of PCOS than Caucasians, and an "Asian phenotype" for the polycystic ovarian syndrome is of interest.[39] The PCOS rate (NIH 1990) for black and white women appears to be comparable: 8.0 and 4.8%, respectively.[4] The prevalence of PCOS under different criteria depending on ethnicity was investigated by Ding and colleagues in 2017 in a systematic review and meta-analysis of 13 eligible studies. It found that the lowest PCOS prevalence (5.6%, 95% CI: 4.4–7.3, Rotterdam 2003) was among the Chinese cohort. The urgent need to create ethnicity-specific guidelines was emphasized in this review in order to prevent under- or overdiagnosis of PCOS.[40] More recently, Kim and Choi also highlighted the importance of accounting for race and ethnicity in order to standardize the diagnosis of PCOS.[41]

Guidelines for Epidemiological Studies of PCOS

To improve the quality and comparability of PCOS prevalence studies, the Androgen Excess and PCOS (AE-PCOS) Society has recently published best-practice guidelines for designing and conducting epidemiologic and phenotypic studies in PCOS.[42] The published document outlines the key recommendations for study design and includes advice on selecting the study population, the diagnostic criteria, the type of observational study and the primary and secondary endpoint(s). The guidelines advocate that it is fundamental to utilize generalizable populations, a broad diagnostic criteria and methods of high sensitivity when assessing the individual PCOS features in prevalence studies. The exact definition of what is "normal" in the population is also essential and strongly recommended. Crucially, the guidelines provide researchers around the world with the tools to conduct epidemiological studies of PCOS of the best quality and validity.[42]

References

1 Diamanti-Kandarakis, E., Kouli, C. R., Bergiele, A. T. et al. A survey of the polycystic ovary syndrome in the Greek island of Lesbos: Hormonal and metabolic profile. *J Clin Endocrinol Metab* 1999; 84(11): 4006–4011.

2 Michelmore, K. F., Balen, A. H., Dunger, D. B. and Vessey, M. P. Polycystic ovaries and associated clinical and biochemical features in young women. *Clin Endocrinol (Oxf)* 1999;51(6): 779–786.

3 Asunción, M., Calvo, R. M., San Millán, J .L., Sancho, J., Avila, S. and Escobar-Morreale, H. F. A prospective study of the prevalence of the polycystic ovary syndrome in unselected Caucasian women from Spain. *J Clin Endocrinol Metab* 2000; 85(7): 2434–2438.

4 Azziz, R, Woods, K. S., Reyna, R., Key, T. J., Knochenhauer, E. S. and Yildiz, B. O. The prevalence and features of the polycystic ovary syndrome in an unselected population. *J Clin Endocrinol Metab* 2004; 89(6): 2745–2749.

5 Vutyavanich, T., Khaniyao, V., Wongtra-Ngan, S., Sreshthaputra, O., Sreshthaputra, R. and Piromlertamorn, W. Clinical, endocrine and ultrasonographic features of polycystic ovary syndrome in Thai women. *J Obstet Gynaecol Res* 2007; 33(5): 677–680.

6 March, W. A., Moore, V. M., Willson, K. J., Phillips, D. I., Norman, R. J. and Davies, M. J. The

prevalence of polycystic ovary syndrome in a community sample assessed under contrasting diagnostic criteria. *Hum Reprod* 2010; 25(2): 544–551.

7 Mehrabian, F., Khani, B., Kelishadi, R. and Ghanbari, E. The prevalence of polycystic ovary syndrome in Iranian women based on different diagnostic criteria. *Endokrynol Pol* 2011; 62(3): 238–42.

8 Tehrani, F. R., Simbar, M., Tohidi, M., Hosseinpanah, F. and Azizi, F. The prevalence of polycystic ovary syndrome in a community sample of Iranian population: Iranian PCOS prevalence study. *Reprod Biol Endocrinol* 2011; 9: 39.

9 Yildiz, B. O., Bozdag, G., Yapici, Z., Esinler, I. and Yarali, H. Prevalence, phenotype and cardiometabolic risk of polycystic ovary syndrome under different diagnostic criteria. *Hum Reprod* 2012; 27(10): 3067–3073.

10 Li, R., Zhang, Q., Yang, D. et al. Prevalence of polycystic ovary syndrome in women in China: A large community-based study. *Hum Reprod* 2013; 28(9): 2562–2569.

11 Zhuang, J., Liu, Y., Xu, L. et al. Prevalence of the polycystic ovary syndrome in female residents of Chengdu, China. *Gynecol Obstet Invest* 2014; 77(4): 217–223.

12 Rashidi, H., Ramezani Tehrani, F., Bahri Khomami, M., Tohidi, M. and Azizi, F. To what extent does the use of the Rotterdam criteria affect the prevalence of polycystic ovary syndrome? A community-based study from the Southwest of Iran. *Eur J Obstet Gynecol Reprod Biol* 2014; 174: 100–105.

13 Goodarzi, M. O., Quiñones, M .J., Azziz, R., Rotter, J. I., Hsueh, W. A. and Yang, H. Polycystic ovary syndrome in Mexican-Americans: Prevalence and association with the severity of insulin resistance. *Fertil Steril* 2005; 84(3): 766–769.

14 Boyle, J. A., Cunningham, J., O'Dea, K., Dunbar, T. and Norman, R. J. Prevalence of polycystic ovary syndrome in a sample of Indigenous women in Darwin, Australia. *Med J Aust* 2012; 196(1): 62–66.

15 Broekmans, F. J., Knauff, E. A., Valkenburg, O., Laven, J. S., Eijkemans, M. J. and Fauser, B. C. PCOS according to the Rotterdam consensus criteria: Change in prevalence among WHO-II anovulation and association with metabolic factors. *BJOG* 2006; 113(10): 1210–1217.

16 Lauritsen, M .P., Bentzen, J. G., Pinborg, A. et al. The prevalence of polycystic ovary syndrome in a normal population according to the Rotterdam criteria versus revised criteria including anti-Müllerian hormone. *Hum Reprod* 2014; 29(4): 791–801.

17 Jalilian, A., Kiani, F., Sayehmiri, F., Sayehmiri, K., Khodaee, Z. and Akbari, M. Prevalence of polycystic ovary syndrome and its associated complications in Iranian women: A meta-analysis. *Iran J Reprod Med* 2015; 13(10): 591–604.

18 Bozdag, G., Mumusoglu, S., Zengin, D., Karabulut, E. and Yildiz, B. O. The prevalence and phenotypic features of polycystic ovary syndrome: A systematic review and meta-analysis. *Hum Reprod* 2016; 31(12): 2841–2855.

19 Skiba, M. A., Islam, R. M., Bell, R. J. and Davis, S. R. Understanding variation in prevalence estimates of polycystic ovary syndrome: a systematic review and meta-analysis. *Hum Reprod Update* 2018; 24(6): 694–709.

20 Farah, L., Lazenby, A. J., Boots, L. R. and Azziz, R. Prevalence of polycystic ovary syndrome in women seeking treatment from community electrologists. Alabama Professional Electrology Association Study Group. *J Reprod Med* 1999; 44(10): 870–874.

21 Azziz, R., Sanchez, L. A., Knochenhauer, E. S. et al. Androgen excess in women: Experience with over 1000 consecutive patients. *J Clin Endocrinol Metab* 2004; 89(2): 453–462.

22 Carmina, E., Rosato, F., Janni, A., Rizzo, M. and Longo, R. A. Extensive clinical experience: Relative prevalence of different androgen excess disorders in 950 women referred because of clinical hyperandrogenism. *J Clin Endocrinol Metab* 2006; 91(1): 2–6.

23 Allen, S. E., Potter, H. D. and Azziz, R. Prevalence of hyperandrogenemia among nonhirsute oligo-ovulatory women. *Fertil Steril.* 1997; 67(3): 569–572.

24 Lowe, P., Kovacs, G. and Howlett, D. Incidence of polycystic ovaries and polycystic ovary syndrome amongst women in Melbourne, Australia. *Aust N Z J Obstet Gynaecol* 2005; 45(1): 17–19.

25 Deshpande, P. S. and Gupta, A. S. Causes and prevalence of factors causing infertility in a public health facility. *J Hum Reprod Sci* 2019; 12(4): 287–293.

26 Kudesia, R., Illions, E. H. and Lieman, H. J. Elevated prevalence of polycystic ovary syndrome and cardiometabolic disease in South Asian infertility patients. *J Immigr Minor Health* 2017; 19(6): 1338–1342.

27 Legro, R. S. Obesity and PCOS: Implications for diagnosis and treatment. *Semin Reprod Med* 2012; 30(6): 496–506.

28 Yildiz, B. O., Knochenhauer, E. S. and Azziz, R. Impact of obesity on the risk for polycystic ovary syndrome. *J Clin Endocrinol Metab* 2008; 93(1): 162–168.

29 Liang, P., Xi, L., Shi, J. et al. Prevalence of polycystic ovary syndrome in Chinese obese women of reproductive age with or without metabolic syndrome. *Fertil Steril.* 2017; 107(4): 1048–1054.

30 Gabrielli, L. and Aquino, E. M. Polycystic ovary syndrome in Salvador, Brazil: A prevalence study in primary healthcare. *Reprod Biol Endocrinol* 2012; 10: 96.

31 Okoroh, E. M., Hooper, W. C., Atrash, H. K., Yusuf, H. R. and Boulet, S. L. Prevalence of polycystic ovary syndrome among the privately insured, United States, 2003–2008. *Am J Obstet Gynecol* 2012; 207(4): 299.e1–299.e2997.

32 Moran, C., Tena, G., Moran, S., Ruiz, P., Reyna, R. and Duque, X. Prevalence of polycystic ovary syndrome and related disorders in Mexican women. *Gynecol Obstet Invest* 2010; 69(4): 274–280.

33 Chang, A. Y., Ayers, C., Minhajuddin, A. et al. Polycystic ovarian syndrome and subclinical atherosclerosis among women of reproductive age in the Dallas heart study. *Clin Endocrinol (Oxf)* 2011; 74(1): 89–96.

34 Ezeh, U., Yildiz, B. O. and Azziz, R. Referral bias in defining the phenotype and prevalence of obesity in polycystic ovary syndrome. *J Clin Endocrinol Metab* 2013; 98(6): E1088–1096.

35 Lizneva, D., Kirubakaran, R., Mykhalchenko, K. et al. Phenotypes and body mass in women with polycystic ovary syndrome identified in referral versus unselected populations: Systematic review and meta-analysis. *Fertil Steril* 2016; 106(6): 1510–1520.e2

36 Kumarapeli, V., Seneviratne, R. de A., Wijeyaratne, C. N., Yapa, R. M. and Dodampahala, S. H. A simple screening approach for assessing community prevalence and phenotype of polycystic ovary syndrome in a semi-urban population in Sri Lanka. *Am J Epidemiol* 2008; 168(3): 321–328.

37 Knochenhauer, E. S., Key, T. J., Kahsar-Miller, M., Waggoner, W., Boots, L. R. and Azziz, R. Prevalence of the polycystic ovary syndrome in unselected black and white women of the southeastern United States: A prospective study. *J Clin Endocrinol Metab* 1998; 83(9): 3078–3082.

38 Chen, X., Yang, D., Mo, Y., Li, L., Chen, Y. and Huang, Y. Prevalence of polycystic ovary syndrome in unselected women from southern China. *Eur J Obstet Gynecol Reprod Biol* 2008; 139(1): 59–64.

39 Huang, Z. and Yong, E. L. Ethnic differences: Is there an Asian phenotype for polycystic ovarian syndrome? *Best Pract Res Clin Obstet Gynaecol* 2016; 37: 46–55.

40 Ding, T., Hardiman, P. J., Petersen, I., Wang, F. F., Qu, F. and Baio, G. The prevalence of polycystic ovary syndrome in reproductive-aged women of different ethnicity: A systematic review and meta-analysis. *Oncotarget* 2017; 8(56): 96351–96358.

41 Kim, J. J. and Choi, Y. M. Phenotype and genotype of polycystic ovary syndrome in Asia: Ethnic differences. *J Obstet Gynaecol Res* 2019; 45(12): 2330–2337.

42 Azziz, R., Kintziger, K., Li, R. et al. Recommendations for epidemiologic and phenotypic research in polycystic ovary syndrome: An androgen excess and PCOS society resource. *Hum Reprod* 2019; 34(11): 2254–2265.

Ovarian Ultrasonography in Polycystic Ovary Syndrome

Heidi Vanden Brink and Marla E. Lujan

Historical Considerations Related to Polycystic Ovarian Morphology on Ultrasonography in the Diagnosis of PCOS

Initial Descriptions of Polycystic Ovaries in PCOS

Polycystic ovary syndrome (PCOS) is a complex endocrine disorder whose diverse clinical manifestation has led to considerable debate regarding which collection of symptoms constitute a diagnosis. Stein and Leventhal first described PCOS in a group of seven women displaying a broad spectrum of clinical findings including amenorrhea, infertility, obesity, hirsutism and acne.[1] The only consistent finding was the combined presence of irregular menses and enlarged bilateral polycystic ovaries. The presence of polycystic ovarian morphology (PCOM) was based on pelvic pneumography – a process in which air injected into the peritoneal cavity allowed for the relative shadowing of organs to be detected by X-ray. PCOM was designated when ovaries appeared to be enlarged to at least ¾ the size the uterine shadow.[1] Stein and Leventhal proceeded to surgically resect ½–¾ of each ovary, which subsequently had the remarkable effect of reinstating regular menstrual cycles in all patients. At the time of surgery, the ovaries were described as being two to four times the size of normal ovaries and appeared distinctly "globular" in shape.[1] Histological examination of the ovarian wedges removed revealed that the ovarian cortex was hypertrophied in all cases and that the ovarian capsule (tunica) was thickened, tough and fibrotic. Histological sections contained numerous small "cysts," varying from 1 to 15 mm in size and were generally confined to the cortex near the surface of the ovary. Approximately 20 to 100 small cysts were identified in each ovarian specimen and the presence of corpora lutea was rare. [1] Later histological assessments by others confirmed the "polyfollicular" nature of PCOM[2] and described a tendency toward excessive follicle maturation with polycystic ovaries containing the same number of primordial follicles as normal ovaries but twice as many developing follicles at the primary, secondary and tertiary (antral) stage. [3] While the precise nature of excessive and untimely follicle maturation in PCOS remains unresolved, the presence of PCOM is a common morphological feature of women with androgen excess and ovulatory dysfunction.[4, 5]

Advent of Ultrasonographic Imaging of Polycystic Ovaries

Pelvic pneumography did not gain popularity in the evaluation of PCOM, and in the years that followed, laparotomy and wedge resection became standard for both diagnosis and treatment of PCOS. Issues of invasiveness when evaluating PCOM were solved with the introduction of B-scanners in the 1960s. Using sound waves in the range of 3.5 MHz, static B-scanners produced relatively accurate 2D images of internal organs. However, the resolution limits of the B-scanners only allowed for a gross appreciation of ovarian size, and individual follicles were difficult to visualize.[6] The advent of real-time scanners (3.5–5.0 MHz) in the early 1980s eventually allowed for visualization and measurement of follicles as small as 2 mm, using a rapid succession of individual B-mode images to produce a moving video display. The earliest real-time scanners were configured for use in transabdominal ultrasonography (TAUS) and had the benefit of no longer requiring the patient to be submerged in water. TAUS descriptions of PCOM correlated well with histological findings,[7] and comparisons with laparoscopic inspection showed high sensitivity (97%) and specificity (100%) to detect PCOM.[8] TAUS was widely superseded by transvaginal ultrasonography (TVUS), which allowed for a more accurate and convenient view of the ovaries owing to the use of higher frequency transducers (> 6 MHz) that provide better resolving power (albeit at the expense of depth of penetration) and avoided the need for the acoustic window provided by a full bladder on TAUS. Further, PCOM detection rates on TVUS approximated 100%, which was substantially higher compared to rates using TAUS wherein failure to optimally visualize the ovaries was documented in up to 42% of cases.[9] As such, TVUS emerged as the gold standard approach for evaluating PCOM.

Polycystic Ovaries on Ultrasonography As a Cardinal Feature of PCOS

Despite the widespread availability of real-time TVUS in the 1990s, the first attempt by experts to generate an international consensus on diagnostic criteria for PCOS resulted in the exclusion of PCOM as a potential marker of the syndrome. According to the National Institutes of Health (NIH) criteria, the diagnosis was to be based on the combined presence of oligo-anovulation and clinical and/or biochemical hyperandrogenism (in the absence of other reasons for androgen excess or anovulatory infertility).[10] While these criteria were an important first step toward characterizing the phenotypic spectrum of PCOS, they overrode standards and practices employed in other nations where morphological diagnoses were a standard. In the years that followed, it became apparent that PCOM represented a relatively consistent finding among women demonstrating biochemical and clinical indices PCOS. Moreover, it was recognized that asymptomatic women with polycystic ovaries demonstrated subtle endocrine and metabolic abnormalities, implicating ovarian dysmorphology in the pathogenesis of PCOS.[11] In 2003, ultrasonographic evidence of PCOM was incorporated in a new set of consensus criteria at a joint meeting of the European Society of Human Reproduction and Embryology (ESHRE) and the American Society for Reproductive Medicine (ASRM) held in Rotterdam, the Netherlands. These "Rotterdam criteria" effectively broadened the phenotypic spectrum of PCOS in allowing a diagnosis when

two of three cardinal features were present: (1) oligo-anovulation, (2) clinical and/or biochemical hyperandrogenism and (3) polycystic ovaries on ultrasound. While there was concern that these criteria were too expansive – particularly in allowing the presence of the syndrome in the absence of androgen excess as judged by the 2006 Androgen Excess and PCOS (AE-PCOS) Society criteria,[12] they did reflect a majority agreement that PCOM is a significant component of the clinical presentation of PCOS. As recently as 2018, the first International Evidence-Based Guideline for the Assessment and Management of PCOS has upheld the use of the Rotterdam criteria to identify PCOS and, by extension, reaffirmed the value of ultrasonographic evaluations of ovarian morphology as a critical determinant in the clinical evaluation of PCOS.

Definitions for PCOM on Ultrasonography in the Detection of PCOS

Early Definition of Polycystic Ovaries on Transabdominal Ultrasonography

The first set of long-standing criteria for PCOM were developed by Adams and colleagues in the 1980s using transabdominal approaches and were largely based on expert opinion (Table 4.1). They described PCOM as having follicle excess, defined by the presence of 10 or more small follicles in a single slice (or cross-section) of the ovary – this metric has come to be abbreviated as FNPS (follicle number in a single slice). They noted two options for follicular arrangement either peripheral or scattered throughout, and although there was some suggestion of ovarian enlargement owing to an increased stroma, no threshold for ovarian enlargement was provided.

Rotterdam Definition of Polycystic Ovaries on Transvaginal Ultrasonography

With the introduction of PCOM as a cardinal feature of PCOS by the Rotterdam consensus, the definition for PCOM was updated to reflect the use of primarily transvaginal approaches (Table 4.1). The definition of follicle excess was revised to reflect 12 or more (2–9mm) follicles

Table 4.1 Definitions for follicle excess and ovarian enlargement in PCOS

Adams et al. (1986)

FNPS	≥ 10 (2–8 mm)	TAUS	Expert opinion [1]	Follicle distribution may be peripheral or scattered throughout an increased stroma

Rotterdam Consensus (2003)

FNPO	≥ 12 (2–9 mm)	TVUS	ROC curve analysis [2]	Stromal characteristics judged as too subjective for inclusion
OV	≥ 10 mL		Expert opinion	PCOM in one ovary is sufficient

AE-PCOS Society Task Force Report (2014)

FNPO	≥ 25 (2–9 mm)	TVUS	ROC curve analyses and 95th percentile of healthy women [3]	
OV	≥ 10 mL			

International Evidence-Based Guideline (2018)

FNPO	≥ 20 (2–9 mm)	TVUS	Clinical consensus recommendation* [4]	FNPO assessments should be limited to TVUS using 8 MHz
OV	≥ 10 mL		Clinical consensus recommendation* [4]	OV should be used when FNPO cannot be reliably assessed (i.e. TAUS and/or poor image quality)

Abbreviations: AE-PCOS, Androgen Excess and PCOS Society; FNPS, follicle number in a single slice; FNPO, follicle number per entire ovary; OV, ovarian volume; ROC curve, receiver operating characteristic curve analysis; TAUS, transabdominal ultrasonography; TVUS, transvaginal ultrasonography.

* Clinical consensus recommendations made by the guideline development group were defined as recommendations informed by evidence in other populations using rigorous and transparent processes based on a paucity of evidence in PCOS populations.

[1] Adams et al. Prevalence of polycystic ovaries in women with anovulation and idiopathic hirsutism. *Br Med J (Clin Res Ed)* 1986; 293: 355–359; [2] Jonard et al. Ultrasound examination of polycystic ovaries: Is it worth counting the follicles? *Hum Reprod* 2003; 18: 598–603; [3] Dewailly et al. Definition and significance of PCOM: A task force report from the Androgen Excess and Polycystic Ovary Syndrome Society. *Hum Reprod Update* 2014; 20: 334–352; [4] Teede et al. Recommendations from the international evidence-based guideline for the assessment and management of polycystic ovary syndrome. *Hum Reprod* 2018; 33: 1–17.

throughout the entire ovary and not just in a single slice. This new metric is abbreviated FNPO (follicle number per entire ovary) and reflected the findings of a single diagnostic test showing this threshold to have 75% sensitivity and 99% specificity to detect PCOS.[13] Further, a threshold for ovarian enlargement at ≥ 10 mL was provided, based on expert opinion.

Controversy over Rotterdam Criteria for Polycystic Ovaries

The Rotterdam criteria for PCOM proved problematic owing to numerous reports of high rates of PCOM in healthy women of reproductive age. This was interpreted as evidence that PCOM lacked specificity, while others proposed that criteria be revisited in light of advancements in ultrasound technology. As part of the 2014 AE-PCOS Society Task Force Report on the Definition and Significance of Polycystic Ovarian

Morphology, we concluded that the Rotterdam definition for follicle excess was obsolete and proposed a new threshold for FNPO at ≥ 25 follicles – that was notably more than double that supported by the Rotterdam consensus (Table 4.1). By contrast, the threshold for ovarian enlargement at 10 mL was corroborated. These recommendations for (re)defining PCOM were based on the assessment of published data for ovarian characteristics in healthy women of reproductive age and reflected a compromise between an estimate of the upper limits of normal of FNPO and OV in healthy women using new technology, as well as the performance of these metrics in diagnostic test studies of PCOS available at the time. Briefly, data were available for more than 1000 women across 6 studies and included community-based populations but also women attending fertility clinics wherein there was sufficient data to corroborate a normal endocrine profile. Ultimately, the 95th percentile of FNPO across studies converged at 23 follicles and OV at 10.8 mL. These values aligned with findings of diagnostic test studies, which showed significant diagnostic potential of FNPO, followed by OV, for the condition of PCOS.[14,15] It was not possible to provide direct evidence that new technology was enabling detection of more follicles and driving increases in FNPO over time, particularly since published reports did not provide information on the age of their equipment. However, when we plotted FNPO in healthy women versus increasing transducer frequency, as a surrogate for technological advancement, an effect of transducer frequency was noted particularly when frequency was greater or equal to 8 MHz.

Current Guideline Recommendations for Defining Polycystic Ovaries

In 2018, the International Evidence-Based Guideline for the Assessment and Management of PCOS provided four Clinical Consensus Recommendations (CCR) and five Clinical Practice Points (CPP) to inform the ultrasonographic evaluation of PCOM (Table 4.2).[16] No evidence-based recommendations (EBR) to define PCOM could be provided as the Guideline concluded that too few data were available on ovarian morphology in unbiased populations on which to base EBR. While there are some community-based data in healthy volunteers, data on ovarian morphology largely stem from women attending infertility clinics. Thresholds based on the 95th percentile were critiqued for their arbitrary nature and uncertainty regarding their clustering with short- or long-term health outcomes in PCOS (i.e. biological relevance). Further, the difficulty in harmonizing data across studies was highlighted. Indeed, there is no consensus on approaches for evaluating ultrasonographic ovarian features, there is confusion on terminology for ultrasonographic metrics and technology varies widely across studies, which theoretically could have an impact.

The Guideline recommends transvaginal (or endovaginal) ultrasonographic imaging as the preferred approach to evaluate ovarian features if sexually active and if acceptable to the individual. Using TVUS whose bandwidth includes

Table 4.2 Guideline recommendations for the ultrasound evaluation of PCOS

Clinical Consensus Recommendations
- Transvaginal approach is preferred in the diagnosis of PCOS, if sexually active and if acceptable to the individual.
- Ultrasound should not be used in those with a gynecological age of < 8 years due to high incidence of multi-follicular ovaries.
- Threshold for polycystic ovarian morphology (PCOM) should be revised regularly with advancing ultrasound technology, and age-specific cutoffs for PCOM should be defined.
- Using transvaginal ultrasonography (bandwidth includes 8 MHz), the threshold for PCOM on either ovary is a follicle number per ovary (FNPO) of ≥ 20 and/or an ovarian volume (OV) of ≥ 10 mL, ensuring no corpus luteum or dominant follicles are present.

Clinical Practice Points
- Ultrasound is not required for those with irregular menstrual cycles and hyperandrogenism but enables the identification of the complete PCOS phenotype.
- If using older ultrasound technology, the threshold for PCOM should be OV ≥ 10 mL on either ovary. Use of FNPO is discouraged.
- If using transabdominal ultrasound, reporting is best focused on OV ≥ 10 mL, given the difficulty in reliably obtaining FNPO.
- Training in careful and meticulous follicle counting per ovary is needed to improve FNPO reporting.
  - Minimum reporting standards when evaluating ovarian morphology include:
  - Approach/route assessed
  - Transducer bandwidth frequency
  - Last menstrual period
  - Endometrial thickness and appearance
  - Follicle number in each ovary (2–9 mm)
  - Three dimensions and volume of each ovary
  - Appearance or absence of other ovarian structures (e.g. ovarian cysts, corpus luteum, dominant follicles ≥ 10 mm)

Clinical consensus recommendations (CCR) made by the Guideline development group were defined as recommendations informed by evidence in other populations using rigorous and transparent processes based on a paucity of evidence in PCOS populations. Clinical practice points (CPP) represent recommendations that arose based on discussions stemming from evidence-based recommendations or CCR. In the case of CPP, evidence was not sought.

Source. Adapted from Teede et al. Recommendations from the international evidence-based guideline for the assessment and management of polycystic ovary syndrome. *Hum Reprod* 2018; 33: 1–17.

8 MHz, the threshold for PCOM on either ovary is an FNPO of ≥ 20 and/or an OV of ≥ 10 mL, ensuring no corpora lutea or dominant follicles are present (Table 4.2). The evidence synthesis related to this revised threshold for follicle excess is not yet published, but it is expected to reveal the position that thresholds should be based primarily on data generated in the most unbiased populations available – with reconsideration of the appropriateness of the 95th percentile to judge the upper limit of normal. If using older technology or TAUS, the Guideline recommends a focus on ovarian enlargement using an OV threshold of ≥ 10 mL on either ovary given the potential difficulty in reliably assessing FNPO. However, we are of the opinion that if you have good visualization of follicles in the largest cross-sectional slice of the ovary using either TVUS or TAUS, a FNPS threshold of 9 or 10 follicles in a single slice can be used. This approach reflects early reports by Adams and colleagues,[17] as well as our more recent work indicating that FNPS increases the diagnostic accuracy OV for PCOS when used in combination.[14, 18] Ultimately, these most recent Guideline recommendations support follicle excess (i.e. FNPO) as the most predictive marker for PCOS, followed by ovarian enlargement. Consistent with previous definitions, identification of PCOM in one ovary is sufficient. Our recent findings of left–right differences in PCOM in women with PCOS support prioritizing the use of FNPO, over FNPS and OV.[19] FNPO showed the strongest correlation between ovaries and, unlike FNPS and OV, there were no differences in the probability of unilateral versus bilateral PCOM in women with PCOS when using FNPO as the defining feature. Last, the Guideline acknowledges that criteria to define PCOM should be expected to change regularly with advancing ultrasound imaging technology.

Other Ultrasonographic or Surrogate Markers of Polycystic Ovarian Morphology

Ovarian Stroma

Stromal hypertrophy was noted by Stein and Leventhal in the earliest descriptions of PCOS.[1]

Likewise, Adams and colleagues commented on the abundance of stroma in their early description of PCOM on ultrasonography.[17] An enlarged central stroma is thought to result from ovarian thecal hyperthecosis secondary to excessive luteinizing hormone (LH) and/or insulin stimulation.[7, 20] For these reasons, stromal enlargement is posited as a specific morphologic indicator of ovarian hyperandrogenism. Stromal area (SA), stromal echogenicity or brightness (SEcho) and the ratio of stromal to total ovarian area (S/A) have all been proposed as ultrasonographic indicators of PCOS – albeit with varying degrees of diagnostic accuracy.[18] We have shown that stromal assessments have no or inferior predictive power for PCOS compared to FNPO and OV.[18] The 2018 Guideline does not support the use of stromal assessments in the evaluation of PCOM in part owing to a perceived redundancy with ovarian size. We have demonstrated that commonly used methods to estimate SA, S/A and SEcho lack reproducibility (unpublished data). Together, there is a need to standardize stromal assessments in order to improve their clinical utility in the ultrasound diagnosis of PCOS.

Follicle Distribution Pattern

Early descriptions of PCOM on ultrasonography also commonly reference the arrangement of ovarian follicles as a "string of pearls," referring to the preponderance of small anechoic follicles situated around the periphery of an enlarged, hyperechoic central stroma.[17] A peripheral accumulation of follicles is thought to be attributed to stromal hypertrophy[3] and may reflect etiological origins of PCOS for a subset of patients. We showed that a peripheral distribution pattern is a highly specific indicator of PCOS [18] – but lacks sensitivity as heterogeneous distribution of follicles is also possible. Similar to stromal measures, assessments of follicle distribution pattern are difficult to standardize. We proposed a scale for grading the degree of peripherally distributed follicles (FDP) and found no association between FDP and reproductive or metabolic features in women with PCOS, unlike other ultrasonographic features (e.g. FNPO and OV).[21] We posit that our suggestion of an intermediate category (peripheral follicle aggregation with > 1 central follicle) for follicle distribution may have introduced an additional layer of subjectivity to the assessment that clouded the physiologic relevance of an overt FDP. Alas, assessments of follicle distribution pattern cannot be considered diagnostic for PCOS at this time.

Vascular Indices

Despite numerous studies evaluating differences in ovarian blood flow using 2D and 3D approaches, no current consensus has been reached regarding the diagnostic or prognostic utility of Doppler imaging in the ultrasonographic evaluation of PCOS. In general, 3D metrics such as the vascularization index (VI), flow index (FI) and vascularization-flow index (VFI) were shown to be consistently higher in women with PCOS, implying increased blood flow within the ovary relative to non-PCOS ovaries.[22, 23] Null or inconsistent findings using 2D metrics (resistivity index, RI; pulsatility index, PI) may be attributed to the reliance on a single blood vessel in the ovary, as opposed to 3D metrics, which encapsulate organ-level perfusion, as has been noted by others.[22] Further, it must be acknowledged that Doppler imaging is more technically challenging than B-mode or grayscale imaging, subject to motion artifacts and additional image optimization considerations that together impact reproducibility.[24] That said, in 2007 Lam and colleagues reported that lean women with PCOS, or women with hirsutism, had increased ovarian vascularity defined by 3D Doppler indices versus their overweight or nonhirsute counterparts, suggesting phenotypic variation and a potentially underlying role of adiposity or accrued androgen exposure on ovarian blood flow.[22] Ultimately, resolving the physiologic relevance for Doppler imaging in the diagnosis and evaluation of PCOS is needed to better justify its future consideration as part of the diagnostic work-up for PCOS.

Anti-Müllerian Hormone (AMH)

Anti-Müllerian hormone (AMH) is a glycoprotein belonging to the transforming growth factor beta (TGF-β) family that is produced by ovarian granulosa cells from the primary stage through to dominance. Small antral follicles contribute substantially to circulating AMH levels and, for this reason, AMH levels correlate with FNPO and antral follicle counts (AFC) made on ultrasonography. Several groups have interrogated the potential for AMH to serve as a proxy for PCOM and numerous thresholds have been proposed – all showing significant predictive power for PCOS.[25] That said, the recent 2018 Guideline concluded that serum AMH levels should not yet be used as an alternative for the detection of PCOM or as a single test for the diagnosis of PCOS.[16] The evidence synthesis on this recommendation was recently published and indicated that no thresholds for AMH to define PCOM could be proposed.[25] Studies reporting on AMH levels in women with PCOS were judged to have moderate to high risk of bias and lacked well-defined study populations. AMH levels reported were significantly heterogeneous across studies and those proposing cutoffs to define PCOM used inconsistent methods to define thresholds. Further, methodological challenges related to the lack of concordance across AMH assays were noted and much of the available data on AMH levels in PCOS were deemed obsolete owing to discontinued assays. That said, the Guideline concluded that AMH shows promise as a surrogate marker for PCOM, particularly if an international standard can be developed for assay harmonization. An endocrine assay with a high degree of reproducibility could represent a convenient alternative to ultrasound wherein challenges related to costs, accessibility and reproducibility admittedly exist. That said, the degree to which AMH is interchangeable with PCOM is still debatable. A better understanding of their biological relevance across the spectrum of PCOS would better delineate the role of AMH as a surrogate or adjuvant to ultrasonographic evaluations of PCOM.

Technical Considerations Related to the Ultrasonographic Evaluation of Polycystic Ovarian Morphology

2D Real-Time Imaging

Ultrasound assessments of ovarian morphology are most commonly made using 2D real-time (2D-RT) imaging. That is, live scanning with the patient or participant. In 2D-RT, an ovary is identified in a reference (scanning) plane – typically

Table 4.3 Overview of ultrasound imaging techniques to evaluate follicle number per ovary (FNPO) and ovarian volume (OV)

	Strengths	Limitations
2D Real-Time Imaging	- Convenient - Enables real-time B-mode and Doppler interrogation of ovarian and para-ovarian structures	- Assessments cannot be audited and are subject to scheduling pressures - Longer scans may lead to user fatigue and patient intolerability - FNPO assessments may be unreliable owing to over- or undercounting - Risk of PCOM misclassification based on FNPO - OV calculations subject to error owing to manual approximation of orthogonal planes
2D Offline Imaging	- Enables auditing and reassessments in questionable cases - Minimizes scanning time - Provides more reproducible estimates of FNPO as follicles can be flagged as they are counted - Preferred approach when more precise evaluations of FNPO and/or follicle size are needed - Reliably classifies PCOM status	- Methods focused on both follicle number and size are time-consuming and may not be feasible in clinical practice - OV calculations subject to error owing to manual approximation of orthogonal planes
3D Imaging	- Enables auditing and reassessments in questionable cases - Reduces live scanning time by capturing datasets for offline analysis - Motorized array enables precise capture of orthogonal planes, which improves accuracy of OV estimates - Simultaneous viewing of orthogonal planes may better delineate ovarian features - Provides adequate assessments of PCOM status when a precise follicle number is not required	- Reproducibility of techniques are not well established - Proprietary software limits functionalities available for assessments of FNPO and OV - Requires substantial training in image analysis

one that captures the long axis of the ovary – and a manual sweep of the transducer enables the live assessment of ovarian features viewed in that one and only scanning plane. The respective orthogonal plane can be approximated by rotating the transducer 90 degrees and repeating a manual sweep to assess the ovary from one margin to the next in this separate plane. Real-time imaging has advantages over offline assessments, including its convenience and ability to resolve intra- and para-ovarian structures by using Doppler interrogation and/or applying variable degrees of pressure with the transducer against the structures in question. By contrast, real-time assessments cannot be audited, are subject to sonographer fatigue, patient discomfort owing to a longer scanning time and scheduling pressures.

Standardized approaches for obtaining AFC in real time have been proposed.[26, 27] In general, they entail performing a scout sweep of the ovary in both the transverse and sagittal planes to determine the optimal scanning plane for visualizing

follicles as well as determining the size of the largest follicle (F1) and presence or absence of a corpus luteum (CL). Once the desired plane is determined, manual adjustments to optimize image quality (i.e. change in gain, focal zone(s), depth) can be made to increase contrast and better delineate between anechoic follicles and the ovarian stroma. All follicles 2–10 mm in diameter identified when scanning from one ovarian margin to the next would yield the FNPO for one particular ovary. In instances where a follicle larger than 10 mm is identified, that follicle is not included in the FNPO estimate. The process is then repeated for the contralateral ovary. In the case of assessments for PCOM, the average of the counts for the left and right ovary yields the final FNPO.

To estimate OV, the ovary is scanned until the largest cross-sectional view of the ovary is identified. A still image of this single slice is captured and the corresponding orthogonal view identified. Most ultrasound systems enable linear measurements of the longitudinal (D1), transverse (D2) and anteroposterior (D3) dimensions to be made while viewing both captured images simultaneously (in adjacent views). Likewise, systems are equipped with volumetric calculators that employ the equation of a prolate ellipsoid to yield OV [$\pi/6$ (D1 × D2 × D3)]. The process is repeated for the contralateral ovary. In the case of assessments for PCOM, the average of the OV measurements for the left and right ovary yields the final OV. In instances where a follicle larger than 10 mm is identified, the convention is to use the measurement of a single ovary – the one without a dominant follicle – to estimate OV.

2D Offline Imaging

Two-dimensional (2D) real-time imaging of the ovaries can be captured in cineloops (videoclips) and later viewed offline. This approach is used for training, resolving uncertainties and auditing purposes in clinical practice. In our experience, recognizing and counting antral follicle in real time is challenging and difficult to reproduce, [28, 29] particularly in the case of PCOM where follicle excess, follicle clustering and/or compromised image quality owing to obesity are common. Figure 4.1 outlines several considerations for the recognition of antral follicles that are, in our experience, particularly helpful when making determinations of FNPO. Use of 2D offline imaging enables the rater to count and measure follicles without the pressures of a live patient. The use of calipers to flag individual follicles as they are counted is a major advantage over real-time

imaging as it minimizes the risk under- or over-counting of follicles thereby improving accuracy. Indeed, a major challenge in PCOM is the sheer number of follicles, which can be daunting when assessing the ovary in its entirety. We have developed a grid method for use in 2D offline imaging that helps to compartmentalize the approach to counting follicles thereby making estimates of FNPO more manageable (Figure 4.2).[29] The method involves superimposing a grid over the ovarian cineloop, which partitions the ovary into two or more sections, depending on user preferences. The rater is then able to scroll through the ovary counting (and marking) all follicles that appear within a given grid section. This process is repeated for each grid section and the FNPO yielded represents a tally of the follicles across all grid sections. This approach is highly reliable but time-consuming, particularly when both the size and the number of follicles are assessed. That said, we recently piloted a real-time approach to the grid method where, instead of measuring or marking each follicle, the investigator simply kept a tally of the follicles observed in 2–6 grid sections. Unlike conventional 2D real-time imaging, this 2D real-time with grid method did not lead to misclassification of PCOM,[30] justifying the additional 1 minute needed to perform the measurement.

3D Imaging

The use of 3D ultrasound systems is expanding widely in primary and specialized healthcare settings. A stark advantage of 3D over 2D imaging is

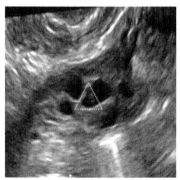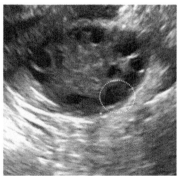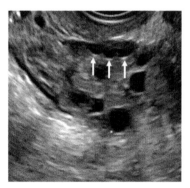

Figure 4.1 Identifying follicles on ultrasonography
Most follicles will appear as round anechoic circular structures. Follicles may also appear (left panel) irregularly shaped or compressed, (middle panel) shaded or not purely anechoic or (right panel) not have discernible walls between adjacent follicles (clustered). The number of clustered follicles may be inferred by bright artifacts of specular reflection (arrows) commonly detected at the base of individual follicles.

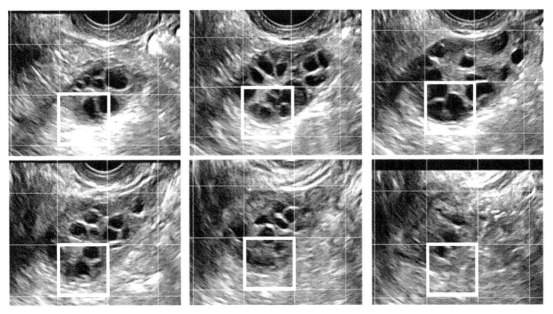

Figure 4.2 2D offline image analysis using the grid method for assessing follicle number per ovary

the ability to simultaneously capture conventional (2D) and 3D views of the ovary within seconds after standard image-optimization procedures. Namely, with a single press of a button, the motorized array within the 3D ultrasound transducer captures serial images throughout the ovary in three planes and obviates the error associated with manual estimates of the orthogonal planes. The volume files generated essentially yield 2D cineloops through the ovary that are no different than those collected using similar frequency 2D transducers but have the benefit of enabling multi-planar views (MPV) of the ovary on which to perform assessments. The ability to capture comprehensive imaging for offline analysis reduces the duration of scans for patients, improving patient tolerability and enhancing clinical workflow similar to other inherent offline 3D imaging modalities such as computerized tomography (CT) and magnetic resonance imaging (MRI). Ultimately, 3D imaging is a convenient way to obtain, analyze and store ovarian data for more reliable offline analyses.

A number of methods are available to obtain follicle counts using 3D offline approaches depending on the functionalities offered by the ultrasound system manufacturer. At minimum, all 3D systems offer MPV wherein a rater can scroll through 2D serial slices of the ovary counting (and measuring) follicles while

simultaneously consulting the additional planes to corroborate the identity and location of follicles (Figure 4.3). Tomographic ultrasound imaging (TUI) enables the simultaneous visualization of serial slices through the ovary (at prespecified slice thickness) in a single plane as an alternative means to obtain follicle counts (Figure 4.3). Further, volumetric rendering algorithms such as sonography-based automated volume count (SonoAVC) enable semiautomated assessments of follicle number and size within an acquired volumetric dataset (Figure 4.3). Use of these methods for obtaining FNPO requires familiarity with the software and the reproducibility of 3D estimates is controversial.[30, 31] In a recent method comparison study evaluating agreement among several 2D and 3D methods to obtain FNPO, we showed that MPV, TUI and SonoAVC adequately categorized PCOM status but resulted in substantial over- or underestimations of FNPO as compared to the offline 2D-grid method, which currently limits their utility when a more precise estimation of FNPO is needed.[30]

Volumetric rendering algorithms are also available to measure OV (Figure 4.4). The use of 3D imaging has a striking advantage over 2D imaging in this regard as rendered estimates of OV make no predetermined assumptions about the shape of the ovary, which commonly deviates

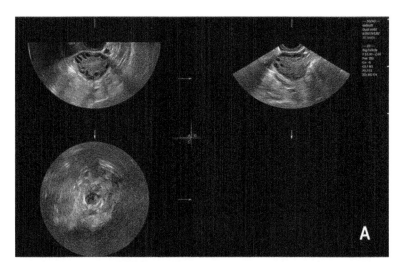

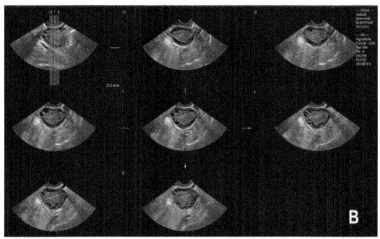

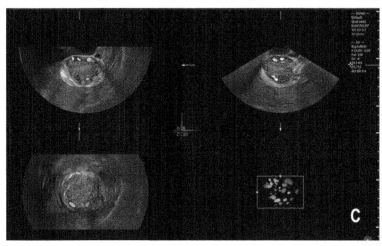

Figure 4.3 3D imaging options for assessing follicle number per ovary: (a) multi-planar view, (b) tomographic ultrasound imaging (TUI) and (c) sonography-based automated volume count (SonoAVC) are shown

from that of a prolate ellipsoid. Even when OV is estimated using MPV, the availability of exact orthogonal dimensions for length, width and height is an advantage over 2D real-time imaging.

Ultimately, 3D estimates of OV likely better reflect the true size of the ovary but normative data and 3D thresholds for ovarian enlargement are not available at this time.

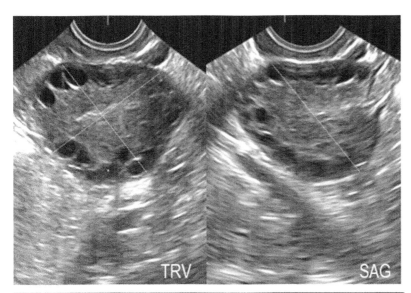

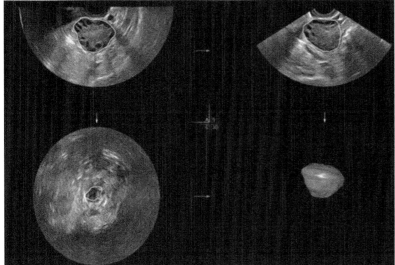

Figure 4.4 Ultrasound imaging options for assessing ovarian volume 2D real-time imaging (top) and 3D virtual organ computer-aided analysis (VOCAL) imaging (bottom) are shown

Physiological Considerations Related to PCOM in the Diagnosis of PCOS

Adolescent Reproductive Transition

Criteria to define PCOM are limited by their failure to account for factors known to influence ovarian morphology such as age and developmental stage. The 2018 Guideline does not recommend ultrasonographic evaluations in those with a gynecological age of less than eight years due to the high incidence of "multi-follicular ovaries" during adolescence when contrasted with ovarian morphology in adult women. The notion of multi-follicular ovaries during this reproductive life stage must be interpreted with caution. Normative data on ovarian morphology during adolescence are limited by their cross-sectional nature and focus on ovarian size, with few studies addressing quantitative evaluations of follicle populations.[32] Application of adult definitions of abnormal morphology to this developmentally unique group is likely inappropriate, and conclusions related to the limited diagnostic accuracy for adolescents with reproductive disturbances are premature given the paucity of normative data. Progress in evaluating adolescent ovarian

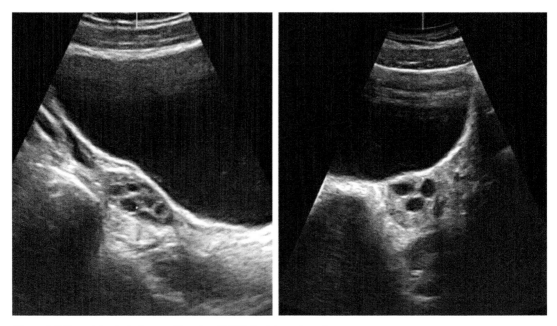

Figure 4.5 Transabdominal ultrasound imaging (TAUS) of adolescent ovaries
Antral follicles are clearly visualized in an adolescent 6 months post-menarche (left) and in another adolescent 1.5 years post-menarche (right).

morphology has also lagged given the historical lack of enthusiasm for the quality of TAUS. However, we and others recently showed the ability to resolve antral follicles as small as 1–2 mm in adolescents using updated TAUS technology and demonstrated the ability to adequately resolve follicle populations (Figure 4.5).[32, 33] Ongoing research by our group and others suggests that, despite the dynamic nature of ovarian morphology during adolescence, differences in ovarian features are apparent in early gynecological life and coincide with menstrual irregularity and other features of PCOS.[34, 35] Ultimately, data delineating the natural trajectory of ovarian morphology in healthy girls from those with sustained reproductive dysfunction are needed to justify development gynecologic age-specific criteria for follicular excess and/or ovarian enlargement.

Reproductive Aging

Ultrasonographic markers of PCOM, including both FNPO and OV, decrease naturally with age in both healthy women and women with PCOS – with a potential for differential rates of decline in some but not all markers.[36] Longitudinal studies show that aging is associated with an amelioration of PCOS symptoms including a decrease in androgen levels and more regular menstrual cycles. This phenomenon may reflect an impact of natural aging on reducing folliculogenesis and steroidogenesis, which translates to an alleviation of the follicle excess and arrest that is characteristic of PCOS. Although current definitions of PCOM have diagnostic potential for PCOS in women older than 35 years, the diagnostic performance of currently recommended thresholds is poorer in women of late reproductive age.[37, 38] Unsurprisingly, the Guideline identified the need to develop reliable and age-specific diagnostic thresholds for PCOM across the reproductive lifespan.[16] Three recent studies confirm that lower thresholds to define PCOM are needed to discriminate women 35 years and older with PCOS from controls.[37, 39, 40] These studies may be considered limited by their dependence on real-time imaging and consideration of predetermined chronological age groups (e.g. < 28.5 years and > 29.5 years [39] or in 5-year increments [37, 38]). Although these bins may not seem arbitrary, biologic features of reproductive aging, rather than chronologic proxies, may provide more physiologic insight into when PCOM thresholds should change as women age. Alas, improved knowledge related to the natural course of PCOM across the lifespan remains a research priority. This is important in aging women with PCOS who, despite an amelioration of PCOS symptoms, show persistent and heightened cardiometabolic risk, independent of adiposity, and require identification and monitoring for PCOS and associated comorbidity progression.[41]

The Ovary As a Biomarker

There is growing interest in expanding the utility of ultrasonographic features of ovarian morphology to inform phenotypic severity and reflect underlying reproductive pathology or metabolic involvement and response to treatment. Efforts to expand the diagnostic utility is premised by the notion that the ovary is an integration site of reproductive and metabolic inputs such that disruptions in ovarian physiology manifest as ultrasonographically distinct morphologic features when assessed cross-sectionally. Ovaries in PCOS are characterized primarily by an excess of small antral follicles (2–5 mm) and ovarian enlargement[16, 42] and reflect the hyperandrogenic anovulatory nature of PCOS. We and others showed that markers of ovarian size and total antral follicle populations (particularly those ≤ 6mm) reflect the magnitude of ovarian hyperandrogenism in women with PCOS.[21, 43] Follicle counts positively associate with biochemical measures of hyperandrogenism, the ratio of luteinizing to follicle-stimulating hormone production (LH:FSH) and menstrual cycle length consistent with ovarian morphology capturing the degree of reproductive dysfunction in women with PCOS.[21] More recently, we corroborated that these associations manifest early, as girls with PCOS show similar associations between ovarian morphology and reproductive dysfunction to their adult counterparts.[33] The ability to reflect the degree of reproductive symptomology could be helpful in screening and/or corroborating diagnoses for women with concerns over ovulatory dysfunction and/or androgen excess, particularly in instances where access to reliable assays are more limited.

The ovary may also capture the degree of metabolic derangement in PCOS, which could help to identify those with increased risk for concurrent comorbidities. In women with PCOS, ovarian enlargement (OV > 9 or > 10cm^3) was recently found to be more likely in women with insulin resistance (HOMA-IR > 4)[44] and showed utility to distinguish between those with or without metabolic syndrome.[45] Likewise, women with higher follicle counts (FNPO) had poorer metabolic profiles, including increased lipids[46] and worse measures of glucoregulation [46,47] versus body mass index (BMI)–matched women who lost their PCOM status owing to decreased thresholds for follicle excess. However, studies directly evaluating relationships between follicle populations and metabolic status have not yielded consistent findings. We showed in both women and adolescents with PCOS that BMI negatively associated with FNPS[33] or AFC,[21] with the latter observation being driven by an excess of small follicles. In addition, we reported inverse associations between small follicles (≤5 mm) with measures of central adiposity, glucoregulatory status, hyperlipidemia and pro-inflammation.[21] Our findings are tempered by reports of a weak positive association between 2–5 mm follicles and fasting insulin levels and no metabolic factor accounting for the number of small (2–5 mm) and medium (6–9 mm) antral follicles by principal component analysis in women with PCOS.[48] We suspect that discrepancies across studies may be attributed to methodological differences in counting and measuring follicles (real-time vs. offline), which highlights the need for standardization of ultrasonographic assessments. That said, there exists the potential for metabolic factors to influence diagnostic performance of ovarian markers to predict PCOS and perhaps necessitate varying thresholds to define PCOM in women with and without obesity. This is an important unresolved question, as studies that have proposed diagnostic thresholds for PCOM have typically included lean healthy women as their comparator to a largely overweight/obese group with PCOS.

Beyond diagnosis and evaluation, ovarian features may also have prognostic potential to monitor or predict response to therapy in women with PCOS. In the case of assisted reproduction, identification of PCOM or follicle number as a continuous metric may be helpful to guide treatment options that optimize ovarian response and reduce the risk of ovarian hyperstimulation syndrome (OHSS).[49, 50] Ovarian features may also predict metabolic treatment outcomes. Two recent randomized controlled trials reported reductions in OV,[51, 52] FNPO[51] and/or stromal size,[52] alongside weight loss, improved glucoregulation and lower free androgens in response to nutritional interventions [51] or insulin-sensitizing therapy,[52] implying that the ovary is responsive to changes in metabolic status in PCOS. Similarly, a chart review of women with and without PCOS who underwent bariatric surgery noted that OV predicted the degree of improvement in glucoregulation, as judged by HbA1C, and circulating triglycerides.[53] Collectively, there is growing evidence to consider leveraging features of ovarian morphology as prognostic indicators in diverse clinical outcomes.

Closing Remarks

The latest international recommendations acknowledge that PCOS continues to be a diagnostic challenge and detection of polycystic ovaries on ultrasonography is a critical part of this debate. PCOM has relevance in defining the phenotypic spectrum of PCOS and has known prognostic value in certain clinical settings. The Guideline supports the careful and meticulous assessment of FNPO and OV to define PCOM on ultrasonography but also encourages more research in order to generate biologically accurate criteria for PCOM. New findings should be based on unbiased and well-defined populations, employing approaches that determine whether PCOM clusters with short- and long-term health outcomes in PCOS. Further, accurate criteria for PCOM that hold up across the reproductive lifespan are needed. That said, ultrasonographic approaches to assess ovarian morphology must be reproducible and efforts to optimize the evaluation of individual features of ovarian morphology are equally important, not different from other assays. Ultimately, we can expect revisions to criteria for PCOM as advances in imaging technology emerge and cross-validation with serum markers enable identification of surrogate or adjunct measures for PCOM on ultrasonography.

References

1 Stein, I. F. and Leventhal, M. L. Amenorrhea associated with bilateral polycystic ovaries. *Am J Obstet Gynecol* 1935; 29(2): 181–191.

2 Goldzieher, J. W. and Green, J. A. The polycystic ovary: I. Clinical and histologic features. *J Clin Endocrinol Metab* 1962; 22: 325–338.

3 Hughesdon, P. E. Morphology and morphogenesis of the Stein-Leventhal ovary and of so-called "hyperthecosis." *Obs Gynecol Surv* 1982; 37(2): 59–77.

4 Maciel, G. A. R., Baracat, E. C., Benda, J. A. et al. Stockpiling of transitional and classic primary follicles in ovaries of women with polycystic ovary syndrome. *J Clin Endocrinol Metab* 2004; 89(11): 5321–5327.

5 Franks, S., Mason, H. and Willis, D. Follicular dynamics in the polycystic ovary syndrome. *Mol Cell Endocrinol* 2000; 163(1–2): 49–52.

6 Swanson, M., Sauerbrei, E. E. and Cooperberg, P. L. Medical implications of ultrasonically detected polycystic ovaries. *J Clin Ultrasound* 1981; 9(5): 219–222.

7 Saxton, D. W., Farquhar, C. M., Rae, T., Beard, R. W., Anderson, M. C. and Wadsworth, J. Accuracy of ultrasound measurements of female pelvic organs. *Br J Obs Gynaecol* 1990; 97(8): 695–699.

8 Eden, J. A., Jones, J., Carter, G. D. and Alaghband-Zadeh, J. A comparison of follicular fluid levels of Insulin-like Growth Factor-1 in normal dominant and cohort follicles, polycystic and multicystic ovaries. *Clin Endocrinol (Oxf)* 1988; 29(3): 327–336.

9 Hull, M. G. R. Epidemiology of infertility and polycystic ovarian disease: Endocrinological and demographic studies. *Gynecol Endocrinol* 1987; 1 (3): 235–245.

10 Zawadzki, J. K. and Dunaif, A. Diagnostic criteria for polycystic ovary syndrome: Towards a rational approach. In A. Dunaif, J. R. Givens, F. P. Haseltine and G. R. Merriam, eds. *Polycystic Ovary Syndrome*. Boston, MA: Blackwell Scientific, 1992: 377–384.

11 Dewailly, D., Lujan, M. E., Carmina, E. et al. Definition and significance of polycystic ovarian morphology: A task force report from the Androgen Excess and Polycystic Ovary Syndrome Society. *Hum Reprod Updat* 2014; 20(3): 334–352.

12 Azziz, R., Carmina, E., Dewailly, D. et al. Positions statement: Criteria for defining polycystic ovary syndrome as a predominantly hyperandrogenic syndrome: An Androgen Excess Society guideline. *J Clin Endocrinol Metab* 2006; 91(11): 4237–4245.

13 Jonard, S., Robert, Y., Cortet-Rudelli, C., Pigny, P., Decanter, C. and Dewailly, D. Ultrasound examination of polycystic ovaries: Is it worth counting the follicles? *Hum Reprod* 2003; 18(3): 598–603.

14 Lujan, M. E., Jarrett, B.Y., Brooks, E. D. et al. Updated ultrasound criteria for polycystic ovary syndrome: Reliable thresholds for elevated follicle population and ovarian volume. *Hum Reprod* 2013; 28(5): 1361–1368.

15 Dewailly, D., Gronier, H., Poncelet, E. et al. Diagnosis of polycystic ovary syndrome (PCOS): Revisiting the threshold values of follicle count on ultrasound and of the serum AMH level for the definition of polycystic ovaries. *Hum Reprod* 2011; 26(11): 3123–3129.

16 Teede, H. J., Misso, M. L., Costello, M. F. et al. Recommendations from the international evidence-based guideline for the assessment and management of polycystic ovary syndrome. *Hum Reprod* 2018; 33(9): 1–17.

17 Adams, J., Polson, D. W. and Franks, S. Prevalence of polycystic ovaries in women with anovulation and idiopathic hirsutism. *Br Med J (Clin Res Ed)* 1986; 293(6543): 355–359.

18 Christ, J. P., Willis, A. D., Brooks, E. D. et al. Follicle number, not assessments of the ovarian stroma, represents the best ultrasonographic marker of polycystic ovary syndrome. *Fertil Steril* 2014; 101(1): 280–287.

19 Jarrett, B. Y., Vanden Brink, H., Brooks, E. D. et al. Impact of right–left differences in ovarian morphology on the ultrasound diagnosis of polycystic ovary syndrome. *Fertil Steril* 2019; 112 (5): 939–946.

20 Barbierit, R. L., Makris, A., Randall, R. W., Daniels, G., Kistner, R. W. and Ryan, K. J. Insulin stimulates androgen accumulation in incubations of Ovarian Stroma Obtained from Women with Hyperandrogenism*. *J Clin Endocrinol Metab* 1986, 62(5): 904–910.

21 Christ, J. P., Vanden Brink, H., Brooks, E. D., Pierson, R. A., Chizen, D. R. and Lujan, M. E. Ultrasound features of polycystic ovaries relate to degree of reproductive and metabolic disturbance in polycystic ovary syndrome. *Fertil Steril* 2015; 103 (3): 787–794.

22 Lam, P. M., Johnson, I. R. and Raine-Fenning, N. J. Three-dimensional ultrasound features of the polycystic ovary and the effect of different phenotypic expressions on these parameters. *Hum Reprod* 2007; 22(12): 3116–3123.

23 Battaglia, C., Battaglia, B., Morotti, E. et al. Two- and three-dimensional sonographic and color Doppler techniques for diagnosis of polycystic ovary syndrome: The stromal/ovarian volume ratio as a new diagnostic criterion. *J Ultrasound Med* 2012; 31(7): 1015–1024.

24 Raine-Fenning, N. J., Campbell, B. K., Clewes, J. S., Kendall, N. R. and Johnson, I. R. The interobserver reliability of three-dimensional power Doppler data acquisition within the female pelvis. *Ultrasound Obs Gynecol* 2004; 23(5): 501–508.

25 Teede, H., Misso, M., Tassone, E. C. et al. Anti-Müllerian hormone in PCOS: A review informing international guidelines. *Trends Endocrinol Metab* 2019; 30(7): 467–478.

26 Coelho Neto, M. A., Ludwin, A., Borrell, A. et al. Counting ovarian antral follicles by ultrasound: A practical guide. *Ultrasound Obstet Gynecol* 2018; 51(1): 10–20.

27 Broekmans, F. J. M., de Ziegler, D., Howles, C. M., Gougeon, A., Trew, G. and Olivennes, F. The antral follicle count: Practical recommendations for better standardization. *Fertil Steril* 2010; 94(3): 1044–1051.

28 Lujan, M. E., Chizen, D. R., Peppin, A. K. et al. Improving inter-observer variability in the evaluation of ultrasonographic features of polycystic ovaries. *Reprod Biol Endocrinol* 2008; 6: 30.

29 Lujan, M. E., Brooks, E. D., Kepley, A. L., Chizen, D. R., Pierson, R. A. and Peppin, A. K. Grid analysis improves reliability in follicle counts made by ultrasonography in women with polycystic ovary syndrome. *Ultrasound Med Biol* 2010; 36(5): 712–718.

30 Vanden Brink, H., Pisch, A. and Lujan, M. A comparison of two and three-dimensional ultrasonographic methods for the evaluation of follicle counts and classification of polycystic ovarian morphology. *Fertil Steril* 2021; 115(3): 761–770.

31 Deb, S., Campbell, B. K., Clewes, J. S. and Raine-Fenning, N. J. Quantitative analysis of antral follicle number and size: A comparison of two-dimensional and automated three-dimensional ultrasound techniques. *Ultrasound Obstet Gynecol* 2010; 35(3): 354–360.

32 Hagen, C. P., Mouritsen, A., Mieritz, M. G. et al. Circulating AMH reflects ovarian morphology by magnetic resonance imaging and 3D ultrasound in 121 healthy girls. *J Clin Endocrinol Metab* 2015; 100 (3): 880–890.

33 Rackow, B. W., Vanden Brink, H., Hammers, L., Flannery, C. A., Lujan, M. E. and Burgert, T. S. Ovarian morphology by transabdominal ultrasound correlates with reproductive and metabolic disturbance in adolescents with PCOS. *J Adolesc Heal* 2018; 62(3): 288–293.

34 Hernandez, M. I., López, P., Gaete, X. et al. Hyperandrogenism in adolescent girls: Relationship with the somatotrophic axis. *J Pediatr Endocrinol Metab* 2017; 30(5): 561–568.

35 Fruzzetti, F., Campagna, A. M., Perini, D. and Carmina, E. Ovarian volume in normal and hyperandrogenic adolescent women. *Fertil Steril* 2015; 104(1): 196–199.

36 Alsamarai, S., Adams, J. M., Murphy, M. K. et al. Criteria for polycystic ovarian morphology in polycystic ovary syndrome as a function of age. *J Clin Endocrinol Metab* 2009; 94(12): 4961–4970.

37 Kim, H. J., Adams, J. M., Gudmundsson, J. A., Arason, G., Pau, C. T., Welt and C. K. Polycystic ovary morphology: Age-based ultrasound criteria. *Fertil Steril* 2017; 108(3): 548–553.

38 Ahmad, A. K., Quinn, M., Kao, C. N., Greenwood, E., Cedars, M. I. and Huddleston, H. G. Improved diagnostic performance for the diagnosis of polycystic ovary syndrome using age-stratified criteria. *Fertil Steril* 2019; 111(4): 787–793.e2.

39 Lie Fong, S., Laven, J. S. E., Duhamel, A. and Dewailly, D. Polycystic ovarian morphology and the diagnosis of polycystic ovary syndrome: Redefining threshold levels for follicle count and serum anti-Müllerian hormone using cluster analysis. *Hum Reprod* 2017; 32(8): 1723–1731.

40 Quinn, M. M., Kao, C. N., Ahmad, A. K. et al. Age-stratified thresholds of anti-Müllerian hormone improve prediction of polycystic ovary syndrome over a population-based threshold. *Clin Endocrinol (Oxf)* 2017; 87(6): 733–740.

41 Cooney, L. G. and Dokras, A. Beyond fertility: Polycystic ovary syndrome and long-term health. *Fertil Steril* 2018; 110(5): 794–809.

42 Jonard, S. and Dewailly, D. The follicular excess in polycystic ovaries, due to intra-ovarian hyperandrogenism, may be the main culprit for the follicular arrest. *Hum Reprod Update* 2004; 10(2): 107–117.

43 Dewailly, D., Lujan, M. E., Carmina, E. et al. Definition and significance of polycystic ovarian morphology: A task force report from the androgen excess and polycystic ovary syndrome society. *Hum Reprod Updat* 2014; 20(3): 334–352.

44 Reid, S. P., Kao, C., Pasch, L., Shinkai, K., Cedars, M. I. and Huddleston, H. G. Ovarian morphology is associated with insulin resistance in women with polycystic ovary syndrome: A cross sectional study. *Fertil Res and Pract* 2017; 3: 8. https://doi.org/10.1186/s40738-017-0035-z

45 Sipahi, M., Tokgöz, V. Y., Keskin, Ö. , Atasever, M., Menteşe, A. and Demir, S. Is ovarian volume a good predictor to determine metabolic syndrome

development in polycystic ovary patients. *J Obstet Gynaecol (Lahore)* 2019; 39(3): 372–376.

46 Kim, J. J., Hwang, K. R., Chae, S. J., Yoon, S. H. and Choi, Y. M. Impact of the newly recommended antral follicle count cutoff for polycystic ovary in adult women with polycystic ovary syndrome. *Hum Reprod* 2020; 35(3): 652–659.

47 Quinn, M. M., Kao, C. N., Ahmad, A. et al. Raising threshold for diagnosis of polycystic ovary syndrome excludes population of patients with metabolic risk. *Fertil Steril* 2016; 106(5): 1244–1251.

48 Peigné, M., Catteau-Jonard, S., Robin, G., Dumont, A., Pigny, P. and Dewailly, D. The numbers of 2–5 and 6–9 mm ovarian follicles are inversely correlated in both normal women and in polycystic ovary syndrome patients: What is the missing link? *Hum Reprod* 2018; 33(4): 706–714.

49 Holte, J., Brodin, T., Berglund, L., Hadziosmanovic, N., Olovsson, M. and Bergh, T. Antral follicle counts are strongly associated with live-birth rates after assisted reproduction, with superior treatment outcome in women with polycystic ovaries. *Fertil Steril* 2011; 96(3): 594–599.

50 Fauser, B. C. J. M., Diedrich, K., Devroey, P. and Evian Annual Reproduction (EVAR) Workshop Group. Predictors of ovarian response: progress towards individualized treatment in ovulation induction and ovarian stimulation. *Hum Reprod Update* 2008; 14(1): 1–14.

51 Kazemi, M., Pierson, R. A., McBreairty, L. E., Chilibeck, P. D., Zello, G. A. and Chizen, D. R. A randomized controlled trial of a lifestyle intervention with longitudinal follow-up on ovarian dysmorphology in women with polycystic ovary syndrome. *Clin Endocrinol (Oxf)* 2020; 92(6): 525–535.

52 Nylander, M., Frøssing, S., Clausen, H. V., Kistorp, C., Faber, J. and Skouby, S. O. Effects of liraglutide on ovarian dysfunction in polycystic ovary syndrome: A randomized clinical trial. *Reprod Biomed Online* 2017; 35(1): 121–127.

53 Christ, J. P. and Falcone, T. Bariatric surgery improves hyperandrogenism, menstrual irregularities, and metabolic dysfunction among women with polycystic ovary syndrome (PCOS). *Obes Surg* 2018; 28(8): 2171–2177.

Chapter 5

The Classification of Polycystic Ovary Syndrome Informed by the International Guideline 2018

Robert J. Norman, Rhonda Garad and Helena Teede

Introduction

The diagnosis of polycystic ovary syndrome (PCOS) has remained controversial over the past several decades with disagreements in defining individual components that make up the diagnostic criteria and significant clinical heterogeneity across the phenotypes, further varied by ethnic differences and changes in clinical features across the life course.[1–3] The earliest definitions (see Chapter 1) were geared around the so-called Stein-Leventhal syndrome, which was classically associated with obesity, significant menstrual abnormality, infertility and large polycystic ovaries, discovered at laparotomy or laparoscopy.[4] With the advent of modern endocrinology, it was discovered that increased androgens, high LH: FSH ratio and hyperinsulinemia with increased glucose intolerance were frequently present. The introduction of new ultrasound modalities applied to gynecological investigation led to visualization of polycystic appearing morphology analogous to the surgical discoveries of the previous era.[5, 6] This led to new definitions, incorporating measurements of hormones, clinical features and ultrasonography.

A National Institutes of Health (NIH) consensus conference agreed that PCOS should be defined on the basis of anovulation and hyperandrogenism, largely predating the advent of modern ultrasound.[7] The Rotterdam (also called ASRM-ESHRE) criteria included ultrasound of the ovaries, so that two out of three of the following were included provided other conditions had been excluded:[8]

1. Irregular anovulatory cycles.
2. Polycystic-appearing ovaries on ultrasound.
3. Clinical or biochemical hyperandrogenemia.

This definition has been widely accepted and forms the basic diagnostic criteria underpinning the evidence-based guideline for PCOS published in 2018 (Figure 5.1).[9] There have been subsequent attempts at varying this definition, including that by the Androgen Excess and PCOS (AE-PCOS) Society, in which various subtypes were introduced.[10] Some countries have also utilized their own definitions that vary somewhat from the Rotterdam criteria, and this includes Chinese and Japanese Society positions. Key to all these definitions, however, are the menstrual cycles, evidence of increased androgenization and the appearance of polycystic ovaries.

Irregular Cycles and Ovulatory Dysfunction

Ovulatory dysfunction is a key diagnostic feature of PCOS, with irregular cycles often reflecting ovulatory dysfunction but recognizing that lack of ovulation can also occur with regular menstrual cycles (Table 5.1).[11] When anovulation needs to

Algorithm and criteria for diagnosing PCOS
Step1: Irregular cycles + clinical hyperandrogenism (hirsutism, acne, alopecia) (exclude secondary causes) = diagnosis
⇩
Step 2: If no clinical hyperandrogenism Test for biochemical hyperandrogenism (exclude secondary causes) = diagnosis

Figure 5.1 Algorithm and criteria for diagnosing polycystic ovaries

Table 5.1 Evaluation of normality in a menstrual cycle

	Strength of evidence	Features
1.1.1	CCR	Irregular menstrual cycles are defined as: • normal in the first year post menarche as part of the pubertal transition • > 1 to < 3 years post menarche: < 21 or > 45 days • >3 years post menarche to perimenopause: < 21 or > 35 days or < 8 cycles per year • > 1 year post menarche > 90 days for any one cycle • Primary amenorrhea by age 15 or > 3 years post thelarche (breast development) When irregular menstrual cycles are present, a diagnosis of PCOS should be considered and assessed according to the guidelines.
1.1.2	CCR	In an adolescent with irregular menstrual cycles, the value and optimal timing of assessment and diagnosis of PCOS should be discussed with the patient, taking into account diagnostic challenges at this life stage and psychosocial and cultural factors.
1.1.3	CPP	For adolescents who have features of PCOS but do not meet diagnostic criteria, an "increased risk" could be considered and reassessment advised at or before full reproductive maturity, 8 years post menarche. This includes those with PCOS features before combined oral contraceptive pill (COCP) commencement, those with persisting features and those with significant weight gain in adolescence.
1.1.4	CPP	Ovulatory dysfunction can still occur with regular cycles and if anovulation needs to be confirmed serum progesterone levels can be measured.

CCR, clinical consensus recommendation; CPP, clinical practice point.

be confirmed, hormonal assessment is relevant if PCOS is clinically suspected and this can often be achieved by measuring progesterone at the appropriate time of the cycle. It is generally thought that if cycles last for more than 35 days or there are fewer than 8 cycles in a 12-month period that this could be considered to be abnormal.[9]

Caution

We know that irregular cycles and ovulatory dysfunction are also normal components of the pubertal and menopausal transitions, and therefore defining abnormality at these life stages can be difficult. The major problem is misclassifying young teenagers as having PCOS on the basis of menstrual abnormality when it may be part of a physiological transition. Maturation of the hypothalamic–pituitary–ovarian axis occurs over time and cycles in adolescence do not often match those of reproductive-aged women. Young women are often put on the oral contraceptive pill and therefore it becomes very difficult to assess a natural ovulatory function of the ovary. Therefore, the international evidence-based guideline considers that irregular menstrual cycles are a normal part of the first years post menarche and should only be fully considered to be a diagnostic *eight years post menarche*. Irregular menstrual cycles before this may be considered to be

a potential diagnostic criterion for PCOS but should not be relied on. It is recommended that, in this situation, discussion should occur with the patient and her family, taking into account diagnostic challenges as at this stage. The psychological and cultural factors may lead to undue distress that come before ascertaining a firm diagnosis. More information is required as to the natural course and maturation of menstrual patterns in young girls of various ethnic background and body weight.

Hyperandrogenism

Hyperandrogenism is a key diagnostic feature of PCOS, affecting 60–100% of women, and features are challenging to assess because they vary by methods of assessment, ethnicity and confounding factors, including excess weight and life stage. Assessment of biochemical hyperandrogenism is hampered by the lack of clarity on which androgens to measure, which assays to use, normal ranges and access and costs issue for high-quality assays.[9] The recommendation from the international guideline is that calculated free testosterone, free androgen index or calculated bioavailable testosterone are the best measures of biochemical hyperandrogenism (Table 5.2). In the absence of the availability of liquid chromatography–mass spectrometry methods for total and free testosterone, dehydroepiandrosterone

Table 5.2 Evaluation of biochemical hyperandrogenism

	Strength of evidence	Features
1.2.1	EBR	Calculated free testosterone, free androgen index or calculated bioavailable testosterone should be used to assess biochemical hyperandrogenism in the diagnosis of PCOS.
1.2.2	EBR	High-quality assays such as liquid chromatography–mass spectrometry (LCMS)/mass spectrometry and extraction/ chromatography immunoassays should be used for the most accurate assessment of total or free testosterone in PCOS.
1.2.3	EBR	Androstenedione and dehydroepiandrosterone sulfate (DHEAS) could be considered if total or free testosterone is not elevated; however, these provide limited additional information in the diagnosis of PCOS.
1.2.4	CCR	Direct free testosterone assays, such as radiometric or enzyme-linked assays, preferably **should not be** used in assessment of biochemical hyperandrogenism in PCOS, as they demonstrate poor sensitivity, accuracy and precision.
1.2.5	CPP	Reliable assessment of biochemical hyperandrogenism is not possible in women on hormonal contraception, due to effects on sex hormone-binding globulin and altered gonadotropin-dependent androgen production.

EBR, evidence-based recommendation; CCR, clinical consensus recommendation; CCP, clinical practice point.

Table 5.3 Evaluation of clinical hyperandrogenism

	Strength of evidence	Features
1.3.1	CCR	A comprehensive history and physical examination should be completed for symptoms and signs of clinical hyperandrogenism, including acne, alopecia and hirsutism and, in adolescents, severe acne and hirsutism.
1.3.2	CCR	Health professionals should be aware of the potential negative psychosocial impact of clinical hyperandrogenism. Reported unwanted excess hair growth and/or alopecia should be considered important, regardless of apparent severity.
1.3.3	CCR	Standardized visual scales are preferred when assessing hirsutism, depending on ethnicity, acknowledging that self-treatment is common and can limit clinical assessment (see recommendations on ethnic variation).
1.3.4	CCR	The Ludwig visual score is preferred for assessing the degree and distribution of alopecia.
1.3.5	CPP	There are no universal accepted visual assessments for evaluating acne.

sulfate (DHEAS) can also be considered if testosterone is not raised. Direct free testosterone assays using immunometric assays should be avoided and androgens measured while the patient is on the contraceptive pill are invalid. Practitioners should be aware that, if markedly elevated androgen levels are obtained, other causes of biochemical hyperandrogenism should be considered.

With respect to clinical hyperandrogenism, virilization is rare, and there is considerable ethnic variation. Much attention has been focused on hirsutism and there are a number of semi-objective scores, including the Ferriman–Gallwey Score (Table 5.3).[12] Most clinical hyperandrogenism occurs with hirsutism in a male pattern in women, largely on the upper lip, chin and neck, upper chest, upper abdomen, lower abdomen, thighs, upper back, lower back and upper arms. Defining abnormal can be difficult and the modified Ferriman–Gallwey Score is considered abnormal if > 3 in white and black women and > 5 in Mongoloid Asian women. More than 50% of women with a modified Ferriman–Gallwey Score in the range 3–5 have elevated androgens and/or PCOS and more than 70% of women will score > 5. Acne can be quite common, depending on ethnic background. A comprehensive history and physical examination should be completed for hyperandrogenism, bearing in mind the potential negative psychosocial impact of clinical hirsutism. Care needs to be taken to not confuse vellus hair density with terminal hairs.

Table 5.4 Evaluation of ovarian ultrasound features

	Strength of evidence	Features
1.4.1	CCR	Ultrasound should not be used for the diagnosis of PCOS in those with a gynecological age of < 8 years (< 8 years after menarche), due to the high incidence of multi-follicular ovaries in this life stage.
1.4.2	CCR	The threshold for PCOM should be revised regularly with advancing ultrasound technology, and age-specific cutoff values for PCOM should be defined.
1.4.3	CCR	The transvaginal ultrasound approach is preferred in the diagnosis of PCOS, if sexually active and if acceptable to the individual being assessed.
1.4.4	CCR	Using endovaginal ultrasound transducers with a frequency bandwidth > 8 MHz, the threshold for PCOM should be on either ovary, a follicle number per ovary of ≥ 20 and/or an ovarian volume ≥ 10ml, ensuring no corpora lutea, cysts or dominant follicles are present.
1.4.5	CPP	If using older technology, the threshold for PCOM could be an ovarian volume ≥ 10 mL on either ovary.

Table 5.5 Evaluation of AMH in diagnosis

	Strength of evidence	Features
1.5.1	EBR	Serum AMH levels should not yet be used as an alternative for the detection of PCOM or as a single test for the diagnosis of PCOS.
1.5.2	CPP	There is emerging evidence that with improved standardization of assays and established cutoff levels or thresholds based on large-scale validation in populations of different ages and ethnicities, AMH assays may become more accurate in the detection of PCOM.

Ultrasound and Polycystic Ovary Morphology

Polycystic ovary morphology (PCOM) was incorporated into the diagnosis for PCOS in the Rotterdam criteria and has been widely accepted despite its limitations. Initially the diagnosis of PCOM in the Rotterdam Criteria was considered to be > 12 follicles measuring 2–9 mm or an ovarian volume of > 10 mL. With improved ultrasound equipment and training, it has become apparent that many women without PCOS easily meet this criterion and have been falsely diagnosed as having PCOS. The evidence-based criteria now maintain the diagnosis of PCOM should not contribute to women with a gynecological age of less than eight years due to the high incidence of multi-follicular ovaries in teenage women.[9] Current recommendations are that the follicle number per ovary of > 20 and/or an ovarian volume of > 10 mL is enough to diagnose PCOM if using a transvaginal approach (Table 5.4). It should be noted that, in patients with irregular cycles and hyperandrogenism, an ovarian ultrasound is not necessary for PCOS diagnosis. In cases where the ovary is difficult to see but can be measured, a volume of > 10 mL is enough to make the diagnosis.

Anti-Müllerian Hormone (AMH)

Because ultrasound is inherently unreliable in inexperienced hands and reporting is often difficult with invasive technology, use of a blood test measuring anti-Müllerian hormone (AMH) has become popular.[6, 13] AMH is secreted by the granulosa cells of the preantral follicle and it has been shown that AMH levels are much higher in women with PCOS compared to normal ovulatory women (Table 5.5).[14] Strong correlations have been demonstrated between circulating AMH and antral follicle count on ultrasound in PCOS. There has generally been a tendency to say that high AMH values indicate the presence of PCOM. However, assays are quite variable and there is no international standard for AMH, and so the evidence-based guideline currently recommends that AMH should not be used as an alternative for the detection of PCOM or as a single test for the diagnosis of PCOS.[9] It is recognized that with improved standardization of assays and established cutoff levels AMH will become much more important in detecting PCOM and reducing the prevalence of use of ultrasound.

Other Factors

Ethnic Variation

While PCOS was originally described in Caucasians, the condition has been shown to be common throughout the world (see Chapter 3). The prevalence of anovulation and PCOM seems to be fairly standard across all ethnic groups but the expression of hyperandrogenism can vary with much more severe hirsutism in Middle Eastern, Hispanic and Mediterranean women. In East Asians, acne is common with less hirsutism. Metabolic features also differ significantly between ethnic groups, independent of high BMI.[15]

Menopausal Life Stage

The criteria for the diagnosis of a PCOS will vary with age; and as cycles become irregular naturally in the perimenopause, the diagnosis can become

much more difficult. PCOS phenotypes are poorly defined and it has proved difficult to make retrospective diagnosis of PCOS in the postmenopausal period. However, postmenopausal persistence of metabolic features of PCOS is likely to continue because of ongoing hyperandrogenism (Table 5.6). However, women presenting with new-onset, severe or worsening hyperandrogenism post menopause, should be investigated for androgen-secreting tumors and ovarian thecosis.[9]

Exclusion of Other Causes

The NIH Consensus Conference, Rotterdam, and the AE-PCOS all emphasize the importance of excluding other causes of polycystic ovary morphology, hyperandrogenism and abnormal endocrinology. Hypothalamic amenorrhea is common among women with weight-related abnormalities, taking certain medications, having a prolactinoma or due to altered physiological states such as eating disorders, excessive exercise and weight loss. Hyperandrogenism can present through a variety of ovarian and adrenal tumors, Cushing's syndrome and late-onset congenital adrenal hyperplasia.[16] A polycystic-type ovary is common in normal young women in the teenage years and in those who have lost significant weight.[17] All of these features need to be considered before attributing a diagnosis of PCOS.

Subclassification of PCOS Phenotypes

One of the benefits of the debate about the classifications of PCOS is the understanding that subclassifications of PCOS are essential for optimal attribution of severity and risk (see Table 5.7).

Table 5.6 Evaluation of PCOS in menopausal situations

	Strength of evidence	Features
1.6.1	CCR	Postmenopausal persistence of PCOS could be considered likely with continuing evidence of hyperandrogenism.
1.6.2	CCR	A diagnosis of PCOS post menopause could be considered if there is a past diagnosis of PCOS, a long-term history of irregular menstrual cycles and hyperandrogenism and/or PCOM, during the reproductive years.
1.6.3	CPP	Postmenopausal women presenting with new-onset, severe or worsening hyperandrogenism, including hirsutism, require further investigation to rule out androgen-secreting tumors and ovarian hyperthecosis.

Table 5.7 All possible phenotypes of PCOS based on common diagnostic features

Features	Potential phenotypes															
	A	B	C	D	E	F	G	H	I	J	K	L	M	N	O	P
Hyperandrogenemia	+	+	+	+	−	−	+	−	+	−	+	−	−	−	+	−
Hirsutism	+	+	−	−	+	+	+	+	−	−	+	−	−	+	−	−
Oligo-anovulation	+	+	+	+	+	+	−	−	−	+	−	−	+	−	−	−
Polycystic ovaries	+	−	+	−	+	−	+	+	+	+	−	+	−	−	−	−
NIH 1990 criteria	✓	✓	✓	✓	✓	✓										
Rotterdam 2003 criteria	✓	✓	✓	✓	✓	✓	✓	✓	✓	✓						
AE-PCOS criteria	✓	✓	✓	✓	✓	✓	✓	✓	✓							

+, presence; −, absence.

This presentation of subtypes is now considered a prerequisite for high-quality clinical care and research publications.

Regional Variations on the Rotterdam Criteria for Diagnosis

Given the wide phenotypic variation in presentation of PCOS, several variations of this classification exist, particularly in ethnic groups with less obesity and different presentation of clinical hyperandrogenism.

Conclusion

There has been criticism by some of the overdiagnosis of PCOS because of allegations of allegedly increased interventions, resulting in psychosocial distress from having a diagnosis associated with an increased risk of diabetes and purported cardiovascular disease. While many of these claims have been overstated, it is wise for the clinician to be cautious in the teenage years about attributing a diagnosis of PCOS until reproductive cycle maturity has been achieved and in situations where there is marginal evidence for abnormalities. Little is lost by repeating investigations or asking the patient to wait for a period of time until her natural cycle and metabolism is established. It is likely that AMH will emerge as an important diagnostic feature in due time and the use of ultrasound may diminish. It is possible that, with time, better assays for the measurement of androgens will be developed and that, with more data, certainty about anovulation and irregular cycles will be clarified. In the interim, it is important not to miss the diagnosis of PCOS, given its emotional, metabolic and reproductive sequelae.

References

1 Norman, R. J., Dewailly, D., Legro, R. S. and Hickey, T. E. Polycystic ovary syndrome. *Lancet* 2007; 370(9588): 685–697. https://doi.org/10.1016/S0140-6736(07)61345-2

2 Azziz, R., Carmina, E., Chen, Z. et al. Polycystic ovary syndrome. *Nat Rev Dis Primers* 2016; 2: 16057. https://doi.org/10.1038/nrdp.2016.57

3 Azziz, R. Polycystic ovary syndrome. *Obstet Gynecol* 2018; 132(2): 321–336. https://doi.org/10.1097/AOG.0000000000002698

4 Azziz, R., Dumesic, D. A. and Goodarzi, M. O. Polycystic ovary syndrome: An ancient disorder? *Fertil Steril* 2011; 95(5): 1544–1548. https://doi.org/10.1016/j.fertnstert.2010.09.032

5 Adams, J., Polson, D. W. and Franks, S. Prevalence of polycystic ovaries in women with anovulation and idiopathic hirsutism. *Br Med J (Clin Res Ed)* 1986; 293(6543): 355–359. https://doi.org/10.1136/bmj.293.6543.355

6 Dewailly, D., Lujan, M. E., Carmina, E. et al. Definition and significance of polycystic ovarian morphology: A task force report from the Androgen Excess and Polycystic Ovary Syndrome Society. *Hum Reprod Update* 2014; 20(3): 334–352. https://doi.org/10.1093/humupd/dmt061

7 Zawadski, J. K. and Dunaif, A. Diagnostic criteria for polycystic ovary syndrome: Towards a rational approach. In A. Dunaif, J. R. Givens, F. P. Haseltine and G. R. Merriam, eds. Polycystic Ovary Syndrome. Boston, MA: Blackwell Scientific Publications, 1992: 377–384.

8 The Rotterdam ESHRE/ASRM-Sponsored PCOS Consensus Workshop Group. Revised 2003 consensus on diagnostic criteria and long-term health risks related to polycystic ovary syndrome (PCOS). *Hum Reprod* 2004; 19(1): 41–47. https://doi.org/10.1093/humrep/deh098

9 Teede, H. J., Misso, M. L., Costello, M. F. et al. Recommendations from the international evidence-based guideline for the assessment and management of polycystic ovary syndrome. *Hum Reprod* 2018; 33(9): 1602–1618. https://doi.org/10.1093/humrep/dey256

10 Azziz, R., Carmina, E., Dewailly, D. et al. The Androgen Excess and PCOS Society criteria for the polycystic ovary syndrome: The complete task force report. *Fertil Steril* 2009; 91(2): 456–488. https://doi.org/10.1016/j.fertnstert.2008.06.035

11 Pena, A. S., Doherty, D. A., Atkinson, H. C., Hickey, M., Norman, R. J. and Hart, R. The majority of irregular menstrual cycles in adolescence are ovulatory: Results of a prospective study. *Arch Dis Child* 2018; 103(3): 235–239. https://doi.org/10.1136/archdischild-2017-312968

12 Ferriman, D. and Gallwey, J. D. Clinical assessment of body hair growth in women. *J Clin Endocrinol Metab* 1961; 21: 1440–1447. https://doi.org/10.1210/jcem-21-11-1440

13 Lie Fong, S., Laven, J. S. E., Duhamel, A. and Dewailly, D. Polycystic ovarian morphology and the diagnosis of polycystic ovary syndrome: Redefining threshold levels for follicle count and serum anti-Mullerian hormone using cluster analysis. *Hum Reprod* 2017; 32(8): 1723–1731. https://doi.org/10.1093/humrep/dex226

14 Teede, H., Misso, M., Tassone, E. C. et al. Anti-Müllerian hormone in PCOS: A review informing international guidelines. *Trends Endocrinol Metab*

2019 ;30(7): 467–478. https://doi.org/10.1016/j.tem.2019.04.006

15 Zhao, Y. and Qiao, J. Ethnic differences in the phenotypic expression of polycystic ovary syndrome. *Steroids* 2013; 78(8): 755–760. https://doi.org/10.1016/j.steroids.2013.04.006

16 Papadakis, G., Kandaraki, E. A., Tseniklidi, E., Papalou, O. and Diamanti-Kandarakis, E. Polycystic ovary syndrome and NC-CAH: Distinct characteristics and common findings. A systematic review. *Front Endocrinol (Lausanne)* 2019; 10: 388. https://doi.org/10.3389/fendo.2019.00388

17 Pena, A. S., Witchel, S. F., Hoeger, K. M. et al. Adolescent polycystic ovary syndrome according to the international evidence-based guideline. *BMC Med* 2020; 18(1): 72. https://doi.org/10.1186/s12916-020-01516-x

Chapter

6

The Relevance of the Anti-Müllerian Hormone in Polycystic Ovary Syndrome Diagnosis and Management

Martina Capuzzo and Antonio La Marca

Introduction

A diagnosis of polycystic ovary syndrome (PCOS) is based on at least two criteria among anovulation/oligo-ovulation, hyperandrogenism and polycystic ovarian morphology (PCOM) as seen on ultrasound.[1] In the past years, however, given the challenges posed by ultrasound in the diagnosis of PCOM, increasing attention has been given to the possibility of using alternative diagnostic markers. Anti-Müllerian hormone (AMH), which has been shown to have a strong correlation with antral follicle count (AFC) on ultrasound in PCOS, is considered a potential one.

AMH is a dimeric glycoprotein belonging to the transforming growth factor beta (TGF-β) superfamily. It takes its name from its role in the sexual differentiation in the fetus: secreted by the Sertoli cells of the male testes, it induces the regression of Müllerian ducts, which, in the absence of AMH, differentiate into the uterus, oviducts and one-third of the vagina.[2] In adult women, AMH is exclusively secreted by the granulosa cells surrounding the growing follicles from early antral to small antral phase.[3] As the pool of small growing follicles is in parallel with the total number of primordial follicles in the ovaries, AMH reflects the so-called ovarian reserve. Its expression continues to increase in the granulosa cells until primordial follicles have developed into small antral follicles approximately 4–6 mm in size. When growing antral follicles reach diameter of 8 mm, AMH levels show a rapid decrease, becoming undetectable during follicle-stimulating hormone (FSH)–dependent stages of follicular recruitment. AMH induces the decrease of FSH-stimulated aromatizing capacity of granulosa cells, with the consequent reduction of estradiol (E2) production until final follicular selection. The follicles producing less AMH show a greater sensitivity to FSH, allowing the progression of growth and thus ovulation.[4]

AMH in the Pathogenesis of Anovulation

As mentioned, in the cellular differentiation AMH acts with a paracrine inhibitory effect on the activation of folliculogenesis, which is sufficient to prevent the selection of a dominant follicle and thus ovulation. AMH has a negative and inhibitory role in many functions of granulosa-lutein cells, including the notorious reduction of the aromatase CYP19A1 expression induced by FSH. Since in PCOS patients there is an increased number of small antral follicles producing AMH, PCOS patients may have an AMH-dominant microenvironment, which interferes with the actions of FSH on follicles, leading to anovulation and amenorrhea. AMH also reduces FSH receptor messenger RNA (mRNA) expression, with a consequent modulation in the ovarian follicular responses to the hormone.

A modulation of the response to luteinizing hormone (LH) has also been shown. FSH and LH seem to act differently at the level of genes involved in the steroidogenesis such as CYP19A1 and P450scc. Both FSH and LH strongly stimulate CYP19A1 mRNA expression and estradiol production in mature granulosa cells, while P450scc mRNA expression and progesterone synthesis are maximally induced by the presence of LH. Studies conducted in vitro on cultured human granulosa cells incubated with AMH, LH and FSH have shown that AMH modulates the mRNA induction of CYP19A1 and P450scc generated by a 24-hour gonadotropin treatment, demonstrating the inhibition of gonadotropin-dependent steroidogenesis induced by AMH.[5]

Another key element in the pathogenesis of PCOS is insulin resistance. Hyperinsulinemia may

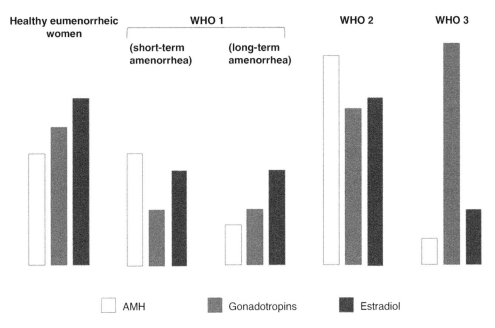

Figure 6.1 Key aspects of the pathogenesis of PCOS
Different factor determining the stockpiling of small antral follicle and the consequent anovulation are shown.

explain the high plasma levels of LH and the altered ovarian and adrenal androgen synthesis typical of this disorder. This hypothesis is supported by the demonstration that insulin-sensitizing drugs such as metformin reduce plasma levels of LH as well as androgen synthesis and improve frequency of menstrual cycle and ovulation.[6]

A central action of AMH on gonadotropin-releasing hormone (GnRH) neurons has also been hypothesized in murine models observing the increased LH pulsatility in many cases of PCOS, in which circulating AMH levels are also often elevated.[7] Key aspects of the pathogenesis of PCOS are shown in Figure 6.1.

Clinical Applications of AMH

The clinical use of AMH has recently been extended and has gained increasing attention in international literature. Its most important application is the correlation with the female reproductive potential. Since its levels reflect the cohort of growing follicles, its value decreases with the increase of female age, correlating with the decrease of the ovarian reserve. After peaking in the mid-20s,[4] AMH shows a longitudinal decline over time. If compared to other markers such as AFC, FSH, inhibin B and estradiol, AMH seems to better reflect the continuous decline of the oocyte/

follicle pool with age.[8] Beside its use as a marker of ovarian reserve, AMH has been efficiently used as a marker to predict the extremes of ovarian response to gonadotropin stimulation in assisted reproductive technologies. High basal AMH levels may predict an increase in a patient's risk of developing ovarian hyperstimulation syndrome (OHSS), while low levels are used to predict poor responders in ovarian stimulation. Another possible clinical use of AMH is the assessment of ovarian function before and after gynecologic surgeries or gonadotoxic agents such as chemotherapy.[4]

AMH in the Differential Diagnosis of Anovulatory Disorders

Anovulatory disorders in women can be various. The main classification in use is adapted from the one proposed by the World Health Organization (WHO) and by the 1995 European Society of Human Reproduction and Embryology (ESHRE) Capri workshop group.[9] In such classification, the possible causes of anovulation are categorized into three groups on the basis of serum levels of gonadotropin and estradiol. WHO 1 anovulatory dysfunction is characterized by low gonadotropin and low estradiol serum levels.[10] The underlining cause is usually a hypothalamic suppression, which occurs in association with weight loss or excessive physical exercise. WHO 2 anovulatory dysfunction, accounting for 80% of all the anovulations, presents normal gonadotropin and estradiol levels: PCOS represents its most frequent example.[11] WHO 3 anovulatory dysfunction is characterized by an ovarian reserve depletion with high gonadotropin and low estradiol levels.[12] Since gonadotropin and estradiol levels are often overlapping in the various forms of anovulation, several other markers have been proposed for the differential diagnosis of anovulatory dysfunctions, such as AMH. In WHO 1 patients, either low, normal or slightly elevated AMH levels have been described. Normal serum AMH levels have been reported in most of the studies on women with central secondary amenorrhea.[13–15] Patients with long-term profound gonadotropin deficiency show significantly lower AMH levels compared with short-term anovulation. AMH has been demonstrated to predict the probability of ovarian function recovery: the higher its level, the higher the probability of menstrual cycle recovery.[16] WHO 3 anovulatory dysfunction is characterized by low or undetectable AMH levels.[17] The follicle pool is depleted with a consequent ovarian insufficiency. Also, in this anovulation disorder AMH levels have a prognostic significance: its levels were shown to be significantly different between incipient ovarian failure, with regular menstrual cycles and elevated FSH, and transitional ovarian failure patients, with

oligomenorrhea and elevated FSH, permitting the identification of the clinical degree of follicle pool depletion.[18] AMH values are also reported to perform as a predictor of follicle presence in ovarian biopsies performed on patients with a premature ovarian failure.[19]

AMH As a Diagnostic Marker in PCOS

When compared with normal ovulatory women, PCOS patients have shown consistently higher levels of serum AMH.[17, 20, 21] There are different reasons behind the elevated serum AMH levels in this category of patients. PCOS women show a stagnation of AMH-producing follicles, with a stockpiling of transitional and classic primary follicles whose differentiation in the subsequent development phases is disrupted.[22] Besides the elevated number of AMH-producing follicles, an increased production of AMH per single follicle has also been observed in these patients, with the mean AMH level 4 times higher in granulosa cells from ovulatory PCOS and 75 times higher in granulosa cells from anovulatory PCOS patients in a study by Pellatt and colleagues, demonstrating a correlation between AMH values and the severity of the syndrome.[23] The correlation between AMH, gonadotropin and estradiol levels in the various forms of anovulation are shown in Figure 6.2.

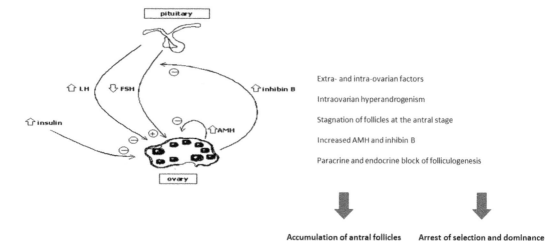

Figure 6.2 Serum AMH, gonadotropins and estradiol levels are shown for healthy eumenorrheic women and for the various forms of anovulation (WHO type 1, 2 and 3)
WHO 1 anovulation disorder is divided between short- and long-term anovulation.

Besides its possible use as a diagnostic marker of PCOS, AMH has also been thought to have a role in the pathogenesis of the disease. The high AMH concentrations present in women with PCOS could play an integral role in causing anovulation due to AMH's inhibitory influence on the actions of FSH that normally promotes follicular development from the small antral stage to ovulation.[2] Factors related to the pathophysiology of PCOS, such as increased LH levels, increased androgen levels and insulin resistance, as discussed, may be also associated with elevated serum AMH levels. LH is known to increase AMH production up to fourfold in granulosa cells of PCOS ovaries and elevates AMH expression in the granulosa cells of oligo- or anovulatory PCOS women, implying a role of LH in excessive AMH expression and follicular arrest. Androgens stimulate the FSH-independent stages of follicular development and may increase AMH production. A positive correlation was noted between fasting insulin and AMH levels, even if the exact relationship between insulin resistance and AMH has not been fully elucidated.[4]

Given the strong implication of AMH in PCOS, AMH level could be used as a biomarker of the diagnosis of PCOS. As serum AMH level reflects excess small follicles not visible on ultrasonography, AMH level would theoretically be more accurate than PCOM as a diagnostic marker. A large debate has been conducted on the possible cutoff value to be used. In a meta-analysis conducted by Iliodromiti and colleagues, the specificity and sensitivity in diagnosing PCOS in the symptomatic women were of 79.4% and 82.8%, respectively, for a cutoff value of AMH of 4.7 ng/mL.[24] Dewailly and colleagues separated asymptomatic women with PCOM from those with normal ovarian morphology in order to better calibrate the cutoff for the AMH value to distinguish patients with PCOS from normal women. A higher specificity (97% vs. 92%) and a better sensitivity (92% vs. 81%) were demonstrated for a cutoff value of AMH of 4.9 ng/mL compared to AFC.[25] However, there is currently no universal and consensual diagnostic threshold for serum AMH in the diagnosis of PCOS. The new ESHRE guidelines, published in 2018, do not recommend the use of serum AMH levels as an alternative for detecting PCOM or as a single test result for the diagnosis of PCOS.[26]

Potential Applications of AMH in PCOS

A possible clinical use for AMH, rather than for the diagnosis of PCOS, is for the characterization of the severity of the syndrome. Higher levels of AMH have been described in PCOS women with amenorrhea rather than in oligomenorrhea, reflecting a more evident impairment in granulosa cell function and follicular development in the ovaries of amenorrhoeic than in those of oligomenorrheic PCOS women. Ultra-high AMH levels (> 10 ng/mL) have been described to have a greater prevalence in women with PCOM, oligomenorrhea and amenorrhea, confirming the correlation between increased AMH levels and PCOS severity.[27]

Thus, AMH has also been proposed as a marker for treatment monitoring in PCOS women. Obese and overweight PCOS patients who, after weight loss, showed improvements in reproductive function had lower baseline AMH levels compared with those who did not respond.[28] Patients with higher AMH levels were also those who responded less to ovulation induction treatments in a study evaluating ovarian response to ovarian stimulation treatments.[29] In patients with functional hypothalamic amenorrhea (FHA) with features of PCOS (increases in serum androgens during gonadotropin administration, PCOM, increased ovarian size), women who had higher levels of AMH (> 4.7 ng/mL) showed minor recovery of their menstrual function.[30] Apart from the studies investigating the correlation between AMH level and IVF outcomes in controlled ovarian stimulation cycles, attention has also been given to the correlation between AMH level with IVF outcomes in minimal ovarian stimulation cycles such as those with clomiphene citrate. Serum AMH levels correlated positively with the number of retrieved oocytes, blastocyst formation rate, blastocyst cryopreservation rate and live birth rate per oocyte retrieval in clomiphene citrate cycles. A low serum AMH level, on the contrary, correlated with low ovarian responsiveness, impaired preimplantation embryonic development and decreased cumulative live birth rate.[31] In a study evaluating transvaginal ovarian drilling followed by controlled ovarian stimulation in PCOS patients, higher AMH levels were shown in poor responder patients.[32]

Future Scenarios: What Is Needed?

As said in the section "AMH As a Diagnostic Marker in PCOS," AMH is currently not recommended by the ESHRE guidelines as a marker for PCOS diagnosis. One of the most important limitations in its use of for such purpose is represented by a different calibration of the values from the existing AMH assays. The optimal performance and stability of the automated AMH assays now in use (the Beckman Coulter Access and the Roche Elecsys), if compared to previous manual assays, are well recognized, with many clinicians assuming that the values derived from those two abovementioned assays are interchangeable.[33] Nevertheless, there is still an ongoing debate in the literature. An international standard is needed to systematize the existing assays before diagnostic cutoffs can be meaningful. A defined study with control populations that are age-specific, as well as biologically relevant cutoff values that reflect clustering of clinical features and are relevant to health outcomes in addition to improved accuracy and standardization of AMH assays, are therefore mandatory before introducing AMH values as a diagnostic marker for PCOS.

References

1 Geisthövel, F. and Rabe, T. The ESHRE/ASRM consensus on polycystic ovary syndrome (PCOS): An extended critical analysis. *Reprod Biomed Online* 2007; 14(4): 522–535. https://doi.org/10.1016/s1472-6483(10)60902-9

2 Visser, J. A. and Themmen, A. P. Anti-Müllerian hormone and folliculogenesis. *Mol Cell Endocrinol* 2005; 234(1–2): 81–86. https://doi.org/10.1016/j.mce.2004.09.008

3 La Marca, A., Pati, M., Orvieto, R., Stabile, G., Carducci Artensio, A. and Volpe, A. Serum anti-Müllerian hormone levels in women with secondary amenorrhea. *Fertil Steril* 2006; 85(5): 1547–1549. https://doi.org/10.1016/j.fertnstert.2005.10.057

4 Oh, S. R., Choe, S. Y. and Cho, Y. J. Clinical application of serum anti-Müllerian hormone in women. *Clin Exp Reprod Med* 2019; 46(2): 50–59. https://doi.org/10.5653/cerm.2019.46.2.50

5 Sacchi, S., D'Ippolito, G., Sena, P. et al. The anti-Müllerian hormone (AMH) acts as a gatekeeper of ovarian steroidogenesis inhibiting the granulosa cell response to both FSH and LH. *J Assist Reprod Genet* 2016; 33(1): 95–100. https://doi.org/10.1007/s10815-015-0615-y

6 La Marca, A., Morgante, G., Palumbo, M., Cianci, A., Petraglia, F. and De Leo, V. Insulin-lowering treatment reduces aromatase activity in response to follicle-stimulating hormone in women with polycystic ovary syndrome. *Fertil Steril* 2002; 78(6): 1234–1239. https://doi.org/10.1016/s0015-0282(02)04346-7

7 Cimino, I., Casoni, F., Liu, X. et al. Novel role for anti-Müllerian hormone in the regulation of GnRH neuron excitability and hormone secretion. *Nat Commun* 2016; 7: 10055. https://doi.org/10.1038/ncomms10055

8 Van Rooij, I. A., Broekmans, F. J., Scheffer, G. J. et al. Serum antimullerian hormone levels best reflect the reproductive decline with age in normal women with proven fertility: A longitudinal study. *Fertil Steril* 2005; 83(4): 979–987. https://doi.org/10.1016/j.fertnstert.2004.11.029

9 Anovulatory infertility. The ESHRE Capri Workshop Group. *Hum Reprod* 1995; 10 (6):1549–1553.

10 Lie Fong, S., Schipper, I., Valkenburg, O., de Jong, F. H., Visser, J. A. and Laven, J. S. The role of anti-Müllerian hormone in the classification of anovulatory infertility. *Eur J Obstet Gynecol Reprod Biol* 2015; 186: 75–9. https://doi.org/10.1016/j.ejogrb.2015.01.007

11 Grinspoon, S., Miller, K., Coyle, C. et al. Severity of osteopenia in estrogen-deficient women with anorexia nervosa and hypothalamic amenorrhea. *J Clin Endocrinol Metab* 1999; 84(6): 2049–2055. https://doi.org/10.1210/jcem.84.6.5792

12 Vescovi, J. D., Jamal, S. A. and De Souza, M. J. Strategies to reverse bone loss in women with functional hypothalamic amenorrhea: A systematic review of the literature. *Osteoporos Int* 2008; 19(4): 465–478. https://doi.org/10.1007/s00198-007-0518-6

13 Wu, C. H., Chen, Y. C., Wu, H. H., Yang, J. G., Chang, Y. J. and Tsai, H. D. Serum anti-Müllerian hormone predicts ovarian response and cycle outcome in IVF patients. *J Assist Reprod Genet* 2009; 26(7): 383–389. https://doi.org/10.1007/s10815-009-9332-8

14 Durlinger, A. L., Visser, J. A. and Themmen, A. P. Regulation of ovarian function: The role of anti Müllerian hormone. *Reproduction* 2002; 124(5): 601–609. https://doi.org/10.1530/rep.0.1240601

15 Weenen, C., Laven, J. S., Von Bergh, A. R. et al. Anti-Müllerian hormone expression pattern in the human ovary: potential implications for initial and cyclic follicle recruitment. *Mol Hum Reprod* 2004; 10(2): 77–83. https://doi.org/10.1093/molehr/gah015

16 Van Elburg, A. A., Eijkemans, M. J., Kas, M. J. et al. Predictors of recovery of ovarian function during

weight gain in anorexia nervosa. *Fertil Steril* 2007; 87(4): 902–908. https://doi.org/10.1016/j.fertnstert.2006.11.004

17 La Marca, A., Pati, M., Orvieto, R., Stabile, G., Carducci Artensio, A. and Volpe, A. Serum anti-Müllerian hormone levels in women with secondary amenorrhea. *Fertil Steril* 2006; 85(5): 1547–1549. https://doi.org/10.1016/j.fertnstert.2005.10.057

18 Knauff, E. A., Eijkemans, M. J., Lambalk, C.B. et al. Dutch Premature Ovarian Failure Consortium: Anti-Mullerian hormone, inhibin B, and antral follicle count in young women with ovarian failure. *J Clin Endocrinol Metab* 2009; 94(3): 786–792. https://doi.org/10.1210/jc.2008-1818

19 Méduri, G., Massin, N., Guibourdenche, J. et al. Serum anti-Müllerian hormone expression in women with premature ovarian failure. *Hum Reprod* 2007; 22(1): 117–123. https://doi.org/10.1093/humrep/del346

20 Pigny, P., Merlen, E., Robert, Y. et al. Elevated serum level of anti-mullerian hormone in patients with polycystic ovary syndrome: Relationship to the ovarian follicle excess and to the follicular arrest. *J Clin Endocrinol Metab* 2003; 88(12): 5957–5962. https://doi.org/10.1210/jc.2003-030727

21 Laven, J. S., Mulders, A. G., Visser, J. A., Themmen, A. P., De Jong, F. H. and Fauser, B. C. Anti-Müllerian hormone serum concentrations in normoovulatory and anovulatory women of reproductive age. *J Clin Endocrinol Metab* 2004; 89(1): 318–323. https://doi.org/10.1210/jc.2003-030932

22 Maciel, G. A., Baracat, E. C., Benda, J. A. et al. Stockpiling of transitional and classic primary follicles in ovaries of women with polycystic ovary syndrome. *J Clin Endocrinol Metab* 2004; 89(11): 5321–5327. https://doi.org/10.1210/jc.2004-0643

23 Pellatt, L., Hanna, L., Brincat, M. et al. Granulosa cell production of anti-Müllerian hormone is increased in polycystic ovaries. *J Clin Endocrinol Metab* 2007; 92(1): 240–245. https://doi.org/10.1210/jc.2006-1582

24 Iliodromiti, S., Kelsey, T. W., Anderson, R. A. and Nelson, S. M. Can anti-Mullerian hormone predict the diagnosis of polycystic ovary syndrome? A systematic review and meta-analysis of extracted data. *J Clin Endocrinol Metab* 2013; 98(8): 3332–3340. https://doi.org/10.1210/jc.2013-1393

25 Dewailly, D., Gronier, H., Poncelet, E. et al. Diagnosis of polycystic ovary syndrome (PCOS): Revisiting the threshold values of follicle count on ultrasound and of the serum AMH level for the definition of polycystic ovaries. *Hum Reprod* 2011;

26(11): 3123–3129. https://doi.org/10.1093/humrep/der297

26 Teede, H. J., Misso, M. L., Costello, M. F. et al. International PCOS Network. Recommendations from the international evidence-based guideline for the assessment and management of polycystic ovary syndrome. *Hum Reprod* 2018; 33(9): 1602–1618. https://doi.org/10.1093/humrep/dey256. [Erratum in: *Hum Reprod* 2019; 34(2): 388.]

27 Tal, R., Seifer, D. B., Khanimov, M., Malter, H. E., Grazi, R. V. and Leader, B. Characterization of women with elevated antimüllerian hormone levels (AMH): Correlation of AMH with polycystic ovarian syndrome phenotypes and assisted reproductive technology outcomes. *Am J Obstet Gynecol* 2014; 211(1): 59.e1–8. https://doi.org/10.1016/j.ajog.2014.02.026

28 Thomson, R. L., Buckley, J. D., Moran, L. J. et al. The effect of weight loss on anti-Müllerian hormone levels in overweight and obese women with polycystic ovary syndrome and reproductive impairment. *Hum Reprod* 2009; 24(8): 1976–1981. https://doi.org/10.1093/humrep/dep101

29 Pellatt, L., Rice, S. and Mason, H. D. Anti-Müllerian hormone and polycystic ovary syndrome: A mountain too high? *Reproduction* 2010; 139(5): 825–833. https://doi.org/10.1530/REP-09-0415

30. Carmina, E., Fruzzetti, F. and Lobo, R. A. Features of polycystic ovary syndrome (PCOS) in women with functional hypothalamic amenorrhea (FHA) may be reversible with recovery of menstrual function. *Gynecol Endocrinol* 2018; 34(4): 301–304. https://doi.org/10.1080/09513590.2017.1395842

31 Ezoe, K., Ni, X., Kobayashi, T. and Kato, K. Anti-Müllerian hormone is correlated with cumulative live birth in minimal ovarian stimulation with clomiphene citrate: A retrospective cohort study. *BMC Pregnancy Childbirth* 2020; 20(740). https://doi.org/10.1186/s12884-020-03446-1

32 Xu, B., Zhou, M., Cheng, M. et al. Transvaginal ovarian drilling followed by controlled ovarian stimulation from the next day improves ovarian response for the poor responders with polycystic ovary syndrome during IVF treatment: A pilot study. *Reprod Biol Endocrinol* 2020; 18(7). https://doi.org/10.1186/s12958-019-0559-7

33 Tadros, T., Tarasconi, B., Nassar, J., Benham, J. L., Taieb, J. and Fanchin, R. New automated antimüllerian hormone assays are more reliable than the manual assay in patients with reduced antral follicle count. *Fertil Steril* 2016; 106(7): 1800–1806. https://doi.org/10.1016/j.fertnstert.2016.08.045

Chapter

7

Origins of Polycystic Ovary Syndrome In Utero

Roy Homburg and Claudia Raperport

Introduction

Polycystic ovary syndrome (PCOS) is the most common metabolic condition, affecting up to 20% of all women of reproductive age. It is difficult to define in premenstrual and postmenopausal years and therefore the diagnosis and management center on women of reproductive age. Many sufferers are diagnosed in adolescence when investigated for symptoms such as persistent acne, hirsutism and oligo- or amenorrhea. Many women may be ignorant of their diagnosis until such time as they seek medical assistance for subfertility.

PCOS is characterized by biochemical and clinical symptoms of hyperandrogenism, menstrual dysfunction and ovaries that have a polycystic morphology on ultrasound. It is also associated with metabolic dysfunction and sufferers carry an increased lifelong risk of cardiovascular disease and type 2 diabetes mellitus and symptoms are exacerbated by obesity. The psychological impacts of the syndrome include increased risk of depression, eating disorders and anxiety.

The endocrine component of this syndrome is closely linked with various metabolic phenomena including increased insulin resistance. Ever since PCOS was first described in 1935, it was noted that obesity and increasing body weight can exacerbate all the symptoms and signs of the syndrome.[1] It is well documented that weight loss of around 5–10% can reduce symptoms and restore ovulation and regular menstrual cycles in overweight affected women. One of the paradoxes involved in this syndrome is the presence of a population of lean women with PCOS who are also hyperandrogenic and anovulatory and may be the most insulin-resistant – irrespective of body mass index.[2] The presence of this group negates the theory that the insulin resistance associated with PCOS is solely driven by increased weight.

This syndrome creates a significant burden on health services, with women often requiring fertility treatment as well as needing medical input for the management of metabolic conditions, cardiovascular complications, obesity-related concerns and associated psychological elements. One of the challenges in proving the etiology of PCOS is the difficulty in defining cases. Diagnostic criteria vary and there is no universally used version. The Rotterdam consensus developed a diagnostic system that specifies that, for diagnosis of PCOS, a woman must have two out of the following three criteria: (1) oligo- or amenorrhea, (2) biochemical or clinical evidence of hyperandrogenism (specifically hirsutism and acne) and (3) typical ultrasound characteristics of a polycystic ovary.[3] The other most common diagnostic classification used is the American National Institutes of Health (NIH) system, which defines PCOS as a combination of ovulatory dysfunction and hyperandrogenism.

Accurate diagnosis is important for research since correct identification of subjects and unaffected controls are vital for accuracy and the different sets of diagnostic criteria can complicate this. It is also important to identify women with the syndrome so that their metabolic and cardiovascular health can be assessed and optimized and their future health risks reduced. The better we can understand the etiology of this syndrome, the more likely we are to find successful prevention or treatments in the future.

Heterogenous diagnostic criteria are one of the factors complicating the search for the etiology of PCOS. Various theories exist supporting the possibility of genetic inheritance or epigenetic alterations related to in utero androgen exposure, which are explored in this chapter.

Genetic Inheritance

Inheritance Patterns

Women with first-degree relatives suffering from PCOS are significantly more likely to be affected themselves.[4] One study looking at familial patterns tested the sisters of affected women and found 22% had undiagnosed PCOS and a further 24% had isolated hyperandrogenism with regular menstrual cycles.[5] Various studies have reported a likely autosomal dominant inheritance pattern when investigating PCOS diagnoses, hyperandrogenism and premature male-pattern baldness (in male relatives) in siblings of women with confirmed PCOS diagnosis.[6, 7]

Although some studies, as mentioned, have suggested an autosomal dominant inheritance pattern, other family studies and twin studies have shown confounding patterns of inheritance and these patterns do not neatly fit into any Mendelian inheritance patterns. One study of twins compared both monozygotic and dizygotic twins and showed a nonsignificant diagnostic concordance of 63% for monozygotic pairs and 67% for the dizygotic pairs.[8] A larger study from the Netherlands showed a significant correlation between PCOS diagnoses in monozygotic twin pairs compared to dizygotic and singleton sisters. However, this study was limited due to diagnostic criteria based on a threshold from a model and relied on self-reported characteristics rather than clinical diagnosis.[9]

Despite the inconclusive results of the twin and family studies, a genetic cause for PCOS seems plausible and widespread research looking for the candidate gene or polymorphism(s) responsible has so far also been inconclusive. The studies detailing these searches have reported heterogenous findings. Several loci have been identified as being related to metabolic traits, including high insulin levels, lipid levels and obesity, supporting a genetic link between these factors and PCOS.[10]

Genetic Findings in Different Phenotypic Subgroups

Interestingly, there is a link shown between genetic predisposition to high body mass index (BMI) and PCOS, and genetic variants that have been associated with PCOS have separately been linked with depression. The genetic loci currently associated with PCOS have links to neuroendocrine, metabolic and reproductive pathways and links with the genetic associations of menopause, metabolic disorders, depression and male-pattern balding.

A 2020 study based on a single genome-wide association study (GWAS) in PCOS sufferers of European ancestry found an interesting division between the two distinct phenotypes of PCOS and their associated genetics. A "reproductive" subtype had increased luteinizing hormone (LH) and sex hormone-binding globulin (SHBG) with lower BMI and insulin levels. A "metabolic" subtype was associated with higher BMI, glucose and insulin levels and a lower LH and SHBG. The same families tended to display the same subtypes. Rare variants of DENND1A were associated with the "reproductive" subtype along with alleles in four other loci identified, whereas the "metabolic" subtype was only associated with one specific allele.[11]

Genetic Findings in Different Ethnic Subgroups

Although similar studies are awaited in women with other ethnic backgrounds, there have been identified ethnic variations in the phenotype associated with this syndrome, with women of Hispanic descent being at higher risk of developing type 2 diabetes and metabolic syndrome, whereas African women are at increased risk of hypertension and cardiovascular complications. [12, 13] Two genetic loci (first identified in a GWAS of Han Chinese women) were also found in women of European ancestry; this finding suggests a possible ancient evolutionary trait. Research into the racial expression of these genetic variants among publicly available genomic databases uncovered evidence that ethnic variations in PCOS are strongly influenced by the genetic background in humans.[14]

Candidate Genes and Polymorphisms

From the current research available it seems that, overall, there are four categories into which the suspected candidate genes fall: (1) those related to insulin resistance, (2) those related to androgen biosynthesis and actions, (3) those responsible for inflammatory cytokine responses and (4) others.

[15] One possible candidate gene was identified in DENND1A, which is a gene involved with regulating ovarian androgen biosynthesis. Common variants in this gene have been associated with reproductive and metabolic traits seen in PCOS sufferers.[11]

The most recent GWAS studies have identified 16 different genetic loci found in groups with self-reported PCOS that also fit the NIH diagnostic criteria. The largest meta-analysis to date, comparing results from 113000 women divided them according to diagnostic groups – Rotterdam, NIH and self-reported PCOS. This study identified 14 genetic loci independently associated with PCOS that applied to all three of the diagnostic groups and persisted after adjustment for age and BMI. Both of the two possible candidate genes discovered were endocrine-related.[10]

Research is ongoing into clarifying both the genes responsible for PCOS and the inheritance patterns. The "risk genes" identified to date only confer a small increase of risk and further research is required to look for rarer variants that may confer a higher risk. The currently identified genes may only account for < 10% of PCOS and they all demonstrate endocrinological mechanisms of action supporting the plausibility of an epigenetic etiology.

Of note, the risk genes identified in extensive GWAS studies for populations with type 2 diabetes show a 23% genetic heritability despite familial studies demonstrating around 50% overall heritability. This further supports the Barker hypothesis that epigenetic mechanisms in utero may play a larger role in the metabolic as well as other health futures of children than currently accepted.[16]

Epigenetic Etiology

Barker Hypothesis

The Barker hypothesis was first described in 1990 when a study showed a link between birthweight and cardiovascular disease risk in adulthood. The theory was that differing states of nutrition in pregnancy altered the future health of the offspring through adaptation mechanisms involving hormone secretion and that the consequences of malnutrition were different in the different trimesters of pregnancy.[16] The hypothesis was then expanded to suggest that the in utero environment altered gene expression and "programmed" future health. With regard to PCOS, the theory is that exposure to excess androgens during the antenatal period could have epigenetic consequences and effectively program the ovaries of a female fetus to predestine her to develop PCOS later in life. This "programming" is thought to be a direct consequence of the actions of androgens on the expression of genes controlling ovarian steroid production, folliculogenesis, gonadotropin-releasing hormone (GnRH) pulsatility and insulin resistance.

Animal studies have supported this hypothesis as detailed in the following section. Human studies have also been attempted, with efforts made to quantify androgen levels in umbilical cord blood, amniotic fluid and antenatal serum levels but studies have been small and results inconclusive.

Animal Models

Background

It is accepted that many of the features of PCOS are directly related to hyperandrogenism. The presence of high circulating free androgen levels can result in a comprehensive set of PCOS traits, including reproductive, metabolic and endocrine. Androgens mediate their actions via androgen receptors (AR) and, in the pathogenesis of PCOS, treatment with flutamide (AR antagonist) can help to restore ovulatory cycles in some PCOS patients.[17] In cases of congenital adrenal hyperplasia and in transsexual female patients treated with exogenous testosterone, the excess androgen secretion has led to all of the symptoms commonly associated with PCOS and the ovarian features of arrested follicular development, polycystic morphology and thickened theca.

There is, fortunately, a large degree of similarity between the reproductive biology of different mammals, specifically surrounding the mechanisms of control of ovulation via the hypothalamic–pituitary–ovarian axis. This has allowed us to learn a huge amount from studies involving rodents and large mammals, where, for ethical reasons, human research is impossible. One example of this is the terminology for congenital adrenal hyperplasia, which was coined after mouse studies confirmed the mechanism of endocrine disruption. PCOS was once thought to be a condition specific to humans, but studies in sheep and rats have shown that these animals can be provoked to display a similar syndrome and rhesus monkeys may suffer from spontaneous PCOS (or an equivalent syndrome). This knowledge has helped hugely in advancing our understanding of this condition.

The theory of in utero androgen exposure resulting in metabolic changes including insulin resistance and a polycystic ovarian morphology has mostly been developed in response to various animal studies where female animals were exposed to exogenous steroid hormones during pregnancy. These studies have shown homogeneous results across various animal species, including sheep, monkeys, mice and rats.

Rodents are ideal research subjects since they reproduce so rapidly, but a limitation of any findings from rodent studies is that they are multi-ovulatory and also complete oocytogenesis in the neonatal period. Sheep are closer to humans in that they are mono-ovulatory and complete oocytogenesis antenatally. Rhesus monkeys are closer still and, like humans, spontaneous hyperandrogenic states have been diagnosed in these primates. The differences in the timing of completion of follicular formation are reflected in the results of the studies, which show that rodents develop PCOS traits when treated with androgens in early neonatal stages, whereas monkeys and sheep have the strongest response to androgen when exposed in utero.

Animal Research Findings

The first research on rats in the 1970s described disordered follicular recruitment and oligo- or anovulatory patterns in rats that had been exposed to exogenous testosterone in utero. Subsequent studies have demonstrated similar outcomes of antenatal androgen administration.[18, 19] Although these studies help validate the hypothesis of fetal androgen exposure being the trigger for "programming" offspring toward a PCOS, as mentioned, rodents have different patterns of oocytogenesis and follicular development and poly-ovulatory cycles.

Sheep are an excellent choice of research subject since their gonadal development follows a quicker but similarly sequenced trajectory. The average length of an ovine gestation is 144–152 days compared to 280 days for humans. Gonadal

differentiation starts in the sheep fetus at day 30 (humans: day 45–62) and antral follicles are present in the fetal ovary by day 135 (humans: day 230). A meta-analysis of the results of all the different antenatal androgen-administered sheep literature was performed and showed that the timing of androgen administration significantly influenced the consequences.[20] When testosterone was given early in the gestation period, virilization of the genitalia occurred. The incidence of anovulatory cycles was highest in ewes exposed to exogenous testosterone between gestation days 50 and 120 compared to earlier and later gestational ages.[21]

Women with PCOS are more likely to be obese and have been shown to have adipocytes that are larger than average and decreased serum adiponectin levels. Abnormal adiposity or adipocyte morphology has been identified in the offspring of mice, sheep and monkeys treated with androgen antenatally.

The results of ovarian biopsies from androgen-exposed sheep were shown on ultrasound to have decreased numbers of primordial follicles and increased numbers of primary follicles, mimicking the pattern of increased recruitment associated with human PCOS.[22, 23] The metabolic traits associated with PCOS were also demonstrated, with insulin resistance also seen in sheep as early as five weeks after birth and continuing into adulthood.[20, 24] Essentially, ewes exposed in utero to exogenous testosterone demonstrated all the changes required to fit a human diagnosis of PCOS.

Regarding fertility, it was noted that, as well as increased anovulatory subfertility, male sheep, when mixed with prenatally androgen-exposed sheep and the control ewes, preferentially chose to mate with the control group.[25]

In support of the ovine and rat findings, Abbott and colleagues carried out seminal work with rhesus monkeys, who were also investigated in similar trials. Pregnant mothers were injected with testosterone at one of two stages during their pregnancies. Rhesus monkeys have a gestational length of 165 days on average and the females were injected daily with testosterone from day 40 to day 80 after free fetal DNA was tested to confirm the absence of a Y chromosome (to ensure all offspring were female).[26]

When followed up to puberty and beyond, the offspring of the injected monkeys demonstrated irregular menstruation, high serum LH levels, insulin resistance and polycystic ovaries. This work not only strengthened the theories of in utero androgen exposure as a cause of PCOS but went further to identify a mid-gestational window within which exposure to testosterone induced the most PCOS-like symptoms in the offspring, including hyperandrogenism, polycystic ovaries, irregular cycles, diminished fertility, increased LH, insulin resistance and adiposity.[26]

Possible Pathogenetic Mechanism

Designed to investigate a possible epigenetic alteration in DNA methylation leading to PCOS, the visceral adipose tissue of adult rhesus monkeys was exposed to prenatal androgen and control subjects. Bayesian classification with singular value decomposition (BCSVD) was used for genome-wide CpG methylation analysis and results showed many differentially methylated loci between the two groups and several modified epigenetic signaling pathways.[26]

One rat study examined the difference between two different doses of prenatal testosterone administration with interesting results. Both groups exhibited hyperandrogenism and polycystic ovaries, but the group administered a lower dose remained ovulatory, whereas the group given a higher dose became anovulatory. The higher dose of testosterone appeared to upregulate the expression of both the steroidogenic acute regulatory protein (StAR) involved in cholesterol availability regulation and the protein expression of peroxisome proliferator-activated receptor gamma (PPAR gamma). In utero androgen exposure induced an antioxidant state. The higher dose of testosterone induced an inflammatory state in the ovary mediated by increased prostaglandin (PG) E levels and expression of COX2 (cyclooxygenase 2), which regulates PG production.[27]

From these animal studies it seems certain that in utero exposure to androgen increases the risk of metabolic and reproductive PCOS traits and that these effects are dose- and timing-dependent.

Human Evidence

Background

Evidence from human studies that elucidate a strong familial association points to a genetic etiology for PCOS but no responsible candidate gene or polymorphism has yet been identified as responsible for a significant proportion of cases. If hormonal factors alter the expression of the "risk genes" it is possible that this could contribute to PCOS pathogenesis and symptom development. Given that the actions of androgen have been shown to cause all of the PCOS-related traits, the assumption would be that the catalyst for epigenetic alteration is maternal androgen levels.

It has previously been assumed that circulating maternal androgen is neutralized by placental aromatase and therefore cannot directly act on the developing fetus. The question then arises, is it maternal androgen acting on the fetus despite aromatase actions or is there another pathway? One alternative is the overproduction of androgen by the fetal ovaries; but what is the stimulus for this overproduction?

Pregnant women with PCOS have raised anti-Müllerian hormone (AMH) and hyperandrogenism that persists throughout pregnancy. Studies have also shown that the female offspring of PCOS mothers have increased ovarian volume and raised AMH levels as infants and this persists into childhood years. Even antenatally, amniotic fluid samples have shown increased testosterone and AMH and decreased SHBG in the pregnancies of PCOS women compared to controls in the mid-gestation period, which appears to be crucial for ovarian "programming."

In the children of PCOS mothers who took metformin during pregnancy, AMH is lower than in the control group, especially if metformin was started before or at conception.[28] Women with non-PCOS hyperandrogenism caused by congenital adrenal hyperplasia or adrenal tumors also have an increased prevalence of PCOS.[29, 30] Combining this evidence with the animal evidence that PCOS traits can be induced in the offspring of hyperandrogenic pregnant mammals, it seems likely that excess androgen from any source is the catalyst for epigenetic alterations leading to increased risk of the various PCOS traits in the future of the offspring.[29, 31]

Amniotic Fluid, Placental and Cord Blood Testing

Clearly there will never be human studies replicating the animal research that expose pregnant mothers to exogenous steroid hormones. Assessing the endogenous hormone levels in the fetal circulation or environment is challenging. Studies have investigated androgen levels in amniotic fluid and have illustrated raised amniotic testosterone in the second trimester of fetuses with PCOS mothers, suggesting increased production of androgen. However, the source of this androgen is difficult to prove.

A study on the epigenetic differences between umbilical cord blood samples from PCOS and control women suggested the existence of a possible "PCOS epigenomic superpathway" with three major components: glucotoxic, lipotoxic and inflammatory. This study was limited in size but suggests that there is a possible "at risk" epigenetic "signature" identifiable from birth.[32] Cord blood samples have also been tested but study results have been variable. It may be possible to quantify in utero androgen exposure by measuring neonatal sebum levels as a surrogate marker but this needs further research.[31]

The difficulty in linking maternal testosterone or androgen levels to fetal programming toward a PCOS picture is the placenta. The unanswered question is, where does the excess androgen originate and what is the mechanism of it reaching and affecting the fetus? Normally, it would be expected that maternal testosterone could not cross the placenta as SHBG should bind testosterone and render it inactive and the placenta has high levels of aromatase enzymes that convert androgens to estrogens. This mechanism has long been attributed to the protection of the fetus from a hyperandrogenic state. The studies on rhesus monkeys showed that, in order to see the PCOS sequelae of excess androgen exposure, levels needed to be equivalent to those seen in male monkeys to overcome the actions of aromatization, binding and inactivation. [33] One small (n = 50) trial biopsied the placental tissue of women with PCOS. Results described reduced p450 aromatase and increased androgen-producing enzyme activity.[34] However, these results need to be reproduced and validated in larger-scale trials.

Roles of AMH and Other Hormones

A more recent development in this search for clarification of the etiology of PCOS is the involvement of AMH. AMH was first understood to be the hormone responsible for sex differentiation of the fetus. It has more recently been found to be secreted by the granulosa cells of the ovarian follicles. Women with PCOS have deranged follicular recruitment patterns leading to multi-follicular ovaries with increased granulosa cell mass and a higher AMH secretion per granulosa cell.[35] This explains the high serum AMH concentrations found in PCOS populations. There is a correlation between the antral follicle count, severity of menstrual irregularities and increased serum levels of AMH. This lends credence to the idea that AMH not only is a marker of the syndrome but potentially has a role in the pathogenesis.[31]

AMH has been shown to interrupt follicular development and has been shown to be as much as 18 times higher in anovulatory women with PCOS compared to normo-ovulatory controls. It inhibits the actions of follicle-stimulating hormone (FSH) and blocks aromatase activity, leading to reduced estradiol levels and a prevention of multi-follicular development, therefore at normal levels it promotes mono-follicular growth and mono-ovulation at normal physiological levels. The significantly increased production associated with PCOS exaggerates this response leading to anovulatory cycles.

It has been shown that high AMH levels in PCOS women persist and increase throughout pregnancy in women compared with weight-matched, non-PCOS controls.[36] This has led to the hypothesis that AMH levels are implicated in the prenatal fetal ovarian "programming" that results in PCOS later in life. A recent murine study provided evidence that excessive AMH levels in pregnancy (as seen in PCOS) can cause hyperandrogenism in their female offspring. Tata and colleagues injected pregnant mice with AMH and demonstrated an increase in maternal testosterone and decreased placental aromatase activity contributing to a hyperandrogenic fetal environment. Establishing a comparable pathogenic PCOS mechanism in humans, however, remains to be demonstrated. It was suggested that the mechanism of action was an upregulation of GnRH receptors by AMH leading to increased LH production, which then stimulates androgen conversion.[36] This theory helps explain the PCOS traits seen in lean women who often have higher AMH and LH than their obese PCOS counterparts but in whom the increased BMI does not contribute to severity of symptoms.

It is yet to be proven whether these findings can be translated into human research. If it can be shown that women with high AMH concentrations have reduced aromatase activity in the placenta, this would explain the increased passage of maternal testosterone to the fetus. Alternatively, it is possible that the high LH levels produced in response to the increased AMH could cross the placenta. Whether the maternal LH or AMH act directly on the fetal ovaries and stimulate androgen production or whether they facilitate increased placental passage of maternal androgen, which then acts directly (or both), is yet to be proven. Tata's work on mice demonstrated higher circulating maternal LH levels in pregnant dams exposed to AMH injection compared to controls ($p < 0.0004$).[36] The studies in rhesus monkeys confirmed that the fetus itself also overproduces LH in response to high circulating androgen and this response was seen rapidly after maternal testosterone injection.[33] These findings have yet to be shown in humans.

Exposure to these hormones appears to be responsible for the epigenetic alteration in development of the fetal ovary. If, in response, the ovaries then began to produce fetal AMH, which in turn blocked aromatase activity, this could further increase the androgen exposure of the fetus. Fetal biopsies through the different trimesters of pregnancy and into the neonatal period demonstrated that AMH is first expressed in male fetuses from 8.5 weeks gestation. The same study did not find AMH in female fetuses until 36 weeks gestation.[37] This suggests that maternal AMH is not present in the fetal circulation (if it crossed the placenta this would likely happen from an earlier gestation and hence result in differentiation of gonads to testes rather than ovaries).

There are clearly epigenetic effects on the developing fetal ovary related to androgen exposure. It is possible that the androgen elicits a response in the ovarian granulosa cells, which,

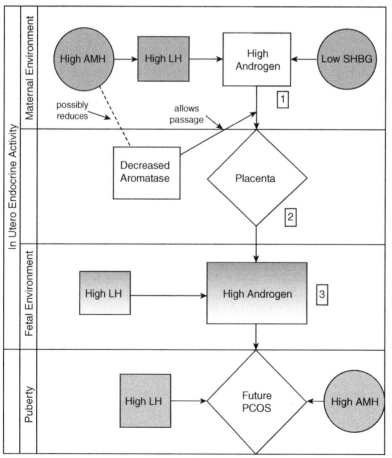

Figure 7.1 The relationship between the hormones involved in PCOS pathogenesis

in a positive feedback cycle, further increases androgen production. Granulosa cell sensitivity to AMH then continues throughout the reproductive lifespan of this offspring (Figure 7.1).

Conclusion

In summary, the etiology of PCOS is still not well understood. Genetic factors clearly play a limited role but have yet to be shown to cause more than a small proportion of cases. Animal studies have demonstrated that androgen exposure in the prenatal period can result in PCOS-like traits in several mammals and that this effect seems to be both dose- and timing-sensitive.

Research is ongoing to definitively prove that the female children of PCOS mothers are exposed to excess androgens, as studies of cord blood and amniotic fluid have not been conclusive and surrogate markers are being investigated, including quantitative neonatal facial sebum levels.[38] The pathway from excess androgen to ovarian dysregulation is also unclear, although several plausible hypotheses have been presented in this chapter.

AMH, LH and androgen are all raised in PCOS mothers compared to controls. There is a reduction in placental aromatase action in PCOS mice compared to controls. AMH appears not to cross the placenta until late gestational periods if at all (possibly any AMH detected at this stage is fetal in origin). If AMH does reduce aromatization of maternal androgen in the placenta as well as stimulate LH production, which in turn increases androgen production, exposure of the fetus to high maternal androgen is inevitable. There seems then to be an epigenetic alteration in function of the fetal ovaries or hypothalamic–pituitary–ovarian axis. The fetal response to this androgen includes an increased sensitivity to AMH leading to disrupted follicular recruitment and therefore reproductive consequences as well as the cascade of androgen-mediated metabolic sequelae recognized as components of PCOS.

References

1   Stein, I. and Leventhal, M. Amenorrhoea associated with bilateral polycystic ovaries. *Am J Obstet Gynecol* 1935; 29: 181–191.

2   Diamanti-Kandarakis, E. and Panidis, D. Unravelling the phenotypic map of polycystic ovary syndrome (PCOS): A prospective study of 634 women with PCOS. *Clin Endocrinol (Oxf)* 2007; 67(5): 735–742.

3   Rotterdam Consensus Consensus on women's health aspects of polycystic ovary syndrome (PCOS). *Hum Reprod* 2012; 27(1): 14–24.

4   Kahsar-Miller, M. D. Prevalence of polycystic ovary syndrome (PCOS) in first degree relatives of patients with PCOS. *Fertil Steril* 2001; 75(1): 53–58.

5   Legro, R. S., Driscoll, D., Strauss, J. F., III, Fox, J. and Dunaif, A. Evidence for a genetic basis for hyperandrogenemia in polycystic ovary syndrome. *Proc Natl Acad Sci USA* 1998; 95(25): 14956–14960.

6   Govind, A., Obhrai, M. S. and Clayton, R. N. Polycystic ovaries are inherited as an autosomal dominant trait: Analysis of 29 polycystic ovary syndrome and 10 control families. *J Clin Endocrinol Metab* 1999; 84(1): 38–43.

7   Carey, A. H., Chan, K. L., Short, F., White, D., Williamson, R. and Franks, S. Evidence for a single gene effect causing polycystic ovaries and male pattern baldness. *Clin Endocrinol* 1993; 38(6): 653–658.

8   Jahanfar, S., Eden, J. A., Warren, P., Seppälä, M. and Nguyen, T. V. A twin study of polycystic ovary syndrome. *Fertil Steril* 1995; 63(3): 478–486.

9   Vink, J. M., Sadrzadeh, S., Lambalk, C. B., and Boomsma, D. I. Heritability of polycystic ovary syndrome in a Dutch twin-family study. *J Clin Endocrinol Metab* 2006; 91(6): 2100–2104.

10 Day, F., Karaderi, T., Jones, M. R. et al. Large-scale genome-wide meta-analysis of polycystic ovary syndrome suggests shared genetic architecture for different diagnosis criteria. *PLoS Genetics* 2018; 14 (12): e1007813.

11 Dapas, M., Lin, F. T. J., Nadkarni, G. N. et al. Distinct subtypes of polycystic ovary syndrome with novel genetic associations: An unsupervised, phenotypic clustering analysis. 2020; *PLoS Med* 17 (6): e1003132.

12 Ehrmann, D. A., Liljenquist, D. R., Kasza, K., Azziz, R., Legro, R. S. and Ghazzi, M. N. Prevalence and predictors of the metabolic syndrome in women with polycystic ovary syndrome. *J Clin Endocrinol Metab* 2006; 91(1): 48–53.

13 Lo, J. C., Feigenbaum, S. L., Yang, J., Pressman, A. R., Selby, J. V. and Go, A. S. Epidemiology and adverse cardiovascular risk profile of diagnosed polycystic ovary syndrome. *J Clin Endocrinol Metab* 2006; 91(4): 1357–1363.

14 Casarini, L. and Brigante, G. The polycystic ovary syndrome evolutionary paradox: A genome-wide association studies-based, in silico, evolutionary explanation. *J Clin Endocrinol Metab* 2014; 99(11): E2412–2420.

15 Deligeoroglou, E., Kouskouti, C. and Christopoulos, P. The role of genes in the polycystic ovary syndrome: Predisposition and mechanisms. *Gynecol Endocrinol* 2009; 25(9): 603–609.

16 Barker, D. J. The developmental origins of adult disease. *J Am Coll Nutr* 2004; 23(6 Suppl): 588s–595s.

17 Rittmaster, R. S. Antiandrogen treatment of polycystic ovary syndrome. *Endocrinol Metab Clin North Am* 1999; 28(2): 409–421.

18 Fels, E. and Bosch, L. R. Effect of prenatal administration of testosterone on ovarian function in rats. *Am J Obstet Gynecol* 1971; 111(7): 964–969.

19 Parker, C. R., Jr. and Mahesh, V. B. Interrelationship between excessive levels of circulating androgens in blood and ovulatory failure. *J Reprod Med* 1976; 17(2): 75–90.

20 Padmanabhan, V. and Veiga-Lopez, A. Sheep models of polycystic ovary syndrome phenotype. *Mol Cell Endocrinol* 2013; 373(1–2): 8–20.

21 Clarke, I. J., Scaramuzzi, R. J. and Short, R. V. Ovulation in prenatally androgenized ewes. *J Endocrinol* 1977; 73(2): 385–389.

22 Forsdike, R. A., Hardy, K., Bull, L. et al. Disordered follicle development in ovaries of prenatally androgenized ewes. *J Endocrinol* 2007; 192(2): 421–428.

23 Smith, P., Steckler, T. L., Veiga-Lopez, A. and Padmanabhan, V. Developmental programming: Differential effects of prenatal testosterone and dihydrotestosterone on follicular recruitment, depletion of follicular reserve, and ovarian morphology in sheep. *Biol Reprod* 2009; 80(4): 726–736.

24 Recabarren, S. E., Padmanabhan, V., Codner, E. et al. Postnatal developmental consequences of altered insulin sensitivity in female sheep treated prenatally with testosterone. *Am J Physiol Endocrinol Metab* 2005; 289(5): E801-806.

25 Steckler, T. L., Roberts, E. K., Doop, D. D., Lee, T. M. and Padmanabhan, V. Developmental programming in sheep: Administration of testosterone during 60–90 days of pregnancy reduces breeding success and pregnancy outcome. *Theriogenology* 2007; 67(3): 459–467.

26 Xu, N., Kwon, S., Abbott, D. H. et al. Epigenetic mechanism underlying the development of polycystic ovary syndrome (PCOS)-like phenotypes in prenatally androgenized rhesus monkeys. *PLoS One* 2011; 6(11): e27286.

27 Amalfi, S., Velez, L. M., Heber, M. F. et al. Prenatal hyperandrogenization induces metabolic and endocrine alterations which depend on the levels of testosterone exposure. *PLoS One* 2012; 7(5): e37658.

28 Crisosto, N., Echiburú, B., Maliqueo, M. et al. Improvement of hyperandrogenism and hyperinsulinemia during pregnancy in women with polycystic ovary syndrome: Possible effect in the ovarian follicular mass of their daughters. *Fertil Steril* 2012; 97(1): 218–224.

29 Dumesic, D. A. and Richards, J. S. Ontogeny of the ovary in polycystic ovary syndrome. *Fertil Steril* 2013; 100(1): 23–38.

30 Yildiz, B. O. and Azziz, R. The adrenal and polycystic ovary syndrome. *Rev Endocr Metab Disord* 2007; 8(4): 331–342.

31 Homburg, R. and Crawford, G. The role of AMH in anovulation associated with PCOS: A hypothesis. *Hum Reprod* 2014; 29(6): 1117–1121.

32 Lambertini, L., Saul, S. R., Copperman, A. B. et al. Intrauterine reprogramming of the polycystic ovary syndrome: Evidence from a pilot study of cord blood global methylation analysis. *Front Endocrinol (Lausanne)* 2017; 8: 352.

33 Abbott, D. H., Barnett, D. K., Levine, J. E. et al. Endocrine antecedents of polycystic ovary syndrome in fetal and infant prenatally androgenized female rhesus monkeys. *Biol Reprod* 2008; 79(1): 154–163.

34 Maliqueo, M., Lara, H. E., Sánchez, F., Echiburú, B., Crisosto, N. and Sir-Petermann, T. Placental steroidogenesis in pregnant women with polycystic ovary syndrome. *Eur J Obstet Gynecol Reprod Biol* 2013; 166(2): 151–155.

35 Catteau-Jonard, S., Jamin, S. P., Leclerc, A., Gonzalès, J., Dewailly, D. and di Clemente, N. Anti-Mullerian hormone, its receptor, FSH receptor, and androgen receptor genes are overexpressed by granulosa cells from stimulated follicles in women with polycystic ovary syndrome. *J Clin Endocrinol Metab* 2008; 93(11): 4456–4461.

36 Tata, B., Mimouni, N. E. H., Barbotin, A. L. et al. Elevated prenatal anti-Müllerian hormone reprograms the fetus and induces polycystic ovary syndrome in adulthood. *Nat Med* 2018; 24(6): 834–846.

37 Rajpert-De Meyts, E., Jørgensen, N., Graem, N., Müller, J., Cate, R. L. and Skakkebaek, N. E. Expression of anti-Müllerian hormone during normal and pathological gonadal development: Association with differentiation of Sertoli and granulosa cells. *J Clin Endocrinol Metab* 1999; 84(10): 3836–3844.

38 Homburg, R., Gudi, A., Shah, A. and Layton, A. M. A novel method to demonstrate that pregnant women with polycystic ovary syndrome hyper-expose their fetus to androgens as a possible stepping stone for the developmental theory of PCOS: A pilot study. *Reprod Biol Endocrinol* 2017; 15(1): 61–65.

Chapter 8

Adrenal and Polycystic Ovary Syndrome

Ozlem Celik and Bülent Okan Yildiz

Introduction

Polycystic ovary syndrome (PCOS) is the most common endocrine disorder in reproductive-aged women, with a prevalence of between 5% and 20%, depending on the diagnostic criteria used.[1] PCOS is a heterogeneous disorder that is defined by a combination of clinical (i.e. hirsutism) or biochemical hyperandrogenism (HA), oligo-anovulation (OA) and polycystic ovarian morphology (PCOM) on ultrasound.[2] Three sets of proposed diagnostic criteria are available for defining PCOS, namely the National Institutes of Health (NIH); European Society of Human Reproduction and Embryology (ESHRE) together with the American Society for Reproductive Medicine (ASRM; or Rotterdam); and Androgen Excess and PCOS (AE-PCOS) Society criteria. All require the exclusion of other mimicking disorders, such as Cushing's syndrome, hyperprolactinemia and non-classic congenital adrenal hyperplasia (NCAH), before making the diagnosis of PCOS. PCOS has four different phenotypes (Phenotypes A–D). Phenotype A is the most common phenotype where patients meet all three diagnostic criteria of PCOS (HA + OA + PCOM). Phenotype B patients have HA and OA without PCOM, whereas Phenotype C patients have HA and PCOM without OA. Phenotype D is the non-hyperandrogenic phenotype that includes OA and PCOM.[2]

The pathophysiology of PCOS is complex and reflects the interactions between genetic, metabolic, fetal, and environmental factors. HA is multifactorial in origin, mainly attributed to the ovary with a substantial contribution of adrenal and to a lesser extent adipose tissue. Around 30% of patients with PCOS show increased adrenal androgens (AAs) basally or in response to adrenocorticotropic hormone (ACTH).[3] In the following, we review steroidogenesis of AAs and their role in PCOS pathophysiology; the prevalence of AA excess; the validity of dehydroepiandrosterone sulfate (DHEAS) as a measure of AA excess; underlying steroidogenic patterns; effects of extra-adrenal factors on adrenal steroidogenesis; and heritability of AA excess in PCOS.

Adrenal Androgen Steroidogenesis

The AAs are primarily secreted by the zonae reticularis of the adrenal cortex (Figure 8.1). Initially steroidogenic pathway starts with the conversion of cholesterol to pregnenolone in two steps, including first the cholesterol side chain cleavage enzyme (P450scc) and then the acute steroidogenic regulatory protein. The resultant pregnenolone is converted to dehydroepiandrosterone (DHEA) in a two-step process catalyzed by cytochrome P450c17α, along the Δ^5-steroid pathway. P450c17α gene expression is dependent on luteinizing hormone (LH) and ACTH as trophic hormones. The Δ^4-steroid pathway, which occurs in parallel, is responsible for the conversion of progesterone, which is derived from pregnenolone, firstly to 17-hydroxyprogesterone (17-HP) and then to androstenedione (A4). In the adrenal gland, 17-HP is converted to either A4 or cortisol (F). A4 requires 17β-hydroxydehydrogenase for conversion to testosterone (T).[4] A significant portion of DHEA is sulfated through the action of DHEA sulfotransferase (DHEA-ST; SULT2A1). The DHEAS is released into the circulation. The activity of the SULT2A1 enzyme depends on the sulfate donor 3′-phosphoadenosine 5′-phosphosulfate (PAPS), which is synthesized by PAPS synthetase (PAPSS). Of the two isoforms, PAPSS1 and PAPSS2, the latter is highly expressed in the major sites of DHEA sulfation, that is, the liver and the adrenal glands.[4]

The adrenal cortex produces these C19 androgen precursors, including DHEA and its sulfate form, Δ^5-androstene-3β, 17β-diol (androstenediol), and 11β-hydroxyandrostenedione

Table 8.1 Relative contribution of ovary, adrenal and peripheral tissues to circulating androgens in women of reproductive age

Androgen	Ovary	Adrenal Gland	Peripheral Tissues
Testosterone	25%	25%	50%
Androstenedione	30%	30%	40%
DHEA	20%	50%	30%
DHEAS		> 95%	< 5%

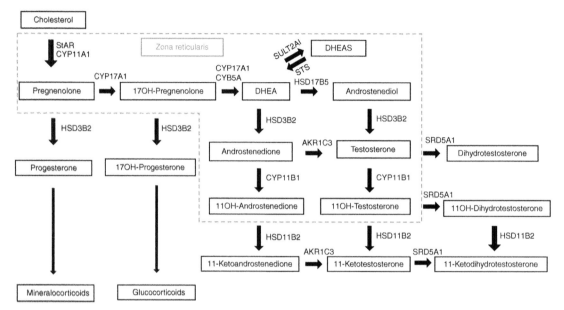

Figure 8.1 Adrenal androgen steroidogenesis including 11-oxygenated androgens
Enzyme's activity/name: steroidogenic acute regulatory protein (StAR), cytochrome P450 cholesterol side chain cleavage (CYP11A1), 3β- hydroxysteroid dehydrogenase/Δ5/4- isomerase type 2 (HSD3B2), cytochrome P450 17A1 (CYP17A1), cytochrome b5 type A (CYB5A), cytochrome P450 11β- hydroxylase (CYP11B1), 5α- reductases (SRD5A), aldo-keto reductase family 1 member C3 (AKR1C3), steroid sulfotransferase type 2A1(SULT2A1), steroid sulfatase (STS), 11β- hydroxysteroid dehydrogenase type 2 (HSD11B2).

(11-OHA4), with variable degrees of androgenic activity. While A4 can also be considered an AA, it is significantly less specific. A4 is the main precursor for the synthesis of T and estrogen in both the ovaries and the adrenal cortex. The adrenal cortex also accounts for about 25% of the circulating T levels (Table 8.1). DHEA can be converted to the most potent of androgens, dihydrotestosterone (DHT), in peripheral tissues once converted to A4 without first requiring formation of T.[3, 4] However, only T and DHT have strong affinity and potency for the androgen receptor (AR), as DHEAS, DHEA and A4 have little to no capacity to bind to the AR and require conversion to T to exert androgenic effects. In healthy women, 80% of T is bound with a high affinity to sex hormone-binding globulin (SHBG), 19% is bound to albumin and only 1% circulates as a free fraction. In contrast, DHEA, DHEAS and A4 are bound to albumin with low affinity and available for peripheral conversion.[5]

Epidemiology of Adrenal Androgen Excess in PCOS

Increased circulating AA levels in PCOS were first reported by Gallagher and colleagues,[6] suggesting adrenocortical hyperfunction in the syndrome. AAs are elevated in 20–50% of women with PCOS depending on the definition used and the age, body mass index (BMI) and race of the participants.[7–9] An observational study of

213 women with PCOS and 182 controls showed that prevalence of DHEAS excess was approximately 20% among White and 30% among Black patients, when using age- and race-adjusted normative values.[9] While BMI and fasting insulin had little impact on circulating DHEAS levels in healthy women, among White PCOS patients these parameters were negatively associated with circulating DHEAS levels in this study.[9] The impact of race on the prevalence of AA excess in PCOS is unclear. In one report, the prevalence of AA excess among PCOS patients was found to be similar among Italian, US Hispanic American and Japanese women.[10] A recent study evaluating 259 nondiabetic patients with PCOS in the USA showed that serum DHEAS levels adjusted for age and BMI were similar across White, Hispanic, Black and Asian women.[11]

AAs begin to decline after the age of 30 years, both in normal women and in those with PCOS. [12] The decrease in DHEAS levels may reflect a decrease in AA production and may partially explain the amelioration in androgen levels and symptoms observable with aging in PCOS patients. We should note, however, that adrenal steroidogenesis remains enhanced in PCOS compared to healthy women up until and beyond menopause.[13]

Validity of DHEAS As a Measure of Adrenocortical Dysfunction in PCOS

Clinically, the measurement of circulating DHEAS, an AA metabolite, has been used to assess AA excess. Because of its high production and low metabolic clearance rates, DHEAS is the second most abundant steroid in blood after F. This hormone is 97–99% of adrenocortical origin, relatively stable throughout the day and the menstrual cycle and easily measured by direct commercial immunoassays. Therefore, it is frequently used as a marker of AA secretion. Only 20–30% of PCOS patients demonstrate elevated DHEAS levels. Nevertheless, DHEAS levels might not always reflect the status of adrenocortical steroidogenesis.[5]

First, the relationship of DHEAS to adrenocortical biosynthesis, as measured by the adrenal steroid production response to ACTH stimulation, is generally weak.[5] Second, the response of DHEAS to extra-adrenal factors may differ from that of AA secretion. For example, when oophorectomized women are treated with exogenous T, the DHEAS to DHEA ratio increases without accompanying change in the adrenocortical secretion of DHEA or A4 in response to ACTH stimulation.[14] In addition, PCOS women treated with a gonadotropin-releasing hormone analogue (GnRH-a) experience a decrease in basal DHEAS levels without accompanying changes in basal DHEA levels, or the steroid response to ACTH stimulation.[15] In vitro studies also support the dichotomy of DHEAS and DHEA production. Insulin within physiologic levels appears to increase DHEAS production while alternatively decreasing the secretion of DHEA.[16] Third, DHEAS levels are not always supranormal in patients with inherited adrenal dysfunction, such as 21-hydroxylase (21-OH) deficient NCAH. For example, a study of 13 patients with untreated 21-OH deficient NCAH showed that 92.3% and 100% of NCAH patients had increased A4 and DHEA basal levels, and 100% had ACTH-stimulated levels of A4 and DHEA above normal. Alternatively, only 53.8% of patients with NCAH had DHEAS levels above normal.[17] Fourth, classifying PCOS patients according to whether they have DHEAS levels above the upper normal limit or not does not clearly distinguish patient groups that have distinct adrenal behaviors. Few differences in steroidogenesis, estimated from the steroid response to ACTH stimulation, were observed between PCOS women with and without DHEAS excess.[5]

Overall, these data suggest that DHEAS levels are loosely associated with the adrenocortical secretion of other adrenal products, basally and in response to ACTH. However, alterations in DHEAS production may also occur independent of changes in adrenocortical steroidogenesis, possibly due to selective effects on adrenal or hepatic DHEA-ST. These data also caution against the artificial classification of PCOS patients into those with and without AA excess based solely on the circulating DHEAS levels, as adrenocortical function appears to represent a continuum and is generally enhanced in PCOS.

11-Oxygenated Adrenal Androgens in PCOS

Most studies on PCOS have focused on classic C19 androgens, their precursors and/or their downstream urinary metabolites for biochemical

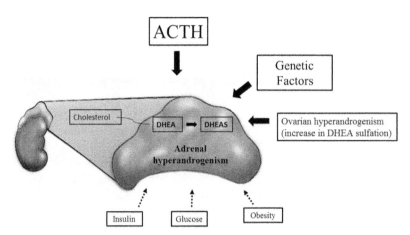

Figure 8.2 Factors contributing to adrenal androgen excess in PCOS

assessment of androgen excess. However, the newly described, adrenal-derived C11-oxy C19 androgen subclass is emerging to be clinically and biochemically significant in the context of PCOS-related androgen excess (Figure 8.1). The C11-oxy C19 androgens are primarily of adrenal origin as this pathway starts with the conversion of A4 to 11OHA4, which can only be catalyzed by 11β-hydroxylase activity of the exclusively adrenally expressed enzyme CYP11B1. C11-oxy C19 androgens are particularly prominent in the serum of women with PCOS as well as in girls with premature adrenarche. O'Reilly and colleagues studied serum androgens by liquid chromatography-tandem mass spectrometry and 24-hour urinary androgen excretion by gas chromatography-mass spectrometry in 114 women with PCOS and 49 healthy controls.[18] As expected, serum concentrations of the classic androgens including T, A4 and DHEA were significantly increased in PCOS. They showed that 11-oxygenated androgens (11β-hydroxyandrostenedione, 11-ketoandrostenedione, 11β-hydroxytestosterone and 11-ketotestosterone) represent the majority of circulating androgens in women with PCOS, with close correlation to markers of metabolic risk. Furthermore, circulating levels of the active C11-oxy C19 androgen 11-ketotestosterone have recently been shown to remain consistent throughout the female lifespan contrary to classic androgen concentrations.[18] However, a recent study demonstrated C19 steroids (A4, T, DHEA) concentrations higher than the combined C11-oxy C19 androgens using ultra-performance-convergence-chromatography-tandem-mass-spectrometry (UPC2-MS/MS). C11-oxy C19 androgens were found to be

similar in patients with PCOS and healthy people.[19] Therefore, more studies on C11-oxy C19 and their downstream metabolites will be needed before a conclusion can be drawn about the roles of C11-oxy C19 AAs compared with the classic androgens.

In Vivo Characterization of Adrenocortical Steroidogenesis in Androgen Excess and PCOS

AA excess in PCOS may represent dysregulation of adrenocortical biosynthesis, principally in response to ACTH stimulation, or abnormalities in the metabolism of adrenal products, including DHEA and F. In the subsections that follow, we review potential abnormalities in steroidogenesis or metabolism of adrenal products. Figure 8.2 shows the factors contributing to AA excess in PCOS.

Abnormalities of Adrenocortical Biosynthesis in PCOS

PCOS women show a generalized hypersecretion of adrenocortical products, basally and in response to ACTH including pregnenolone, 17-HPREG, DHEA, A4 and possibly F. In vivo and in vitro studies showed that ACTH stimulates the adrenocortical release of androgens and glucocorticoids. Because there is an excess of ACTH receptors within the adrenal cortex we generally perform intravenous administration of ACTH-(1–24) to evaluate adrenocortical enzymatic activities in vivo. Commercially available doses of 0.25 mg provide maximum adrenal stimulation, regardless of body weight.[20] The AA excess of PCOS may result from generalized adrenocortical hyperresponsivity to normal levels of ACTH. Evaluating hypothalamic–pituitary–adrenal (HPA) axis sensitivity and responsivity after corticotropin-releasing hormone (CRH) stimulation 12 PCOS women with DHEAS excess, 12 without DHEAS excess and 12 controls, Azziz and colleagues reported that AA excess in PCOS patients is related to an exaggerated secretory response of the adrenal cortex for DHEA and A4 but not to an altered pituitary responsivity to CRH or to increased sensitivity of these AAs to ACTH stimulation. Whether the increased responsivity to ACTH for these steroids is secondary to increased zonae reticularis mass or to differences in P450c17α activity remains to be determined.[21]

Previous studies reported that there are no specific adrenal steroidogenic defects among women with PCOS.[22] Despite the inconsistencies between in vitro and in vivo studies, several studies have shown dysregulation of P450c17α activity in women with PCOS. The exaggerated 17-hydroxylase activity observed in PCOS women with DHEAS excess may also reflect a functional abnormality in P450c17 function, the enzyme determining both 17-hydroxylase and 17,20-lyase activity. Exaggerated 17-hydroxylase activity might be related to various extra-adrenal factors such as obesity and insulin and glucose levels.

The enzyme 3β-HSD, negatively correlated with AA levels, is expressed in adrenal and ovary. Previously, in some PCOS patients presenting with high DHEAS levels and an exaggerated 17-HPREG to 17-HP ratio after ACTH stimulation, the presence of a genetic defect of 3β-HSD activity was postulated, although not all agreed.[22] Carbunaru and colleagues investigated 3β-HSD deficiency in hyperandrogenic females with insulin-resistant PCOS and girls with premature pubarche.[23] They demonstrated the absence of inherited defects in their 3β-HSD B2 gene, and it was likely that the descending 3β-HSD B phenotype was associated with a variant of insulin-resistant PCOS. Further studies are needed to clarify the potential role of the 3β-HSD enzyme activity in AA excess of women with PCOS.

Peripubertal AA excess is associated with the development of PCOS-like symptomatology in patients with 21-OH deficient NCAH.[24] Patients with PCOS have a greater incidence of exaggerated AA secretion during the peripubertal period. Premature and/or exaggerated adrenarche is reported to be associated with the development of PCOS in a number of studies.[22] Increased DHEAS serum concentrations and biochemical evidence of an exacerbated adrenarche were observed in daughters of women with PCOS, suggesting that these features are an early step in the development of PCOS.[25]

Limited data are available regarding AA excess in different subphenotypes of PCOS. In order to determine whether adrenocortical function varies among PCOS phenotypes, we studied 119 nonobese PCOS patients, 24 women with HA only and 39 age- and BMI-matched healthy controls. We measured baseline DHEAS levels and 17-HP, A4, DHEA and F levels in response to ACTH stimulation. We found that PCOS patients and women with HA only have similar and higher basal and stimulated AA levels than controls and all three hyperandrogenic subphenotypes of PCOS (Phenotypes A–C) exhibit similar and higher basal and stimulated AA secretion patterns compared to non-hyperandrogenic subphenotype (Phenotype D).[26]

Abnormalities in the Metabolism of Cortisol in PCOS

An interesting proposition is that AA excess and the enhanced adrenocortical function observed in PCOS is the result of increased peripheral metabolism of F. The principal pathways for metabolism of F include enhanced inactivation of this steroid by 5α-reductase (5α-RA) type 1 and 5β-reductase (5β-RA) and impaired reactivation of F from cortisone by 11β-HSD1.[5] Previously, Stewart and colleagues studied 11 patients with PCOS, without evidence of 21-OH or 3β-HSD deficiency.[27] Urinary total F metabolites were higher in patients than controls, with a high ratio of 5α to 5β F metabolites in the urine. These data suggested that PCOS women studied had abnormal F metabolism, potentially indicating enhanced 5α-RA and/or impaired 5β-RA activity. These investigators did not find an abnormality in the interconversion of F to cortisone in their patients and later on reported confirmatory findings in an extended cohort of women with PCOS. [28] Similar results were reported by other investigators.[29]

In contrast, most studies on basal and stimulated serum F concentrations showed unaltered production with some reporting decreased or increased levels.[5, 22] Part of the discrepancies may be attributed to differences in age and BMI between patients and controls, because these factors are important determinants of the ACTH–F axis.[5]

The interconversion of F and hormonally inactive cortisone is catalyzed by at least two isoforms of 11β-HSD. The type 2 11β-HSD (11β-HSD2) is found predominantly in the placenta and kidneys and converts F to cortisone. Type 1 enzyme (11β-HSD1) is found predominantly in the liver and gonads and exerts 11-reductase activity converting cortisone back to F. Consequently, dysregulation of the activity 11β-HSD1 could induce decreased F production/reactivation, which would result in increased adrenocortical function in PCOS.[5]

Rodin and colleagues measured the 24-hour urinary excretion of steroid hormone metabolites by high-resolution capillary gas chromatography in 65 women with PCOS and 45 normal women matched for BMI.[30] The urinary excretion of T and A4 metabolites was 1.9 times higher in the women with PCOS than in the normal women, and the excretion of DHEA metabolites (C19 steroid sulfates) and F metabolites was 1.5 and 1.3 times higher, respectively, after adjustment for BMI. Women with PCOS also had significantly higher ratios of 11-oxo (oxygenated) metabolites to 11-hydroxy metabolites of F and of 11-oxo to 11-hydroxy metabolites of corticosterone. They suggested that their results could be explained by either enhanced 11β-dehydrogenase activity or impaired 11β-reductase activity causing increased oxidation of F to cortisone, which could not be accounted for by obesity.[30]

Abnormality in F metabolism could not be explained by the presence of endogenous inhibitors of 11β-HSD1 activity. Whether these abnormalities represent a primary or a secondary abnormality is unclear. For example, the expression of 11β-HSD1 is highly regulated, including by sex steroids and growth hormone and insulin. Stewart and Edwards suggested that the findings of 11βHSD1 dysregulation might reflect the increased android obesity of patients with PCOS.[31] These investigators reported that 11β-HSD1 activity is reduced in patients who have android or central obesity but not in those with gynoid obesity, regardless of gender. However, Tsilchorozidou and colleagues observed both enhanced 5α-RA and reduced

11β-HSD1 activities among 18 lean PCOS women compared with 19 lean controls. They observed that insulin seemed to enhance the 5α-reduction of steroids in PCOS but was not associated with the reduced 11β-HSD1 activities observed in their lean PCOS women.[29] Nonetheless, sex steroids may be playing a role in the observed abnormalities of F metabolism.

Overall, although total F production rate is generally normal in women with PCOS, increased peripheral metabolism of F has been observed. The interpretation of these data has been complicated by the confounding extra-adrenal factors including obesity, insulin and glucose levels and ovarian secretions.

Effects of Extra-Adrenal Factors on Adrenal Steroidogenesis

A number of extra-adrenal factors may play a role in the AA excess of PCOS, including ovarian products and factors related to insulin action and/or obesity.

Interaction of the Ovary and Adrenal in PCOS

Limited evidence showed that ovarian factors may be increasing AA secretion in PCOS, possibly including androgens and estrogens. Azziz and colleagues showed that T administration to oophorectomized women did not significantly change the response of A4, DHEA or F to ACTH stimulation; however, it was associated with elevations in the ratio of DHEAS to DHEA.[14] They suggested that ovarian HA may increase DHEA sulfation and consequently the circulating levels of DHEAS.[14] In vitro studies reported that T had no predictable effect on the production of DHEA, DHEAS or F in human adrenal tissue.[16] Accordingly, T appears to have only a modest effect on AA, primarily increasing the sulfation of DHEA to DHEAS.

Some investigators, but not all, evaluating the effect of ovarian suppression with GnRH-a reported decreased DHEAS levels, suggesting an effect of the ovary on the adrenal in PCOS.[5,32] Studies in hypoestrogenic women have suggested that exogenous estrogen administration can alter the adrenocortical response to ACTH stimulation, although there is little consensus as to the extent, significance or type of alteration.[32]

Ditkoff and colleagues observed that transdermal estradiol (E2) replacement for one week in long-acting GnRH-a treated PCOS patients with AA excess was sufficient to restore the hyper-responsiveness of androgens to ovine corticotropin-releasing hormone (oCRH) stimulation.[33] Azziz and colleagues determined the steroid responses to a continuous incremental ACTH-(1–24) infusion (20–1280 ng/1.5 m^2 per hour), followed by an ACTH (1–24) bolus of 0.25 mg, before and after 3 months of transdermal E2 therapy (0.05 mg/day) in 14 postmenopausal women. Estradiol administration had no effect on basal, post-dexamethasone or maximally stimulated serum levels of F, DHEA, A4 or 17-HP. Furthermore, E2 did not affect adrenal sensitivity or responsiveness to ACTH-(1–24) stimulation. [20] Studying the adrenocortical response to acute ACTH stimulation before and after bilateral oophorectomy, the same group reported no differences in basal DHEAS or basal or stimulated DHEA levels.[34]

Taken together, these data suggest that the ovarian sex steroids have a limited impact on the adrenocortical response to stimulation in PCOS and a modest contribution to circulating DHEAS levels, possibly by enhancing hepatic or adrenal DHEA-ST.

Effect of Abnormalities of the Glucose–insulin Axis

Approximately 50–70% of patients with PCOS have insulin resistance (IR) and hyperinsulinemia and many have evidence of glucose intolerance. [35] Hyperinsulinemia in PCOS stimulates androgen secretion by ovarian theca cells and increases the hormonally active free androgen fraction by reducing the hepatic production of SHBG. Although the relationship between IR, hyperinsulinemia and resultant increased ovarian androgen production is well recognized in PCOS, the association between IR, hyperinsulinemia and AA production is less well understood.

Insulin levels appear to be negatively correlated with, or to actually acutely suppress, circulating DHEAS levels in normal women and men.[36] During oral glucose tolerance testing (OGTT), in women with PCOS acute glucose-induced hyper-insulinemia was found either to have no effect or to decrease DHEAS levels. Azziz and colleagues compared seven hyperandrogenic severely

hyperinsulinemic (i.e. peak insulin levels during a 2-hour oral glucose tolerance test (OGTT) > 500 mU/mL) women with eight hyperandrogenic normoinsulinemic (i.e. peak insulin levels during a 2-hour OGTT < 190 mU/mL) patients and nine healthy BMI-matched controls. Basal A4, DHEA and DHEAS circulating levels were higher in the severely hyperinsulinemic patients, although the difference in DHEA did not reach statistical significance in this study. These responses did not change before and after ACTH stimulation.[37]

In order to determine whether more subtle abnormalities of insulin action are related to the adrenocortical dysfunction of PCOS, a few small studies used frequently sampled intravenous glucose tolerance test (FSIVGTT). Falcone and colleagues examined T, A4 and DHEA levels during the three hours of FSIVGTT, finding that DHEA levels decreased in controls and insulin sensitive women with PCOS, but did not change in insulin-resistant women with PCOS.[38] Farah-Eways and colleagues studied nine women with PCOS and nine BMI-, age- and race-matched controls using FSIVGTT and ACTH stimulation tests.[39] Neither insulin sensitivity nor acute insulin response to glucose was found to correlate with basal DHEAS or basal or ACTH-stimulated AA production. The main finding was that glucose effectiveness (the ability of glucose to promote its own removal from the bloodstream) was correlated with DHEAS and basal and stimulated steroids in women with PCOS.[39] These data suggested adrenocortical dysfunction in PCOS may be more closely linked to those mechanisms underlying glucose-mediated glucose disposal.

Ovarian and AAs have been reported to have opposing effects on body weight and insulin levels in women with PCOS but the results are controversial. Previous studies reported that there is a beneficial impact of AAs on the metabolic phenotype and early cardiovascular disease in women with PCOS. Brennan and colleagues found that elevated DHEAS concentrations have been inversely correlated with IR, estimated by homeostatic model assessment for insulin resistance (HOMA-IR), in a cohort including 352 women with PCOS after correction for age, BMI and waist-to-hip ratio (WHR).[40] This relationship was stronger than that of free T and SHBG in the multivariate analysis.[40] Carmina and colleagues reported increased DHEAS levels have been associated with a favorable lipid profile along with improved insulin sensitivity in PCOS patients with AA excess when matched to patients with similar age and BMI and normal AAs.[41] Moreover, Chen and colleagues demonstrated in 318 women with PCOS that, despite a positive correlation of DHEAS levels with T, high DHEAS levels were positively associated with a beneficial metabolic phenotype, including parameters such as abdominal obesity, IR and dyslipidemia.[42] Lerchbaum and colleagues confirmed that high levels of circulating AAs and lower levels of ovarian androgens exert a beneficial effect on metabolic disturbances in a large cohort of women with PCOS using OGTT and DHEAS to FT ratio.[43] More recently, Paschou and colleagues reported that women with PCOS and adrenal HA do not exhibit any deterioration in IR and lipid profile despite the higher levels of total androgens. [44] Alpañés and colleagues studied the impact of AA excess on cardiometabolic risk factors in 298 women with PCOS, of whom 120 were obese and 178 nonobese (BMI < 30 kg/m^2). In contrast to other studies, they found that AA excess in women with PCOS is associated with reduced insulin sensitivity and increased blood pressure but may have a beneficial impact on the lipid profile.[45]

The underlying mechanisms of the potential impact of AAs are not clear but may reflect a direct effect of DHEAS on insulin and lipid metabolism. DHEA might have an effect on insulin action. DHEA decreases gluconeogenesis by suppressing the activity and expression of glucose-6-phosphatase and phosphoenolpyruvate carboxykinase. DHEA increases glucose uptake in hepatocytes and increases insulin binding to its receptor. Also, insulin and glucose were experimentally reported to enhance DHEAS synthesis in the adrenal gland.[22] A small preliminary study using human adrenal minces reported that insulin in physiologic levels resulted in an increase in DHEAS and a decrease in DHEA, with no change in F secretion.[16] These data suggest that insulin might primarily increase the activity of DHEA-ST.

Additional evidence that insulin resistance–associated factors play a role in regulating adrenocortical biosynthesis arises from studies examining the effect of insulin sensitizers. Firstly, Azziz and colleagues reported that the circulating DHEAS levels decreased 18–26% with troglitazone at 600 mg/day, regardless of

basal DHEAS level in women with PCOS.[46] Thiazolidinediones (TZDs) have also been demonstrated to improve insulin sensitivity and hyperandrogenemia in women with PCOS. [22]. Smaller studies treating PCOS women with pioglitazone found no effect on basal or ACTH-stimulated DHEAS, whereas ACTH-stimulated A4 and 17-HP were reduced after treatment. Alternatively, metformin does not appear to have a similar effect.[5] There is evidence TZDs were more effective than metformin in reducing the levels of free testosterone and DHEAS. It is possible that the effect of TZDs observed on steroid levels may be the result of direct inhibition of steroid biosynthesis such as P450c17 and 3β-HSD by these drugs.[47] In 2011, a meta-analysis of 10 trials using metformin in PCOS showed that DHEAS levels were not significantly reduced by metformin.[48]

Overall, there are conflicting data regarding the interaction between the insulin–glucose axis and adrenocortical dysfunction in PCOS. Insulin itself may have a modest stimulatory effect on DHEA-ST but may actually result in steroidogenic changes reducing the adrenal production of DHEA.

Effect of Obesity on Adrenocortical Steroidogenesis

Although obesity affects approximately 50–60% of PCOS patients, the relationship of AA excess and BMI is also poorly understood. Obesity may impact adrenocortical function by decreasing insulin sensitivity and increasing circulating insulin levels. However, obesity may also alter adrenal function through the secretion of adipocytokines and other inflammatory products and by increasing the circulating levels of estrogens through increased aromatization by adipose tissue stromal cells.[5] Studying 30 normal-weight and 27 obese healthy, eumenorrheic, nonhirsute female volunteers, Azziz and colleagues reported higher free T levels, higher DHEAS to DHEA ratio and an almost twofold higher net increment of A4 in response to ACTH in obese volunteers with no other differences between the groups for basal or adrenal response measures.[49] In contrast, Vicennati and colleagues, studying 12 women with abdominal and 13 with peripheral obesity and 7 healthy normal-weight women reported no significant differences in basal or stimulated serum levels of DHEA, A4 and 17-HP among the three groups, without any correlation between basal and stimulated androgen levels and BMI. Although basal F levels were similar, the response of F (as area under the curve) to ACTH stimulation was higher in women with abdominal obesity than the other two groups in this study.[50] A number of other investigators also observed a greater degree of F secretion and metabolism in obese subjects with visceral adiposity.[5]

A negative association between DHEAS and BMI or fasting insulin among PCOS patients has been reported suggesting that the proportion of AA excess may be higher in nonobese PCOS patients. Studying 136 reproductive-aged PCOS patients and 42 controls, Moran and colleagues reported that the A4 and DHEAS levels were significantly higher in nonobese than in obese PCOS patients, with a significant correlation between LH and A4 in nonobese group.[51]

Lean PCOS patients present with less IR, which suggests that the pathogenesis in this group may differ from that of obese PCOS patients.[51] More recently, Deng and colleagues evaluated differences in the steroidogenic pathway between obese and nonobese women PCOS using liquid chromatography coupled with tandem mass spectrometry (LC-MS/MS).[52] The lean PCOS patients showed increased DHEAS, 17-HP and estrone levels compared with both the lean controls and the obese PCOS patients, while a lower free androgen index (FAI) was found in the lean PCOS patients compared with the obese PCOS patients. In addition, the lean PCOS patients showed increased activity of P450c17α, P450aro and 3βHSD2, as well as decreased activity of P450c21. Furthermore, there was a higher frequency of CYP21A2 (encoding P450c21) c.552 C > G (p.D184E) in the lean PCOS patients compared with the obese PCOS patients.[52] Accordingly, AA excess might be playing different roles in lean and obese PCOS patients, represented as different enzyme activity in the steroidogenic pathway.

Overall, these findings suggest that the adrenal in obese healthy women may secrete high F, and possibly A4 and DHEA, in response to ACTH, although not all investigators agree. Whether this is due to hyperinsulinemia in obese individuals or whether this reflects the effects of adipocyte generated adipocytokines or similar factors remains unknown. Circulating DHEAS levels appear to be inversely correlated with adiposity. However, future studies need to more clearly document the effect of obesity on adrenocortical function, including the production and metabolism of glucocorticoids, differences in the steroidogenic pathways, the effect of body fat distribution, the effect of weight loss, the mechanisms underlying such relationships and their role in the adrenocortical hyper-responsivity of PCOS.

Heritability of Adrenal Steroidogenesis in PCOS

There is growing evidence that inheritance plays a significant role in determining the circulating AA levels in normal individuals. Various investigators have observed a significant degree of heritability for the AA metabolite DHEAS, with the relative basal levels of DHEA and DHEAS varying little over time.[5] Whether this represents the inheritance of factors regulating adrenocortical biosynthesis or of factors determining AA metabolism or clearance is unclear. We prospectively studied 23 untreated PCOS patients and 7 age- and BMI-matched control women on two occasions 3–5 years apart.[53] We showed that the adrenocortical secretion of AAs or F in PCOS, similar to healthy women, remains stable over time, suggesting an inherited basis for AA secretion in PCOS as well. We observed a decrease in DHEAS levels over time only among PCOS patients whose initial levels of this metabolite were above the group median, suggesting that the activity of sulfotransferase in these patients may be upregulated by factors other than those affecting adrenocortical biosynthesis and that such regulatory influences attenuate over time.[53]

Although there is no evidence of the heritability of DHEA, the heritability estimates of DHEAS ranges from 26% (European American adult men) to 65% (Chinese girls) in twin studies.[22] Evidence for genetic contribution includes a well-documented familial clustering of PCOS, as well as increased prevalence of its components, including HA, and T2DM in first-degree relatives of women with PCOS.[25] Early studies showed that DHEAS was under genetic control in PCOS documenting elevated DHEAS levels in brothers of women with PCOS.[54] We found that there is a sister–sister correlation between the serum DHEAS levels of PCOS probands and their sisters. Sixteen of the 69 (23.2%) sisters were affected by PCOS. Among 62 women with PCOS and their 69 sisters, the heritability of DHEAS was 44%, suggesting a significant familial component for DHEAS.[25]

Several candidate gene studies focusing on AA excess have been carried out in PCOS cohorts. Conversion of DHEA to DHEAS and reciprocal reaction is controlled by the enzymes SULT2A1 and steroid sulfatase (STS). Genetic variants in genes encoding these enzymes might influence their activity and as such might contribute to the higher levels of androgens in patients with PCOS. One study reported that single nucleotide polymorphism (SNP) rs182420 in SULT2A1 was associated with DHEAS levels in PCOS cases but not controls, whereas variants within STS were not associated with DHEAS.[55] Another study found no association of SNPs in SULT2A1, PAPSS2 and STS with PCOS. In this study, one variant, SNP rs2910397, which was mapping to SULT2A1, was highly associated with the DHEAS to DHEA ratio in PCOS patients.[56]

Interaction of several genetic variants in genes encoding enzymes in the steroidogenesis might contribute to the variation in AA levels in PCOS.[22] The 3β-HSD type 1 and type 2 enzymes are responsible for the conversion of DHEA to A4 in peripheral and adrenal tissue, respectively. Increased expression of these enzymes might lead to an increase of the conversion of DHEA to A4 and, subsequently, an elevation of the DHEAS to DHEA ratio. Genetic variation in the 11β-HSD1 gene was observed to enhance F clearance and resulted in increased DHEAS levels independently of BMI in PCOS patients.[4] Studies of the genes coding the enzymes involved in DHEA synthesis, including CYP11A and CYP17A1, have generally been negative for association with PCOS or DHEAS levels. Also variants of CYP21A2 have not been found to be predictive of ovarian or adrenal HA in PCOS.[57] In candidate gene analyses, no single gene (fibrillin-3, genes involved in insulin metabolism [insulin, IR, and IRS1], transcription factor 7 like 2, calpain 10, the fat mass and obesity-associated gene [FTO], SHBG and the FSH receptor gene) has been successfully identified and replicated as truly causative across all studies in patients with PCOS.[57]

A number of genome-wide association studies (GWAS) have focused on circulating levels of sex hormones such as DHEAS, T and SHBG. A meta-analysis of GWAS from 7 cohorts, including more than 14,000 Caucasian individuals each with ~2.5 million SNP genotypes, identified 8 independent SNPs highly associated with DHEAS levels.[58] These SNPs explain only a small amount of the variation in DHEAS between subjects, about 4% of the total variance in DHEAS and 7% of the genetic variance.

Taken together, several studies have documented that DHEAS is highly regulated by genetic factors. Candidate gene and GWAS studies in the PCOS and general population have identified less than 10 independent genetic regions that regulate DHEAS levels, leaving a substantial amount of its heritability unexplained. There are several limitations, including small sample size, diagnostic heterogeneity, population stratification, failure to examine the entire candidate gene, not correcting for multiple testing and confounding phenotypes (e.g. obesity). Further well-designed studies are needed to fully characterize the genetic control of AAs levels.

Summary

PCOS is a heterogeneous condition of multifactorial origin and reflects the interactions between genetic, metabolic, fetal and environmental factors. HA is multifactorial in origin and mainly attributed to the ovary, with a substantial contribution of adrenal and to a lesser extent adipose tissue. Overall, between 20% and 30% of patients with PCOS demonstrate AA excess, as reflected by the circulating DHEAS levels. However, a wide variation in the ability of the adrenal to secrete DHEA, basally and in response to ACTH, is present in the normal population. Whether this populational variance in the production of DHEA is due to the effect of inherited factors or alternatively due to the ability of extra-adrenal factors to affect AA secretion remains to be determined. We should note that alterations in DHEAS levels do not necessarily reflect changes in adrenocortical steroidogenesis, possibly due to selective effects of extra-adrenal factors on adrenal or hepatic sulfotransferase. In general, extra-adrenal factors, including obesity, insulin and glucose levels, as well as ovarian secretions, play a limited role in the increased AA production observed in PCOS. Owing to the genetic and phenotypic heterogeneity of the syndrome and the lack of sufficiently large cohorts, studies to date have failed to identify specific genetic defects in adrenocortical dysfunction of PCOS. Further well-designed studies are needed to fully characterize the genetic control of AA steroidogenesis and to determine the influence of AA excess on metabolic dysfunction and cardiovascular risk of PCOS.

References

1 Yildiz, B. O., Bozdag, G., Yapici, Z., Esinler, I. and Yarali, H. Prevalence, phenotype and cardiometabolic risk of polycystic ovary syndrome under different diagnostic criteria. *Hum Reprod* 2012; 27(10): 3067–3073.

2 Azziz, R., Carmina, E., Chen, Z. et al. Polycystic ovary syndrome. *Nat Rev Dis Primers* 2016; 11(2): 16057.

3 Baskind, N. E. and Balen, A. H. Hypothalamic-pituitary, ovarian and adrenal contributions to polycystic ovary syndrome. *Best Pract Res Clin Obstet Gynaecol* 2016; 37: 80–97.

4 Miller, W. L. and Auchus, R. J. The molecular biology, biochemistry, and physiology of human steroidogenesis and its disorders. *Endocr Rev* 2011; 32(1): 81–151.

5 Yildiz, B. O. and Azziz, R. The adrenal and polycystic ovary syndrome. *Rev Endocr Metab Disord* 2007; 8(4): 331–342.

6 Gallagher, T. F., Kappas, A., Hellman, L., Lipsett, M. B., Pearson, O. H. and West, C. D. Adrenocortical hyperfunction in idiopathic hirsutism and the Stein-Leventhal syndrome. *J Clin Invest* 1958; 37(6): 794–799.

7 Wild, R. A., Umstot, E. S., Andersen, R. N., Ranney, G. B. and Givens, J. R. Androgen parameters and their correlation with body weight in one hundred thirty-eight women thought to have hyperandrogenism. *Am J Obstet Gynecol* 1983; 146(6): 602–606.

8 Hoffman, D. I., Klove, K. and Lobo, R. A. The prevalence and significance of elevated dehydroepiandrosterone sulfate levels in anovulatory women. *Fertil Steril* 1984; 42(1): 76–81.

9 Kumar, A., Woods, K. S., Bartolucci, A. and Azziz, R. Prevalence of adrenal androgen excess in patients with the polycystic ovary syndrome (PCOS). *Clin Endocrinol (Oxf)* 2005; 62(6): 644–649.

10 Carmina, E., Koyama, T., Chang, L., Stanczyk, F. Z. and Lobo, R. A. Does ethnicity influence the prevalence of adrenal hyperandrogenism and insulin resistance in polycystic ovary syndrome? *Am J Obstet Gynecol* 1992; 167(6): 1807–1812.

11 Ezeh, U., Ida Chen, Y. D. and Azziz, R. Racial and ethnic differences in the metabolic response of polycystic ovary syndrome. *Clin Endocrinol (Oxf)* 2020; 93(2): 163–172.

12 Azziz, R. and Koulianos, G. Adrenal androgens and reproductive aging in females. *Semin Reprod Endocrinol* 1991; 9: 249–260.

13 Puurunen, J., Piltonen, T., Jaakkola, P., Ruokonen, A., Morin-Papunen, L. and Tapanainen, J. S. Adrenal androgen production capacity remains high up to menopause in women with polycystic ovary syndrome. *J Clin Endocrinol Metab* 2009; 94(6): 1973–1978.

14 Azziz, R., Gay, F. L., Potter, S. R., Bradley, E., Jr. and Boots, L. R. The effects of prolonged hypertestosteronemia on adrenocortical biosynthesis in oophorectomized women. *J Clin Endocrinol Metab* 1991; 72(5): 1025–1030.

15 Azziz, R., Rittmaster, R. S. and Fox, L. M. Role of the ovary in the adrenal androgen excess of hyperandrogenic women. *Fertil Steril* 1998; 69(5): 851–859.

16 Hines, G. A., Smith, E. R. and Azziz, R. Influence of insulin and testosterone on adrenocortical steroidogenesis in vitro: Preliminary studies. *Fertil Steril* 2001; 76(4): 730–735.

17 Huerta, R., Dewailly, D., Decanter, C., Knochenhauer, E. S., Boots, L. R. and Azziz, R. 11beta-hydroxyandrostenedione and delta 5-androstenediol as markers of adrenal androgen production in patients with 21-hydroxylase deficient nonclassic adrenal hyperplasia. *Fertil. Steril* 1999; 72(6): 996–1000.

18 O'Reilly, M. W., Kempegowda, P., Jenkinson, C. et al 11-Oxygenated C19 steroids are the predominant androgens in polycystic ovary syndrome. *J Clin Endocrinol Metab* 2017; 102(3): 840–848.

19 Swart, A. C., du Toit, T., Gourgari, E. et al. Steroid hormone analysis of adolescents and young women with polycystic ovarian syndrome and adrenocortical dysfunction using UPC2-MS/MS. *Pediatr Res* 2021; 89(1): 118–126.

20 Azziz, R., Bradley, E., Jr., Huth, J., Boots, L. R., Parker, C. R., Jr. and Zacur, H. A. Acute adrenocorticotropin-(1–24) (ACTH) adrenal stimulation in eumenorrheic women: Reproducibility and effect of ACTH dose, subject weight, and sampling time. *J Clin Endocrinol Metab* 1990; 70(5): 1273–1279.

21 Azziz, R., Black, V., Hines, G. A., Fox, L. M. and Boots, L. R. Adrenal androgen excess in the polycystic ovary syndrome: Sensitivity and responsivity of the hypothalamic-pituitary-adrenal axis. *J Clin Endocrinol Metab* 1998; 83(7): 2317–2323.

22 Goodarzi, M. O., Carmina, E. and Azziz, R. DHEA, DHEAS and PCOS. *J Steroid Biochem Mol Biol* 2015; 145: 213–225.

23 Carbunaru, G., Prasad, P., Scoccia, B. et al.The hormonal phenotype of Nonclassic 3 beta-hydroxysteroid dehydrogenase (HSD3B) deficiency in hyperandrogenic females is associated with insulin-resistant polycystic ovary syndrome and is not a variant of inherited HSD3B2 deficiency. *J Clin Endocrinol Metab* 2004; 89(2): 783–794.

24 Moran, C., Azziz, R., Carmina, E. et al. 21-Hydroxylase-deficient nonclassic adrenal hyperplasia is a progressive disorder: A multicenter study. *Am J Obstet Gynecol* 2000; 183(6): 1468–1474.

25 Yildiz, B. O., Goodarzi, M. O., Guo, X., Rotter, J. I. and Azziz, R. Heritability of dehydroepiandrosterone sulfate in women with polycystic ovary syndrome and their sisters. *Fertil Steril* 2006; 86(6): 1688–1693.

26 Cinar, N., Harmanci, A., Aksoy, D. Y., Aydin, K. and Yildiz, B. O. Adrenocortical steroid response to ACTH in different phenotypes of non-obese polycystic ovary syndrome. *J Ovarian Res* 2012; 5(1): 42.

27 Stewart, P. M., Shackleton, C. H., Beastall, G. H. and Edwards, C. R. 5 alpha-reductase activity in polycystic ovary syndrome. *Lancet* 1990 335(8687): 431–433.

28 Vassiliadi, D. A., Barber, T. M., Hughes, B. A. et alIncreased 5 alpha-reductase activity and adrenocortical drive in women with polycystic ovary syndrome. *J Clin Endocrinol Metab* 2009; 94(9): 3558–3566.

29 Tsilchorozidou, T., Honour, J. W. and Conway, G. S. Altered cortisol metabolism in polycystic ovary syndrome: Insulin enhances 5alpha-reduction but not the elevated adrenal steroid production rates. *J Clin Endocrinol Metab* 2003; 88(12): 5907–5913.

30 Rodin, A., Thakkar, H., Taylor, N. and Clayton, R. Hyperandrogenism in polycystic ovary syndrome: Evidence of dysregulation of 11 beta-hydroxysteroid dehydrogenase. *N Engl J Med* 1994; 330(7): 460–465.

31 Stewart, P. M. and Edwards, C. R. Hyperandrogenism in polycystic ovary syndrome. *N Engl J Med* 1994; 331(2): 131–132.

32 Gonzalez, F., Hatala, D. A. and Speroff, L. Adrenal and ovarian steroid hormone responses to gonadotropin-releasing hormone agonist treatment in polycystic ovary syndrome. *Am J Obstet Gynecol* 1991; 165(3): 535–545.

33 Ditkoff, E. C., Fruzzetti, F., Chang, L., Stancyzk, F. Z. and Lobo, R. A. The impact of estrogen on adrenal androgen sensitivity and secretion in polycystic ovary syndrome. *J Clin Endocrinol Metab* 1995; 80(2): 603–607.

34 Azziz, R., Chang, W. Y., Stanczyk, F .Z. and Woods, K. Effect of bilateral oophorectomy on adrenocortical function in women with polycystic ovary syndrome. *Fertil Steril* 2013; 99(2): 599–604.

35 Legro, R. S., Kunselman, A. R., Dodson, W. C. and Dunaif, A. Prevalence and predictors of risk for type 2 diabetes mellitus and impaired glucose tolerance in polycystic ovary syndrome: A prospective, controlled study in 254 affected women. *J Clin Endocrinol Metab* 1999; 84(1): 165–169.

36 Nestler, J. E., Usiskin, K. S., Barlascini, C. O., Welty, D. F., Clore, J. N. and Blackard, W. G. Suppression of serum dehydroepiandrosterone sulfate levels by insulin: An evaluation of possible mechanisms. *J Clin Endocrinol Metab* 1989; 69(5): 1040–1046.

37 Azziz, R. and Owerbach, D. Molecular abnormalities of the 21-hydroxylase gene in hyperandrogenic women with an exaggerated 17-hydroxyprogesterone response to shortterm adrenal stimulation. *Am J Obstet Gynecol* 1995; 172(3): 914–918.

38 Falcone, T., Finegood, D. T., Fantus, I. G. and Morris, D. Androgen response to endogenous insulin secretion during the frequently sampled intravenous glucose tolerance test in normal and hyperandrogenic women. *J Clin. Endocrinol Metab* 1990; 71(6): 1653–1657.

39 Farah-Eways, L., Reyna, R., Knochenhauer, E. S., Bartolucci, A. A. and Azziz, R. Glucose action and adrenocortical biosynthesis in women with polycystic ovary syndrome. *Fertil Steril* 2004; 81(1): 120–125.

40 Brennan, K., Huang, A. and Azziz, R. Dehydroepiandrosterone sulfate and insulin resistance in patients with polycystic ovary syndrome. *Fertil Steril* 2009; 91(5): 1848–1852.

41 Carmina, E., Gonzalez, F., Chang, L. and Lobo, R A. Reassessment of adrenal androgen secretion in women with polycystic ovary syndrome. *Obstet Gynecol* 1995; 85(6): 971–976.

42 Chen, M. J., Chen, C. D., Yang, J. H et al. High serum dehydroepiandrosterone sulfate is associated with phenotypic acne and a reduced risk of abdominal obesity in women with polycystic ovary syndrome. *Hum Reprod* 2011; 26(1): 227–234.

43 Lerchbaum, E., Schwetz, V., Giuliani, A., Pieber, T. R. and Obermayer-Pietsch, B. Opposing

effects of dehydroepiandrosterone sulfate and free testosterone on metabolic phenotype in women with polycystic ovary syndrome. *Fertil Steril* 2012; 98(5): 1318–1325.

44 Paschou, S. A., Palioura, E., Ioannidis, D. et al. Adrenal hyperandrogenism does not deteriorate insulin resistance and lipid profile in women with PCOS. *Endocr Connect* 2017; 6(8): 601–606.

45 Alpañés, M., Luque-Ramírez, M., Martínez-García, M. Á., Fernández-Durán, E. and Álvarez-Blasco, F. Escobar-Morreale HF Influence of adrenal hyperandrogenism on the clinical and metabolic phenotype of women with polycystic ovary syndrome. *Fertil Steril* 2015; 103(3): 795–801.

46 Azziz, R., Ehrmann, D. A., Legro, R. S., Fereshetian, A. G., O'Keefe, M. and Ghazzi, M. N. PCOS/Troglitazone Study Group: Troglitazone decreases adrenal androgen levels in women with polycystic ovary syndrome. *Fertil Steril* 2003; 79(4): 932–937.

47 Arlt, W., Auchus, R. J. and Miller, W. L. Thiazolidinediones but not metformin directly inhibit the steroidogenic enzymes P450c17 and 3beta-hydroxysteroid dehydrogenase. *J Biol Chem* 2001; 276(20): 16767–16771.

48 Li, X. J., Yu, Y. X., Liu, C. Q. et al.Metformin vs thiazolidinediones for treatment of clinical, hormonal and metabolic characteristics of polycystic ovary syndrome: A meta-analysis. *Clin Endocrinol (Oxf)* 2011; 74(3): 332–339.

49 Azziz, R., Zacur, H. A., Parker, C. R., Jr., Bradley, E. L., Jr., Boots, L. R. Effect of obesity on the response to acute adrenocorticotropin stimulation in eumenorrheic women. *Fertil Steril* 1991; 56(3): 427–433.

50 Vicennati, V., Calzoni, F., Gambineri, A. et al. Secretion of major adrenal androgens following ACTH administration in obese women with different body fat distribution. *Horm Metab Res* 1998; 30(3): 133–136.

51 Moran, C., Arriaga, M., Arechavaleta-Velasco, F. and Moran, S. Adrenal androgen excess and body mass index in polycystic ovary syndrome. *J Clin Endocrinol Metab* 2015; 100(3): 942–950.

52 Deng, Y., Zhang, Y., Li, S. et al. Steroid hormone profiling in obese and nonobese women with polycystic ovary syndrome. *Sci Rep* 2017;7 (1):14156.

53 Yildiz, B. O., Woods, K. S., Stanczyk, F., Bartolucci, A. and Azziz, R. Stability of adrenocortical steroidogenesis over time in healthy women and women with polycystic ovary syndrome. *J Clin Endocrinol Metab* 2004, 89(11): 5558–5562.

54 Legro, R. S., Kunselman, A. R., Demers, L., Wang, S. C., Bentley-Lewis, R. and Dunaif, A. Elevated dehydroepiandrosterone sulfate levels as the reproductive phenotype in the brothers of women with polycystic ovary syndrome. *J Clin Endocrinol Metab* 2002; 87(5): 2134–2138.

55 Goodarzi, M. O., Antoine, H. J. and Azziz, R. Genes for enzymes regulating dehydroepiandrosterone sulfonation are associated with levels of dehydroepiandrosterone sulfate in polycystic ovary syndrome. *J Clin Endocrinol Metab* 2007; 92(7): 2659–2664.

56 Louwers, Y. V., de Jong, F. H., van Herwaarden, N. A. et al. Variants in SULT2A1 affect the DHEA sulphate to DHEA ratio in patients with polycystic ovary syndrome but not the hyperandrogenic phenotype. *J Clin Endocrinol Metab* 2013; 98(9): 3848–3855.

57 Dumesic, D. A., Oberfield, S. E., Stener-Victorin, E., Marshall, J. C., Laven, J. S. and Legro, R. S. Scientific statement on the diagnostic criteria, epidemiology, pathophysiology, and molecular genetics of polycystic ovary syndrome. *Endocr Rev* 2015; 36(5): 487–525.

58 Zhai, G., Teumer, A., Stolk, L. et al. Eight common genetic variants associated with serum DHEAS levels suggest a key role in ageing mechanisms. *PLoS Genet* 2011; 7(4): e1002025.

Polycystic Ovary Syndrome and Environmental Toxins

Eleni A. Kandaraki and Olga Papalou

Introduction

Polycystic ovary syndrome (PCOS) is now globally recognized as the most common endocrinopathy in women of reproductive age and has a prevalence of 5–21% depending on the criteria used (National Institutes of Health (NIH), Rotterdam or Androgen Excess Society).[1] What is special about the syndrome is its dual entity involving both the reproductive and the metabolic profile of the women affected. As a result, any intrinsic or extrinsic factors affecting both these components could lead to pathophysiological alterations that characterize PCOS. In fact, the heterogenicity of the syndrome suggests that, apart from the genetic background, the role of the environment and a person's lifestyle are equally important. In particular, during the last twenty years, interest has been drawn to the impact of certain environmental toxins, referred to by the terms "endocrine disruptors" or "endocrine disruptive chemicals" (EDCs), which may modify both reproductive and metabolic pathways. Western civilization advancements in industrial products and food processing have led to increased daily exposure to plasticizers, such as bisphenol A (BPA) and phthalates, as well as dietary glycotoxins, such as advanced glycation end products (AGEs), which may exert adverse effects on reproduction and metabolism throughout the female lifespan.[2]

Endocrine Disruptive Chemicals (EDCs)

Terminology and History

The term "endocrine disruptive chemicals" (EDCs) is now broadly used to determine "an exogenous substance or mixture of substances that alters function(s) of the endocrine system and consequently causes adverse health effects in an intact organism, or its progeny, or (sub)populations," based on the International Programme on Chemical Safety (IPCS) and World Health Organization (WHO) definition,[3] or "an exogenous agent that interferes with synthesis, secretion, transport, metabolism, binding action, or elimination of natural blood-borne hormones that are present in the body and are responsible for homeostasis, reproduction, and developmental process" according to the US Environmental Protection Agency.[4] In other terms, any substance that can enter the human body via a broad spectrum of routes and derange the physiological endocrine pathways can be defined as an endocrine disruptor.

Research has come a long way since the publication of Rachel Carson's book in 1962, which was the first to raise awareness about the use of pesticides. Today, serious scientific concerns have been raised about a vast variety of environmental compounds due to their possible toxic effects on the human body, including male and female reproduction, thyroid function, cancer, metabolism and cardiovascular derangements. The Endocrine Society's first scientific statement in 2009, followed by its second statement in 2015, provided a wake-up call regarding the possible deleterious effects of EDCs, the different mechanisms of action and the various ways of exposure. [4, 5] In fact, this group of chemicals is highly heterogenous and can emerge from different sources, such as industrial solvents, plastics, plasticizers, storage containers, pesticides and fungicides, pharmaceutical agents, highly processed foods, cigarettes smoking, textiles and personal care products (Table 9.1).

Sources of Exposure

Historically, the commonest means of penetration into the human body was through air, soil and groundwater pollution, which subsequently

Table 9.1 Common EDCs and products they can be found in

Common EDCs	Found in
Dichlorodiphenyltrichloroethane (DDT) Methoxychlor Chlorpyrifos Atrazine 2,4-Dichlorophenoxyacetic acid Glyphosate Vinclozolin Thiram Hexachlorobenzene (HCB)	Pesticides/fungicides

Polychlorinated biphenyls (PCBs),
  Polybrominated biphenyls (PBBs),
  Dioxins/2,3,7,8-Tetrachlorodibenzo-
  p-dioxin (TCDD)
	Industrial solvents/lubricants, flame retardants, surfaces overlays

Bisphenols/Bisphenol A (BPA)	Plastics, epoxy resins, food storage containers, cans, water tubes, cooking utensils, baby bottles, dye on thermal paper (receipts, tickets, etc.), CDs/DVDs
Diethylstilbestrol (DES)	Pharmaceutical agents
Phytoestrogens Genistein Coumestrol	Natural chemicals found in human and animal food, soy
Heavy metals Lead Cadmium Mercury	Paint, oil and toy industries Batteries, metallic pigments Contaminated fish (mainly from Japan, the Northern Atlantic and Canada)
Phthalates DEHP (diethyl-hexyl phthalate) BBP (benzyl-butyl phthalate) DBP (dibutyl phthalate) Parabens	Plasticizers, cosmetics, sunscreens, children's toys/pacifiers, medical equipment (syringes, blood bags)

Advanced glycation end products (AGEs)/
  dietary glycotoxins/N-(carboxymethyl)
  lysine (CML) and Methylglyoxal (MG)
  derivatives
	High-temperature processed foods (100–200ºC), fast-food meals, cigarettes smoking, diet products

Perfluorochemicals/perfluoroalkyl substances (PFASs)	Textiles, food wrappers, microwave popcorn bags
Triclosan	Detergents, dental care materials

would directly contaminate plants and the drinking water or indirectly contaminate animals via consumption of both plants and water, and which would eventually reach humans through the food chain. Rapidly, the increased demands of modernized ways of living have driven the use of EDCs in a large variety of products that come into direct contact with and enter the human body via skin penetration. These include detergents, lubricants, surfaces overlays, cosmetics, dental care materials, thermal papers, clothing and even children's toys and pacifiers. Additionally, EDCs can be transferred rapidly through food storage and preparation. Plastics have been used to coat the inner surface of food containers, cans, water tubes and cooking utensils and allow contamination, especially with heating.

Moreover, AGEs – which are known to accumulate endogenously during various conditions, such as aging, diabetes, renal failure and Alzheimer's disease – have now been shown to also be absorbed through exogenous sources. Cigarette smoking, diet products, and westernized food habits, namely fast-food meals, microwave usage and rapid cooking under very high temperatures, lead to the increased absorption and deposition of non-enzymatic glycated products in human tissues and particularly the ovaries,[2] interfering with their homeostasis and thus fitting the definition of potential endocrine disruptors (Figure 9.1).[6]

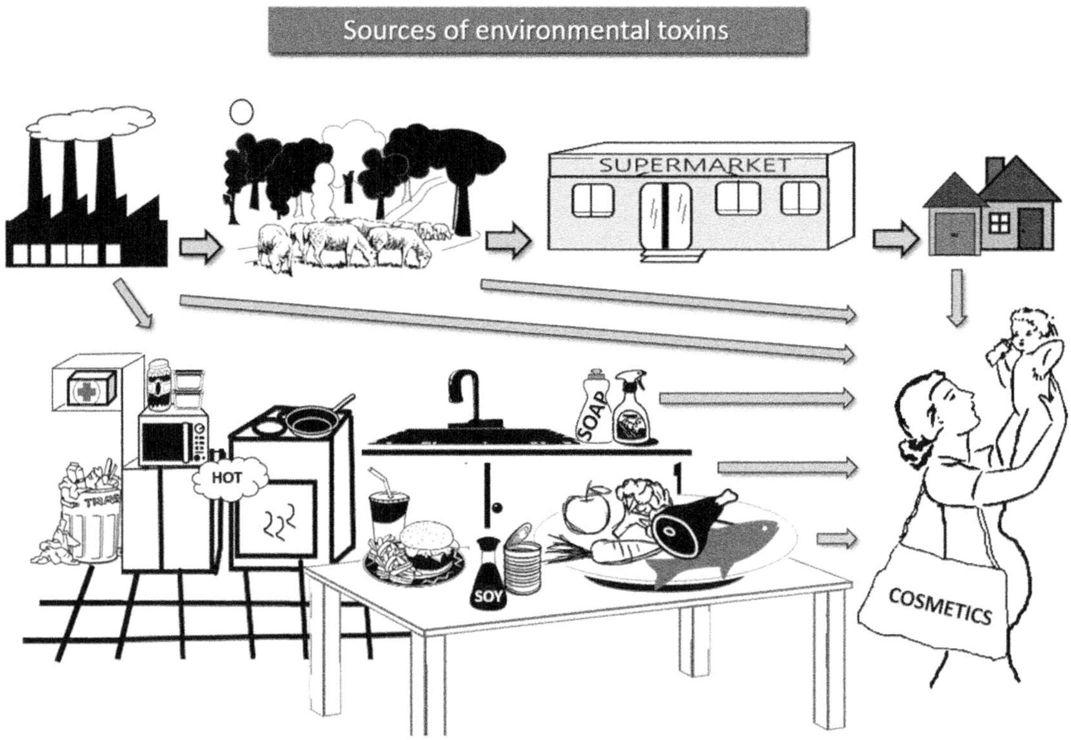

Figure 9.1 Illustration of the various sources from which environmental toxins can reach the human body

Chemical Particularities: Metabolism and Actions

In this heterogenous group of chemicals, many of them have a long half-life and can be detected long after use and many miles away from the original source of contamination due to soil, water or animal transfer.[7] In fact, EDCs that were banned years ago can still be found in the environment. On the other hand, a long half-life may contribute to revealing a causal relationship with regard to adverse reactions, especially in the case of serious contamination incidents, such as was seen with Yusho disease in 1968, which was caused by the consumption of rice contaminated with high levels of polychlorinated biphenyls (PCBs) and dioxins.[8] In most cases, identification of the exact effect that an environmental toxin may have is more complex due to the simultaneous contamination of ecosystems by numerous EDCs. In addition, those with a shorter half-life may be undetectable by the time of examination and cannot be directly linked to the toxic effects they may have caused.

In vitro metabolism is actively linked to EDCs' half-lives, as well as their activity and effects. Dioxins and dichlorodiphenyltrichloroethane (DDT) have a very slow rate of metabolism due to their extensive number of chlorine atoms that remain unconjugated leading to those compounds' long half-life and persistent adverse effects. In contrast, substances such as bisphenols are metabolized more quickly mainly through glucuronidation and do not seem to act on endocrine receptors, whereas their oxidative metabolites do.[9] Phthalates have a similar metabolic pathway as bisphenols, while methoxychlor follows the route of demethylation and hydroxylation by cytochrome P450 and it seems that the metabolic product hydroxyphenyltrichloroethane is a 100-fold more potent estrogenic chemical.

The food industry, in an effort to enrich the taste of food products, as well as to enhance the shelflife and aromas of processed foods, has utilized several physical and chemical methods that have led to the formation of intermediate potentially harmful molecules, such as N-(carboxymethyl)lysine (CML) and Methylglyoxal (MG), the major precursors of dietary glycotoxins (AGEs). They are products of the nonenzymatic reaction between sugars and the free amino groups of proteins, nucleic acids and lipids. AGEs accumulate in tissue and act mainly via their receptor (RAGE, or receptor for advanced glycation end products) to promote oxidative stress and inflammation. With regard to metabolism, they are cleared through the scavenging enzymatic system of glyoxalase I and II. Interestingly, it has been shown that the higher the food consistency in dietary glycotoxins, the lower the enzymatic activity of glyoxalase I, leading to their increased accumulation.[10]

The heterogenicity of EDCs is based on their different chemical structures and reflects on the different actions and effects involving multiple endocrine axes, such as the pituitary, thyroid, glucose metabolism and male and female reproductive system. In fact, other than being substances of small molecular weight (< 1000 Daltons), they rarely share structural similarities. However, some of them, like PCBs, polybrominated biphenyls (PBBs), dioxins and dioxin-like compounds, are composed of a phenolic segment that can mimic the action of a steroid hormone on its receptor. In fact, one of the main paths through which EDCs can alter the signal transmission is via agonistic or antagonistic interaction with nuclear hormone receptors, such as estrogen (ERs), androgen (Ars) and thyroid receptors (TRs). Other modes of action include nonnuclear steroid hormone receptors (membrane estrogen receptors [ERs]), nonsteroid receptors (neurotransmitters such as serotonin and dopamine), enzymatic cascades of steroid biosynthesis and metabolism.[11]

The Challenging Task to Limit Exposure

A challenging field is to identify which EDCs actually cause clinically significant damage to the directly affected or next generation and what measures can actually be implemented to reduce exposure. Current difficulties include the variability among measurement methods and safety levels, adverse effects that may take years to show and conflicting financial interests. In the case of the notorious example of diethylstilbestrol (DES), a synthetic estrogen initially administered as a therapeutic agent to women during pregnancy in the 1940s, it took 30 years to prove its catastrophic consequences for the women's daughters and to finally be banned by the US Food and Drug Administration (FDA).[12] It is not surprising that the chemically similar compound bisphenol A (BPA) is still in extended use in the plastics industry and has been since the 1930s. Recently, the European Chemicals Agency (ECHA) has classified BPA as toxic for reproduction and hazardous to human health. It is also known that it passes through to fetuses during gestation and has been found in breast milk during lactation. Its use in baby bottles has been banned since 2011 and has now also been restricted in thermal papers and materials in contact with food, but a lower limit (up to 0.1 mg/l) is still allowed in children's toys, even if they may come into contact with children's mouths. Currently, efforts are in progress to substitute BPA for safer metabolites, with the aim to limit industrial evolution at the expense of health and particularly reproduction.[13]

EDCs and PCOS

PCOS comprises different phenotypes, reflecting the complex pathogenesis and the synergistic effect of various causative factors, including genetic as well as environmental ones. Considering all the criteria used, this endocrinopathy is overall characterized by two main pillars of women's health: reproductive, which would include the presence of hyperandrogenism (clinical and/or biochemical) and metabolic. The limited data on direct effects on humans embrace the available evidence from in vitro and animal studies to support the claim that lifestyle choices and exposure to environmental toxins seem to have an important impact on both parameters (Figure 9.2).

EDCs and PCOS: Focus on Female Reproduction

The hormonal derangements in PCOS women, mainly an altered androgen to estrogen ratio, are linked to reproductive abnormalities such as menstrual irregularities, anovulatory cycles and infertility. These characteristics usually require a susceptible genetic background, but they may be revealed or exacerbated under the influence of a variety of environmental factors.

Hyperandrogenism

Hyperandrogenism, a common feature of the syndrome defined by high levels of serum androgens, contributes to the relevant clinical signs

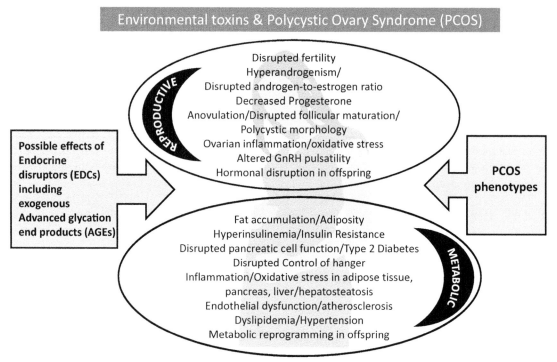

Figure 9.2 Environmental toxins and PCOS
Many of the PCOS features leading to the various PCOS phenotypes coincide with the effects of environmental toxins on female reproduction and metabolism. These PCOS characteristics usually require a susceptible genetic background, but they may be revealed or exacerbated under the influence of EDCs, including the exogenously absorbed advanced glycation end products (AGEs).

(hirsutism, acne and alopecia) and reduced fertility. Several studies have found positive associations between PCOS women and adolescents with high levels of EDCs in their biological fluids. In fact, increased serum BPA was observed in hyperandrogenemic PCOS females compared to healthy controls.[14] Potential interactions between BPA and androgens synthesis and metabolism are being explored. Higher levels of bisphenol A may have a direct effect on ovarian theca cells, leading to increased mRNA expression, 17α-hydroxylase activity and testosterone synthesis. Additionally, BPA may act as a potential sex hormone-binding globulin (SHBG) ligand, allowing more free testosterone to be available and disrupting the androgen to estrogen ratio. Simultaneously, increased androgen levels may interfere with BPA hepatic metabolism, by decreasing BPA clearance, possibly by down-regulation of UDP-glucuronosyltransferase activity, thus closing a vicious circle.[2]

Actions on the Ovary

EDCs with molecular similarities to endogenous steroids, such as BPA and its metabolites, DDT, methoxychlor or phytoestrogens, can have an agonistic and antagonistic action on native androgen, estrogen and progesterone receptors, leading to altered hormonal equilibrium and reproductive dysfunction.[15] Several EDCs even with weak estrogenic activity could have a synergistic and cumulative result and seem to act via a variety of pathways, including classical (ERα/ERβ) and nonclassical (membrane) ERs, G-protein coupled receptors (GPR30), transcription factors (PPARγ, C/EBP, Nrf2, HOX, HAND2) and epigenetic changes, such as DNA methylation.[16] The integrity of these pathways is essential to preserve ovarian steroidogenesis and oocyte maturation. Similarly, in vitro and animal studies have shown the effect of other EDCs, such as phthalates on intrafollicular environment, disequilibrium of androgen/estrogen, decreased progesterone levels and anovulation. Dioxins and PCBs seem also to disrupt ovarian steroidogenesis. However, effects are often subject to dose and the experimental model, so results need to be interpreted with caution. On the other hand, human studies are very few and have limitations but they do enrich our knowledge on EDCs' harmful reactions. Exposure of women to pesticides, such as heptachlor epoxide, was shown to alter hormonal levels and lead to a shorter luteal phase. BPA has been associated with premature ovarian failure and early menopause in women.[5] Moreover, in patients undergoing in vitro fertilization, BPA was linked to a low estrogen curve prior to ovulation as well as a decreased follicle count and fewer oocytes retrieved.[17] Interestingly, the effects of BPA on follicular growth does not seem to be mediated through the estrogen receptors but mostly by interference in steroidogenesis, the aryl hydrocarbon receptor (AHR) pathway and cell cycle regulators. Apart from BPA, other EDCs, such as methoxychlor, dioxin, 2,3,7,8-Tetrachlorodibenzo-p-dioxin (TCDD), phthalates and genistein, have been shown to affect follicular maturation and may contribute to premature or permanent infertility.[18]

AGEs are also known to have a significant impact on reproduction. They seem to exert their effects mainly via crosslinking and AGE–RAGE interaction, promoting oxidative stress and inflammation in the ovarian environment. However, novel data have been collected in investigating the direct or indirect effects on hormonal pathways and interference with hormonal receptors, as high levels of dietary AGEs have been associated with worsening PCOS characteristics and hyperandrogenemia. [6] PCOS women who consumed a diet rich in AGEs were found to have higher androgen levels and ovulatory dysfunction compared to those given a low AGEs diet. Similar results have been reported with in vivo and in vitro experimental models. Apart from high testosterone and androstenedione, lower levels of estradiol and progesterone – all essential hormones to maintain normal cycle and future egg implantation – were measured in female Wistar rats fed a diet high in AGEs. They also seem to have a role in further increasing AMH levels in PCOS women and possibly worsen anovulation.[6]

Actions on the Hypothalamus–Pituitary–Ovarian Control

Although the reproductive homeostasis depends on a variety of pathways that cross-talk with each other, and thus it may be difficult to pinpoint the exact level of dysregulation, EDCs seem to directly affect the ovary as well as indirectly affect the neuroendocrine control of the hypothalamus–pituitary–ovarian (HPG) axis.[19] Derangement of the HPG axis is a key feature in the pathogenesis of PCOS, showing altered pulsatility of the gonadotropin-releasing hormone (GnRH), leading to increased levels of luteinizing hormone (LH) and decreased levels of follicular-stimulating hormone (FSH). In vivo and vitro experimental data show that common EDCs, such as BPA, methoxychlor, genistein, vinclozolin and PCBs, may act directly on the pituitary, as well as on the hypothalamus, affecting the expression of both GnRH neurons and neuropeptides (kisspeptin, galanin) important for GnRH pulsatility.[19, 20] Moreover, dietary glycotoxins seem to alter gonadotropin pulsatility and affect normal follicular maturation via the ERK1/MAPK pathway.[21]

Perinatal Exposure

The time of EDC exposure, especially during early life stages, is crucial to the neuroendocrine development and integrity of the reproductive axis later in life. Prenatal exposure and during infancy has been associated with dimorphic effects in brain development and reproductive abnormalities, which affect fertility in adulthood. For example, estrogenic pesticides given to rodents at a single embryonic age showed permanent changes in their sexual behavior in adulthood. Early postnatal administration of genistein to female rats led to altered pubertal onset and early reproductive failure.[20] Interestingly, exposure to EDCs such as phthalates and BPA to the parental experimental generation has been found to cause epigenetic changes transmitted up to the third generation, leading to the "epigenetic transgenerational inheritance theory."[2] Moreover, neonatal exposure to BPA has been linked to high levels of testosterone and estradiol, low progesterone and altered GnRH pulsatility with polycystic ovarian morphology and reduced fertility in adulthood, resembling a PCOS-like phenotype.[22] Exposure of rhesus monkeys during late gestation to dihydrotestosterone or diethylstilbestrol (DES) led to hyperandrogenism and reproductive abnormalities similar to PCOS later in life.[5] Although data in humans are limited, multiple studies have found environmental pollutants such as dioxins, PCBs, PBBs and BPA to be present in various human fluids, including amniotic fluid and breast milk, in levels higher than those considered safe, which indicates the potential risk to human offspring of exposure during the perinatal period.[12, 18, 23] There are contradicting results regarding the association of BPA with precocious puberty in girls, whereas some evidence supports the association of perfluorooctanoic acid exposure during gestation in Danish women with the timing of puberty in their daughters, which is worrying enough to merit further research in the future. On the other hand, antenatal exposure to phthalates seems to be PCOS-protective in Australian adolescent girls.[5] As mentioned, it can be challenging to examine the actions of separate EDCs, as in reality they usually act synergistically and the effect of one can be influenced by the presence of others. Studies in female rats showed that triclosan, a dental care substance, can interact with BPA in vivo and enhance its effects on the ovary.[5]

Perinatal exposure to dietary glycotoxins (AGEs) seems to affect the reproductive and metabolic parameters of the next generation. In a recent US study, mice exposed to a diet high in AGEs during pregnancy showed low birth weight, delayed puberty and disrupted folliculogenesis in their female offspring.[24]

Remarks

It is worth noting that other reproductive abnormalities linked to EDCs, such as anatomical anomalies, endometriosis, uterine fibroids and even male reproductive derangements, have been reported but are not related to PCOS, and thus are not included in this chapter. Sadly, despite the available data regarding the possible adverse effects of EDC exposure to female reproduction, it seems that healthcare professionals, particularly those involved in perinatal care, do not feel well informed and confident enough to educate patients, as emerged in a recent French multicenter survey.[25]

EDCs and PCOS: Focus on Metabolism

Apart from the reproductive aspect of PCOS, the metabolic parameters are commonly affected as part of the pathophysiology of the syndrome,

involving a disturbed glucose metabolism, insulin resistance, visceral obesity, dyslipidemia and high blood pressure, all features leading to an increased risk of cardiovascular disease. Wide-ranging evidence from experimental and human studies supports the impact of environmental pollutants on female metabolism.

Obesity

Abdominal and visceral obesity is a key feature in the pathophysiology of PCOS, intercalated with insulin resistance and androgen excess. It is a chronic noncommunicative endocrine-related disease, and its prevalence is increasing dramatically in the modern world. With regard to its etiology, it seems to be multifactorial, combining both genetic and environmental factors.[2] Since 2002, the parallel rise in obesity with exposure to environmental toxins is suspected to have been noncoincidental, leading to the "developmental obesogen hypothesis" in 2012 as part of the National Toxicology Program (NTP) workshop.[26]

Several EDCs, such as DES, BPA, phthalates, parabens, PBBs, phytoestrogens and pesticides, have been linked to an increased risk of adiposity and subsequently type 2 diabetes, owing to the effects on both the peripheral adipocyte differentiation and the central control of eating behavior, involving genomic and nongenomic mechanisms of action. Particular emphasis has been given to exposure during the in utero or neonatal period and the consequences on fat distribution postnatally or in adulthood (the developmental obesogen hypothesis).[27] Perinatal exposure to toxins such as phthalates, BPA, DDT-metabolites, hexachlorobenzene (HCB) and PCBs, led to increased birth weight and obesity development, supporting the disruption of metabolic signaling later in life.[2, 28] Although human studies are limited, a stronger link has been found between BPA and phthalates and childhood and adult obesity, which seems to be age- and gender-dependent according to a recent meta-analysis.[29] Multiple birth cohorts have also linked prenatal exposure to perfluoroalkyl substances (PFASs) with child adiposity.[30]

In vitro studies exploring the actions of BPA showed increased adipogenic gene induction and promotion of adipose cell differentiation through interaction with the ER. Both BPA and phthalates seem to interact with the peroxisome proliferator-activated receptors (PPARs) pathway, which has a key role in adipogenesis and lipid metabolism. Epidemiological studies express a possible link between weight gain and phthalate exposure through the PPARγ mechanism. Similarly, higher urinary BPA has been linked to an increased risk of obesity and high waist circumference. Other factors contributing to the pathogenesis would be the reactive oxygen species (ROS) formation and inflammatory cytokine release, which would promote adiponectin suppression and a decrease in lipoprotein lipase activity. Also, the possible antagonistic action on the thyroid receptor (TR) could comprise an additional route of metabolic suppression and promote adiposity.[31]

Little is known regarding the role of EDCs on neuroendocrine control of appetite and increased energy intake. There is some evidence in rodents to support the interference with neuropeptide Y (NPY) expression and the endocannabinoid pathway.[31] Additionally, serum levels of BPA have been linked to levels of the hormones ghrelin and leptin, both of which are secreted by the adipose tissue and regulate hunger. Similarly, parabens exposure has been found in mice to increase levels of leptin.[27]

Dietary AGEs also have been associated with obesity and insulin resistance/type 2 diabetes, which will be analyzed in the subsections that follow. They act as obesity promoters, as shown by the increased body weight that results after the consumption of highly processed food rich in dietary glycotoxins. AGEs seem to act directly on fat accumulation by touching off inflammatory pathways and interfering with orexigenic and anorexigenic hypothalamic control of energy balance.[32] They seem to activate macrophages, promote adipocytokines secretion and adipocytes hypertrophy. Maternal AGEs levels have been correlated with serum AGEs, adiponectin and leptin levels in infants. AGEs-proteins have been found to be recognized as ligand by adipocytes receptor CD36, leading to downregulation of leptin expression. This information supports the disruption of energy metabolism by these glycotoxins and their role in the development of obesity.[6]

Glucose Homeostasis

Deranged glucose metabolism and insulin resistance is a feature that affects up to 80% of women with PCOS, increasing the risk of diabetes mellitus and cardiovascular complications. The hyperinsulinemic stimulation of the ovarian theca cells will lead to hyperproduction of androgens, contributing to anovulation and reproductive dysfunction. EDCs have been linked to disrupted glucose homeostasis either indirectly via promoting obesity or by direct action on the pancreatic b-cells.[2] Most of the available evidence places BPA at the center of attention for the "diabetogenic hypothesis."[30, 33] In fact, some of the first human data linking urinary BPA to type 2 diabetes derived from the National Health and Nutrition Examination Survey (NHANES).[34]

In vivo experiments exploring possible underlying mechanisms showed an exaggerated production of insulin after BPA administration, without affecting islet morphology. Interestingly, short-term administration provoked hypoglycemia, whereas after four days both insulin and glucose levels were permanently increased, mimicking a diabetic effect via an ER-dependent pathway.[35] Furthermore, BPA seems to act on K+ ion channels' expression of mice b-cells and alter membrane potentials, possibly contributing to a BPA-induced diabetogenic effect.[36] BPA also seem to act on pancreatic a-cells and alter glucagon secretion. Other possible pathways could be adipocytokines-related, as BPA in environmental doses was shown to suppress adiponectin production and possibly predispose people to metabolic syndrome and diabetes type 2.[4] Disappointingly, there seems to be a diabetic association found with other bisphenols being tried to replace BPA in aluminum cans and thermal paper receipts.[30]

Apart from BPA, other EDCs have been also examined with regards to causality on obesity and diabetes and seem to affect both insulin secretion from b-cells and insulin action on a receptor and post-receptor level.[26, 37] Animal and epidemiological studies have reported association between the risk of disrupted glucose metabolism and environmental toxicants, such as dioxins, DDT, PCBs, organochlorine pesticides and hexachlorobenzene. Heavy metals such as arsenic and mercury seem to have a blocking and toxic effect on pancreatic b-cells respectively, impairing the glucose–insulin coordinated secretion.[5] A positive association has been also reported between phthalates concentration in children and adolescents with glucose levels in a recent meta-analysis.[28] The evidence for EDCs exposure and development of gestational diabetes remains controversial, with a stronger link toward PFASs, whereas for others, such as bisphenols and parabens, more studies are needed to clarify a solid association.[30]

The damaging role of AGEs on glucose metabolism, including insulin resistance and diabetes has also been shown in multiple animal studies. As in the case of the ovary, food glycotoxins accumulate in various other tissues, such as the pancreas and liver and exert their toxic effects by promoting oxidative stress and inflammation.[6] Low-grade chronic inflammation seems to interfere with insulin signaling pathways (JNK, IKK/NF-κB) affecting the phosphorylation of insulin-related substrates (IRS) and altering skeletal muscle insulin sensitivity by downregulating GLUT-4. In humans, a low AGEs diet has been linked to improved insulin sensitivity, whereas a diet high in AGEs concentration has been related to insulin impairment, as expressed by the homeostasis model assessment of insulin resistance (HOMA-IR) index in nondiabetics.[32] Moreover, perinatal exposure to exogenous AGEs may promote metabolic reprogramming to the offspring and show a positive correlation of maternal serum AGEs levels and infant plasma insulin concentration.[6, 32] Consequently, the abovementioned data support the damaging effect of dietary AGEs in the disruption of metabolic pathways and rightfully classify them as EDCs holding the potential to promote metabolic complications in PCOS patients.

Cardiometabolic Risk

PCOS women have been linked to increased cardiovascular risk during their reproductive life. [38] Visceral obesity, dyslipidemia, hypertension, impaired glucose homeostasis and particularly insulin resistance, which is an independent risk factor even in lean PCOS women,[39] are associated with higher risk of cardiovascular disease (CVD). As discussed, EDCs seem to be associated separately with obesity and impaired glucose metabolism, which would promote the occurrence of CVD. However, as research progressed more data supported a direct effect of EDCs on cardiometabolic risk, independent of obesity or diabetes.[5] In fact, in a large meta-analysis where various EDCs were examined, a direct relation of EDCs with cardiovascular risk was found. PCBs, BPA, phthalates and organo-chlorine pesticides were all associated with CVD risk.[40]

A link between urinary BPA levels and CVD was found early on in the pioneer NHANES data.[34] In animal models, BPA exposure seems to induce arrhythmias by interfering with Ca+ influx on myocytes, promote atheromatic aortic changes, increase low-density lipoprotein (LDL) and induce hypertension.[5] There are also data supporting the claim that early-life exposure to BPA alters epigenetic programming on hepatocytes and induces steatosis in animals. Considering that liver steatosis is a feature of metabolic syndrome and PCOS, this information could also contribute to the cardiometabolic risk of PCOS women.[19] However, in human studies, a direct association between BPA and dyslipidemia is controversial. A recent meta-analysis did not find an association with total cholesterol (TC) or LDL,[40] whereas a recent five-year prospective study found a positive association between BPA and LDL cholesterol, in addition to a higher prevalence of reduced high-density lipoprotein (HDL).[41]

Other EDCs have also been related to components of increased cardiometabolic risk. In a recent study, serum phthalates have been associated with dyslipidemia and insulin resistance in PCOS adolescents, regardless of obesity, although no difference was found regarding phthalates levels compared to controls.[42] Furthermore, organochlorine pesticides have been linked to hypertriglyceridemia, whereas different compounds of the PCBs family have been correlated with atherogenicity and hypertension. Environmental toxins that disrupt lipid metabolism promote the accumulation of lipids in the subendothelial space, resulting in inflammatory changes, the formation of atheromatic plaques and an increase in CVD risk.[37]

Likewise, it looks like EDCs can interfere in various mechanisms controlling blood pressure and promote the development of hypertension and CVD risk. Catecholamines contribute in blood pressure regulation by acting on adrenergic receptors and may transmit their signal via adenylate cyclase (AC) activation, which converts ATP to cAMP and increases cardiac muscle contractility. Neonatal exposure to environmental pollutants such as organophosphorus pesticides have been found to increase AC activity in rodents. Similarly, in vivo exposure to atrazine has been shown to potentiate cAMP signaling, which could augment the action of catecholamines on blood pressure. Another possible mechanism could be through interference in the glucocorticoid pathways and promotion of their hypertensive effect. Pesticides such as thiram and heavy metals such as cadmium have been linked to inhibition of the cortisol deactivating enzyme hydroxysteroid dehydrogenase type 2 (11ß-HSD -2) and consecutively may augment cortisol action on the mineralocorticoid receptors, thus leading to hypertension. Furthermore, sex hormones have a role in lipid metabolism and all the environmental toxins disrupting the estrogen/androgen signaling could be linked to altered lipid profile and atherogenesis.[37]

AGEs have also been implicated in CVD. Endogenous AGEs have been known to accumulate in conditions with cardiovascular complications, such as aging, diabetes or renal diseases. Research on exogenously absorbed AGES in animal and in vitro studies has also shown a link to cardiometabolic consequences, either by promoting obesity and deranged glucose metabolism or by mechanisms affecting endothelial dysfunction and atherosclerosis. [6, 32] In humans, data are limited, but a recent meta-analysis gathering 17 randomized controlled trials resulted in a positive association between a low AGEs diet and improvement in insulin resistance, TC, LDL cholesterol, inflammation and vascular markers.[43] Tobacco smoking, which apart from other chemicals is a known source of exogenous AGEs, also contributes to inflammation and atherosclerosis and seems to have a transgenerational effect. Exposure of women to nicotine during gestation showed increased blood pressure in their offspring.[37]

Cardiometabolic risk factors in PCOS women include obesity, dysglycemia, dyslipidemia, hypertension and vascular dysfunction as expressed by markers of structural and functional changes.[44] Despite some controversies possibly due to age, ethnicity or genetic differences and the necessity of long-term population-based studies to establish a direct causality, it is reasonable to assume that any exogenous factor contributing to the development of these features could contribute to a PCOS-like cardiometabolic phenotype (Figure 9.2).

Conclusions

PCOS is a multigenic entity composed of a specific spectrum of features, including clinical and/or biochemical hyperandrogenism, anovulation, deranged hypothalamic–pituitary–gonadal control, alterations in metabolism and insulin resistance, leading to reduced fertility and possible cardiovascular implications. Experimental models link EDCs to PCOS characteristics and seem to support a transgenerational effect when the exposure occurs during the perinatal period. Nevertheless, human studies are limited but do seem to promote the expression of a PCOS-affected genetic background. Evidence so far shows a stronger association of PCOS women with bisphenol A (BPA) and perfluorochemicals (PFASs). Data on other environmental toxins, such as phthalates, triclosan, dioxins and biphenyls, are still to be explored in order to draw conclusions.[30] Considering that all these environmental substances are found in our day-to-day lives and can come into contact with the human body via multiple sources, exposure is constant, cumulative and may be detrimental to present and future generations.

References

1 Diamanti-Kandarakis, E., Polycystic ovarian syndrome: Pathophysiology, molecular aspects and clinical implications. *Expert Rev Mol Med* 2008; 10: e3.

2 Rutkowska, A. Z. and Diamanti-Kandarakis, E. Polycystic ovary syndrome and environmental toxins. *Fertil Steril* 2016; 106(4): 948–58.

3 World Health Organization, United Nations Environment Programme, Inter-Organization Programme for the Sound Management of Chemicals et al. *State of the Science of Endocrine Disrupting Chemicals 2012: Summary for Decision-Makers.* Geneva: WHO, 2013; https://apps.who.int/iris/handle/10665/78102

4 Diamanti-Kandarakis, E., Bourguignon, J.-P., Guidice, L. C. et al. Endocrine-disrupting chemicals: An Endocrine Society scientific statement. *Endocr Rev* 2009; 30(4): 293–342.

5 Gore, A. C., Chappell, V. A., Fenton, S. E. et al. EDC-2: The Endocrine Society's Second Scientific Statement on Endocrine-Disrupting Chemicals. *Endocr Rev* 2015; 36(6): E1–E150.

6 Ravichandran, G., Lakshmanan, D. K., Karthik, R. et al. Food advanced glycation end products as potential endocrine disruptors: An emerging threat to contemporary and future generation. *Environ Int* 2019; 123: 486–500.

7 Van den Berg M, Sanderson, T., Kurihara, N. and Katayama, A., Role of metabolism in the endocrine-disrupting effects of chemicals in aquatic and terrestrial systems. *Pure Appl. Chem* 2003; 75(11–12): 1917–1932.

8 Aoki, Y., Polychlorinated biphenyls, polychlorinated dibenzo-p-dioxins, and polychlorinated dibenzofurans as endocrine disrupters: What we have learned from Yusho disease. *Environ Res* 2001; 86(1): 2–11.

9 Gramec Skledar, D. and Peterlin Masic, L. Bisphenol A and its analogs: Do their metabolites have endocrine activity? *Environ Toxicol Pharmacol* 2016; 47: 182–199.

10 Kandaraki, E., Chatzigeorgiou, A., Piperi, C. et al. Reduced ovarian glyoxalase-I activity by dietary glycotoxins and androgen excess: A causative link to polycystic ovarian syndrome. *Mol Med* 2012; 18: 1183–1189.

11 Sifakis, S., Androutsopoulos, V. P., Tsatsakis, A. M. and Spanidos, D. A. Human exposure to endocrine disrupting chemicals: Effects on the male and female reproductive systems. *Environ Toxicol Pharmacol* 2017; 51: 56–70.

12 Tang, Z.R., Xu, X. L., Deng, S. L., Lian, Z. X. and Yu, K. Oestrogenic endocrine disruptors in the placenta and the fetus. *Int J Mol Sci* 2020; 21(4): 1519.

13 European Chemicals Agency. Bisphenol A. European Chemicals Agency (website). https://echa.europa.eu/hot-topics/bisphenol-a

14 Kandaraki, E., Chatzigeorgiou, A., Livadas, S. et al. Endocrine disruptors and polycystic ovary syndrome (PCOS): Elevated serum levels of bisphenol A in women with PCOS. *J Clin Endocrinol Metab* 2011; 96(3): E480–E484.

15 Lee, H.R., Jeung, E. B., Cho, M. H., Kim, T. H., Leung, P. C. K. and Choi, K. C. Molecular mechanism(s) of endocrine-disrupting chemicals and their potent oestrogenicity in diverse cells and tissues that express oestrogen receptors. *J Cell Mol Med* 2013; 17(1): 1–11.

16 Cimmino, I., Fiory, F., Perruolo, G. et al. Potential mechanisms of bisphenol A (BPA) contributing to human disease. *Int J Mol Sci* 2020; 21(16): 5761.

17 Piazza, M. J. and Urbanetz, A. A. Environmental toxins and the impact of other endocrine disrupting chemicals in women's reproductive health. *JBRA Assist Reprod* 2019; 23(2): 154–164.

18 Patel, S., Zhou, C., Rattan, S. and Flaws, J. A. Effects of endocrine-disrupting chemicals on the ovary. *Biol Reprod* 2015; 93(1): 20.

19 Palioura, E. and Diamanti-Kandarakis, E. Polycystic ovary syndrome (PCOS) and endocrine disrupting chemicals (EDCs). *Rev Endocr Metab Disord* 2015; 16(4): 365–371.

20 Gore, A. C. Neuroendocrine targets of endocrine disruptors. *Hormones (Athens)* 2010; 9(1): 16–27.

21 Kandaraki, E. A., Chatzigeorgiou, A., Papageorgiou, E. et al. Advanced glycation end products interfere in luteinizing hormone and follicle stimulating hormone signaling in human granulosa KGN cells. *Exp Biol Med (Maywood)* 2018; 243(1): 29–33.

22 Fernandez, M., Bourguignon, N., Lux-Lantos, V. and Libertun, C. Neonatal exposure to bisphenol a and reproductive and endocrine alterations resembling the polycystic ovarian syndrome in adult rats. *Environ Health Perspect* 2010; 118(9): 1217–1222.

23 van den Berg, M., Kypke, K., Kotz, A. et al. WHO/UNEP global surveys of PCDDs, PCDFs, PCBs and DDTs in human milk and benefit-risk evaluation of breastfeeding. *Arch Toxicol* 2017; 91(1): 83–96.

24 Merhi, Z., Du, X. Q. and Charron, M. J. Perinatal exposure to high dietary advanced glycation end products affects the reproductive system in female offspring in mice. *Mol Hum Reprod* 2020; 26(8): 615–623.

25 Marguillier, E., Beranger, R., Garlantezec, R. et al. Endocrine disruptors and pregnancy: Knowledge, attitudes and practice of perinatal health professionals. A French multicentre survey. *Eur J Obstet Gynecol Reprod Biol* 2020; 252: 233–238.

26 Thayer, K. A., Heindel, J. J., Bucher, J. R. and Gallo, M. A. Role of environmental chemicals in diabetes and obesity: A National Toxicology Program workshop review. *Environ Health Perspect* 2012; 120(6): 779–789.

27 Darbre, P. D. Endocrine disruptors and obesity. *Curr Obes Rep* 2017; 6(1): 18–27.

28 Golestanzadeh, M., Riahi, R. and Kelishadi, R. Association of exposure to phthalates with cardiometabolic risk factors in children and adolescents: A systematic review and meta-analysis. *Environ Sci Pollut Res Int* 2019; 26 (35): 35670–35686.

29 Ribeiro, C.M., Beserra, B. T. S., Silva, N. G. et al. Exposure to endocrine-disrupting chemicals and anthropometric measures of obesity: A systematic review and meta-analysis. *BMJ Open* 2020; 10(6): e033509.

30 Kahn, L.G., Philippat, C., Nakayama, S. F., Slama, R. and Trasande, L. Endocrine-disrupting chemicals: Implications for human health. *Lancet Diabetes Endocrinol* 2020; 8(8): 703–718.

31 Stojanoska, M. M., Milosevic, N., Milic, N. and Abenavoli, L. The influence of phthalates and

bisphenol A on the obesity development and glucose metabolism disorders. *Endocrine* 2017; 55(3): 666–681.

32 Sergi, D., Boulestin, H., Campbell, F. M. and Williams, L. M. The role of dietary advanced glycation end products in metabolic dysfunction. *Mol Nutr Food Res* 2020; e1900934.

33 Hwang, S., Lim, J. E., Choi, Y. and Jee, S. H. Bisphenol A exposure and type 2 diabetes mellitus risk: A meta-analysis. *BMC Endocr Disord* 2018; 18(1): 81.

34 Lang, I. A., Galloway, T. S., Scarlett, A. et al. Association of urinary bisphenol A concentration with medical disorders and laboratory abnormalities in adults. *JAMA* 2008; 300(11): 1303–1310.

35 Alonso-Magdalena, P., Morimoto, S., Ripoll, C., Fuentes, E. and Nadal, A. The estrogenic effect of bisphenol A disrupts pancreatic beta-cell function in vivo and induces insulin resistance. *Environ Health Perspect* 2006. 114(1): 106–112.

36 Martinez-Pinna, J., Marroqui, L., Hmadcha, A. et al. Oestrogen receptor beta mediates the actions of bisphenol-A on ion channel expression in mouse pancreatic beta cells. *Diabetologia* 2019; 62(9): 1667–1680.

37 Kirkley, A. G. and Sargis, R. M. Environmental endocrine disruption of energy metabolism and cardiovascular risk. *Curr Diab Rep* 2014; 14(6): 494.

38 Ramezani Tehrani, F., Amiri, M., Behboudi-Gandevani, S., Bidhendi-Yarandi, R. and

Carmina, E. Cardiovascular events among reproductive and menopausal age women with polycystic ovary syndrome: A systematic review and meta-analysis. *Gynecol Endocrinol* 2020; 36(1): 12–23.

39 Zhu, S., Zhang, B., Jiang, X. et al. Metabolic disturbances in non-obese women with polycystic ovary syndrome: A systematic review and meta-analysis. *Fertil Steril* 2019; 111(1): 168–177.

40 Fu, X., Xu, J., Zhang, R. and Yu, J. The association between environmental endocrine disruptors and cardiovascular diseases: A systematic review and meta-analysis. *Environ Res* 2020; 187: 109464.

41 Li, R., Yang, S., Gao, R. et al. Relationship between the environmental endocrine disruptor bisphenol a and dyslipidemia: A five-year prospective study. *Endocr Pract* 2020; 26(4): 399–406.

42 Akin, L., Kendirci, M., Narin, F., Kurtoglu, S., Hatipoglu, N. and Elmali, F. Endocrine disruptors and polycystic ovary syndrome: Phthalates. *J Clin Res Pediatr Endocrinol*; 2020; 12(4): 393–400.

43 Baye, E., Kiriakova, V., Uribarri, J., Moran, L. J. and de Courten, B. Consumption of diets with low advanced glycation end products improves cardiometabolic parameters: Meta-analysis of randomised controlled trials. *Sci Rep* 2017; 7(1): 2266.

44 Kakoly, N.S., Moran, L. J., Teede, H. J. and Joham, A. E. Cardiometabolic risks in PCOS: A review of the current state of knowledge. *Expert Rev Endocrinol Metab* 2019; 14(1): 23–33.

Chapter 10

Lifestyle in Polycystic Ovary Syndrome

Rhonda Garad, Siew Lim, and Lisa Moran

In the recent international guideline on polycystic ovary syndrome (PCOS), healthy lifestyle behaviors and weight management (prevention of excess weight gain, modest weight loss and weight maintenance) are recommended for all girls and women diagnosed with PCOS as the first-line treatment. Current studies indicate a range of health benefits with weight and lifestyle management, including improved reproductive and metabolic health, optimized hormonal outcomes, improved emotional well-being and enhanced quality of life.

Health practitioners play a critical role in the provision of evidence-based, targeted and individualized information and support to optimize healthy lifestyle behaviors across the lifespan. Healthy lifestyle behaviors facilitated through education, self-empowerment and multidisciplinary care for the prevention or management of excess weight are important in improving health outcomes.

This chapter provides guidance on the benefits of multicomponent lifestyle interventions (comprising diet, physical activity and behavioral therapy) and weight management for women affected by PCOS. It also highlights the role of health literacy on social and information supports to motivate, engage and sustain health lifestyle behaviors in affected women.

Introduction

PCOS is a common and complex endocrine disorder impacting reproductive, metabolic and psychological features and affecting between 8% and 13% of reproductive-aged women [1]. PCOS is a highly heritable condition, with phenotypic heterogeneity in reproductive, metabolic and psychological features.[2] The etiology is currently considered to be an interplay of genetic and environmental factors that may be mediated by optimal lifestyle behaviors.[3]

The heterogeneity in the expression of PCOS creates challenges in the assessment and management of affected women and for health systems that are fragmented into specialty silos. Women report difficulties in achieving a timely diagnosis as the condition extends beyond the boundaries of medical specialty areas.[4] Overdiagnosis is also a concern following the adoption of the Rotterdam criteria; however, explicit guidance in the recent PCOS Guideline (2018) on diagnosis in adolescents, has largely addressed this issue.[5] PCOS treatment is also complex as practitioners address the range of symptoms presented.

Lifestyle is fundamental in chronic disease prevention and management, and it has been recommended as a first-line treatment for girls and women with PCOS.[5] Best practice models of care indicate that an integrated and multidisciplinary team approach provides optimal care outcomes.[6] Lifestyle interventions are central to effective PCOS management, with a focus on weight management (weight gain prevention, modest weight loss where required and weight maintenance) and sustained healthy lifestyle (diet and physical activity) behaviors.[7]

This chapter is based on recommendations in the international evidence-based guideline for the assessment and management of polycystic ovary syndrome 2018.[5] The lifestyle recommendations were formed by a lifestyle guideline development group that included multidisciplinary, international experts. The development process followed the Appraisal of Guidelines for Research and Evaluation II and the Grading of Recommendations, Assessment, Development and Evaluation frameworks. Extensive communication and meetings addressed six prioritized clinical questions through five reviews. Evidence-based recommendations were formulated before consensus voting within the panel. Evidence shows the benefits of multicomponent lifestyle intervention, efficacy of exercise and weight-gain prevention with no specific diet recommended.

Lifestyle management is the first-line management in the intervention hierarchy in PCOS. Multicomponent lifestyle intervention, including diet, exercise and behavioral strategies, is central to PCOS management with a focus on weight and healthy lifestyle behaviors.

PCOS, Metabolic Health and Insulin Resistance

Women with PCOS suffer poor metabolic health, which is exacerbated by, but independent of, obesity. Glycemic clamp studies have reported women with PCOS have poor glucose homeostasis and insulin resistance (IR) with fasting hyperinsulinemia and higher insulin levels in response to an oral glucose load as well as a 25% reduction in insulin sensitivity.[2] Girls and women show early onset of risk factors of poor metabolic health such as a higher body mass index (BMI) in adolescence and rapid weight gain, central obesity, hypertension and poor glycemic control up to a decade earlier when compared to non-PCOS peers. IR is a principal driver of PCOS symptomatology and the reproductive features. It is present in the majority of women with PCOS in a form that is mechanistically distinct to obesity-associated IR.[2, 8] Weight gain can then exacerbate IR and the features and complications of PCOS. IR is also a precursor to chronic disease development such as risk factors for heart disease and type 2 diabetes. [5] Women with PCOS have higher prevalence of gestational diabetes, impaired glucose tolerance and type 2 diabetes with risk independent of, yet exacerbated by, obesity. Although pharmacological treatment, diet and physical activity do not normalize IR, lifestyle modification and weight management may improve the symptoms of PCOS through reducing IR.[5]

PCOS, Weight and Obesity

Women with PCOS are commonly overweight or obese, with excess weight exacerbating clinical features. Most women who seek treatment for PCOS are overweight or obese,[9] with rates of weight gain appearing to be higher in women with PCOS. Studies have found that BMI increases of 1 kg/ht2 are associated with a 9% higher prevalence of PCOS.[7] Excess weight in women with PCOS starts at an earlier age, increases at a greater rate and is commonly centrally located, when compared to women without PCOS. Weight and higher rates of weight gain result from a combination of genetic susceptibility and lifestyle. Obesity influences the phenotypic expression of PCOS, exacerbating metabolic, reproductive and psychological features.[10]

Women and girls with PCOS are at higher risk of a high BMI trajectory, which is strongly correlated with gestational diabetes mellitus (GDM) and other long-term weight-related health sequelae.[11] They have a higher BMI at an earlier age when compared to a non-PCOS population and have increased rates of weight gain and greater prevalence of excess weight.[7] A systematic review reported that excess weight, obesity and central obesity had significant effects on reproductive, metabolic and psychological features of PCOS.[12] The authors found that overweight or obese women with PCOS had decreased sex hormone-binding globulin (SHBG), increased total testosterone, free androgen index, hirsutism, fasting glucose, fasting insulin, homeostatic model assessment-insulin resistance index and worsened lipid profile. Furthermore, obesity significantly worsened all metabolic and reproductive outcomes measured, except for hirsutism, when compared to normal-weight women with PCOS, and central obesity was associated with higher fasting insulin levels.

Women with PCOS are at greater risk of obesity. However, the complex pathophysiology and clinical heterogeneity of PCOS has hindered a clear understanding of interactions between PCOS, excess body weight and body fat distribution. Obesity, particularly central obesity, increases IR and hyperandrogenism, may increase PCOS prevalence and exacerbates the clinical features of PCOS. It is also of significant concern to women with PCOS and a key target for prevention and management in this condition. The degree of increased risk of excess weight and the impact on prevalence and severity of features of PCOS remain unclear.

Regular weight monitoring (considering ethnic-specific BMI and waist circumference) is recommended for all women with PCOS. In addition to weight monitoring, weight management through lifestyle interventions is also recommended with a focus initially on weight-gain prevention and maintenance. Women within the unhealthy weight or obese weight range should be encouraged to lose 5–10% of their total body weight (often a few kilos). To achieve weight loss, reducing calorific intake by 30%, or 500–750 kcal/day (1200 to 1500 kcal/day

93

Table 10.1 Recommendations: obesity and weight assessment

CCR Health professionals and women should be aware that women with PCOS have a higher prevalence of weight gain and obesity, presenting significant concerns for women, impacting on health and emotional well-being, with a clear need for prevention.

CCR All those with PCOS should be offered regular monitoring for weight changes and excess weight.

CPP When assessing weight, related stigma, negative body image and/or low self-esteem need to be considered and assessment needs to be respectful and considerate. Beforehand, explanations on the purpose and how the information will be used and the opportunity for questions and preferences need to be provided, permission sought and scales and tape measures adequate. Implications of results need to be explained and where this impacts on emotional well-being, support provided.

CPP Prevention of weight gain, monitoring of weight and encouraging evidence-based and socioculturally appropriate healthy lifestyle is important in PCOS, particularly from adolescence.

Note. Categories of the PCOS Guideline recommendations: CCR, Clinical Consensus Recommendation; CCP, Clinical Practice Point.

intake total), could be recommended for these women. There is also a need to consider individual energy requirements, body weight and physical activity levels when recommending energy restrictions (Table 10.1).

Healthy Lifestyle Behaviors

Healthy lifestyle behaviors encompass healthy eating, regular physical activity and behavioral strategies that can support achieving healthy diet and physical activity. Prior to the recent publication of the PCOS Guideline (2018), there was considerable uncertainty on effectiveness and optimal components of lifestyle intervention for affected girls and women. Here we elaborate on a multicomponent approach to healthy lifestyle behaviors that includes dietary interventions, lifestyle management, behavioral components of lifestyle interventions, behavioral interventions and exercise interventions.

Dietary Interventions

No one specific diet has been found to be more beneficial for women with PCOS. A general, balanced healthy diet is recommended, with energy

restriction if women have a BMI in the unhealthy weight range. The Australian dietary guidelines recommend a varied diet comprised of core foods (vegetables and legumes/beans; fruit; grain (cereal) foods mostly wholegrain and/or high cereal fiber varieties; lean meats and poultry, fish, eggs, nuts and seeds; and milk, yogurt, cheese and/or alternatives) and to limit discretionary foods (foods high in saturated fat such as many biscuits, cakes, pastries, pies, processed meats, commercial burgers, pizzas, fried foods, potato chips, crisps and other savory snacks).[9] There are a number of benefits in recommending general healthy eating principles such as lower cost, ease of access to a variety of foods and not having to prepare separate meals for other members of the household. Additionally, women are more likely to adhere to a general healthy diet over the life course compared to those on strict dietary plans.

The limited studies that have compared different diets in women with PCOS have generally found no difference in anthropometric, metabolic, fertility and non-fertility outcomes or quality of life and emotional well-being outcomes. However, the overall findings were that a diet aimed at reducing weight was of benefit to women with PCOS. These findings are consistent with studies in the general population that show no benefit of any one diet type long-term but that a reduction in overall energy intake resulting in weight reduction has health benefits in women who are overweight.

While no one diet was found to be of benefit, there is evidence that multidisciplinary support in adolescences may contribute to positive outcomes such as short-term weight stabilization and weight loss.[10] In managing PCOS, interactions with a range of practitioners, such as health psychologists and dietitians, appear to be important in successful weight control, addressing emotional well-being and providing nutritional expertise. It is also important that dietary plans are individualized and flexible enough to take into consideration individual food preferences, cultural requirements and socioeconomic factors. Practitioners need to avoid recommending overly restrictive or unbalanced diets as women with PCOS are at increased risk of disordered eating (Table 10.2).[13]

Lifestyle Management

Health professionals should advise all patients with PCOS to adopt healthy lifestyle behaviors that

Table 10.2 Recommendations: dietary intervention

CCR	A variety of balanced dietary approaches could be recommended to reduce dietary energy intake and induce weight loss in women with PCOS and excess weight and obesity, as per general population recommendations.
CCR	General healthy eating principles should be followed for all women with PCOS across the life course, as per general population recommendations.
CPP	To achieve weight loss in those with excess weight, an energy deficit of 30% or 500–750 kcal/day (1200 to 1500 kcal/day) could be prescribed for women, also considering individual energy requirements, body weight and physical activity levels.
CPP	In women with PCOS, there is no or limited evidence that any specific energy equivalent diet type is better than another, or that there is any differential response to weight management intervention, compared to women without PCOS.
CPP	Tailoring of dietary changes to food preferences, allowing for a flexible and individual approach to reducing energy intake and avoiding unduly restrictive and nutritionally unbalanced diets, are important, as per general population recommendations.

Note. Categories of the PCOS Guideline recommendations: CCR, Clinical Consensus Recommendation; CCP, Clinical Practice Point.

include healthy eating and regular physical activity. A team-based approach with referrals to allied health professionals (including dietary and exercise specialists and psychologists) where required is also highly recommended. Given the heterogeneity in the expression of PCOS, a range of expertise is required to meet the needs of affected women. A best practice approach includes (but is not limited to) a multidisciplinary model of care, including health providers such as general practitioners, gynecologists, endocrinologists, exercise physiologists, dietitians and psychologists.

When supporting women and girls with PCOS, health professionals need to be sensitive to the individual circumstances and social contexts of their patients. Issues such as personal sensitivities, social marginalization and weight-related stigma are ideally managed using an individualized, patient-centered care approach. The features of PCOS can be particularly difficult for young women. For example, increased body hair, particularly on the face, can negatively impact body image

and lead to fear of social disapproval. In addition, acne may be severe and may reduce social confidence and lead to poor body image. Girls and women with PCOS may also have experienced, or fear, weight-related stigma. International guidelines highlight the importance of avoiding stigmatization and managing the psychological aspects of weight management, such as improving self-esteem, body image and quality of life.[14] Health practitioners who employ a strengths-based and empowerment approach are likely to observe a higher level of patient engagement. Women with PCOS report the same motivators to exercise as the general population, such as weight control, health improvements, increased energy, stress reduction and health maintenance.[15]

While women with PCOS have similar motivators, they report both common and unique barriers to the uptake and sustaining of exercise regimes.[15] Common barriers include a lack of time and fatigue when exercising. Unique barriers, when compared to women without PCOS, are a lack of confidence regarding their ability to maintain exercise and fear of injury and physical limitations. Health resources and supports need to recognize and address these unique barriers to encourage commencement and perseverance in affected women, as well as titrating exercise regimes in close partnership, which is likely to maintain engagement.

Recommended lifestyle modifications need also to be accommodating of cultural, socioeconomic and health literacy considerations. Cultural taboos such as discussing or acknowledging the presence of health issues, particularly a health condition such as PCOS that encompasses reproductive health, may create barriers to open communication and engagement. Furthermore, lack of agency on dietary choices and/or exercise regimes needs to be sensitively managed. Additionally, financial constraints may mean gym memberships or purchase of specialist support services may not be possible for some patients. Working with patients to accommodate cultural and socioeconomic contexts will achieve better outcomes.[16]

Behavioral Components of Lifestyle Interventions

Use of effective behavior modification strategies are also important both to build the PCOS health literacy of patients and to achieve sustained lifestyle changes. It is also recommended that affected women use SMART (Specific, Measurable, Achievable, Realistic and Timely) goal-setting and self-monitoring. It is important to set achievable lifestyle goals to build the confidence of women with PCOS in goal attainment. Realistic goals include small weight loss of 5–10% in those with excess weight that results in significant clinical improvements. Health professionals can assist patients in understanding the link between improved lifestyle changes and symptom reduction and improvements in outcome measures (reproductive, metabolic and psychological). Improved PCOS health literacy is linked to sustained lifestyle changes over the longer term.[16]

Further studies show that combining behavioral and cognitive behavioral weight-loss components with intensive interventions, including very low calorie diets and weight-loss medications, also improves weight loss more than these interventions alone.[19–21] Guidelines highlight the need for resources (e.g. written, audiovisual) and the potential for e-health to supplement face-to-face support, with strategies including goal-setting, self-monitoring, stimulus control, problem-solving, assertiveness training, slowing the rate of eating, reinforcing changes and relapse prevention. Continued contact after treatment (face-to-face or telephone) also improves weight-loss maintenance. More intensive behavioral interventions induce greater weight loss.[22] In the general population, behavioral and cognitive behavioral interventions have strong empirical support and are recommended in international guidelines on the treatment of excess weight.

It is essential that health professionals consider that affected girls and women have increased barriers to the adoption of healthy lifestyle behaviors. Barriers such as heightened perceived stress, body dissatisfaction, low self-esteem, disordered eating, anxiety and depression could undermine their engagement with lifestyle intervention.[13, 17, 18] Health practitioners additionally need to monitor the emotional well-being and psychological health of their patients and provide education on the link between healthy lifestyle and improved emotional well-being. Referral of women for psychological support and encouraging them to seek social support may assist in engagement and adherence to lifestyle interventions. Lifestyle management relies on women with PCOS being informed, equipped and supported. Unfortunately, the literature indicates that women's needs in these areas are often unmet by their healthcare experiences and the information available (Table 10.3).

Behavioral Interventions

To improve adherence and engagement in lifestyle interventions, behavioral strategies to optimize weight management, healthy lifestyle and emotional well-being may be effective. Women are likely to also benefit from support in developing a range of skills such as goal-setting, self-monitoring, stimulus control, problem-solving, assertiveness training, slower eating, reinforcing changes and relapse prevention.

In addition, referral to practitioners to provide comprehensive health behavioral or cognitive behavioral interventions could be considered to increase support, engagement, retention, adherence and maintenance to a healthy lifestyle and improving health outcomes in women with PCOS. Guidelines highlight the need for accessible resources and the potential for e-health to augment face-to-face support with strategies, including goal-setting, self-monitoring, stimulus control, problem-solving, assertiveness training, slowing the rate of eating, reinforcing changes and relapse prevention. Ongoing support following or in tandem with treatment also improves weight-loss maintenance. More intensive behavioral interventions induce greater weight loss.[19] In the general population, behavioral and cognitive behavioral interventions are supported by evidence and are recommended in international guidelines on the treatment of excess weight (Table 10.4).

Exercise Interventions

Regular exercise provides a range of beneficial outcomes in girls and women with PCOS, such as weight management and excess weight prevention, optimized hormonal outcomes, improved emotional well-being and enhanced quality of life.[5] Unfortunately, there are few high-quality studies exploring the type of exercise that best targets the clinical features of PCOS.[20] However, exercise and physical activity have been shown to impact cardiometabolic and reproductive features of PCOS.[21–23] Additionally, there is moderately strong evidence to show important clinical improvements induced by exercise interventions on cardiovascular risk factors, glycemic control, biomarkers of reproductive health, quality of life and functional

Table 10.3 Recommendations: lifestyle interventions

CCR   Healthy lifestyle behaviors encompassing healthy eating and regular physical activity should be recommended in all those with PCOS to achieve and/or maintain healthy weight and to optimize hormonal outcomes, general health and quality of life across the life course.

EBR   Lifestyle intervention (preferably multicomponent, including diet, exercise and behavioral strategies) should be recommended in all those with PCOS and excess weight, for reductions in weight, central obesity and insulin resistance (IR).

CPP   Achievable goals should be set, such as 5–10% weight loss in those with excess weight, which yields significant clinical improvements and is considered successful weight reduction within six months. Ongoing assessment and monitoring are important during weight loss and maintenance in all women with PCOS.

CPP   SMART (Specific, Measurable, Achievable, Realistic and Timely) goal-setting and self-monitoring can enable achievement of realistic lifestyle goals.

CPP   Psychological factors, such as anxiety and depressive symptoms, body image concerns and disordered eating, need consideration and management to optimize engagement and adherence to lifestyle interventions.

CPP   Health professional interactions around healthy lifestyle, including diet and exercise, need to be respectful, patient-centered and value women's individualized healthy lifestyle preferences and cultural, socioeconomic and ethnic differences. Health professionals need to also consider personal sensitivities, marginalization and potential weight-related stigma.

CPP   Adolescent and ethnic-specific BMI and waist circumference categories need to be considered when optimizing lifestyle and weight.

CPP   Healthy lifestyle may contribute to health and quality-of-life benefits in the absence of weight loss.

CPP   Healthy lifestyle and optimal weight management appear equally effective in PCOS as in the general population and are the joint responsibility of all health professionals partnering with women with PCOS. Where complex issues arise, referral to suitably trained allied health professionals needs to be considered.

CPP   Ethnic groups with PCOS who are at high cardiometabolic risk require greater consideration in terms of healthy lifestyle and lifestyle intervention.

Note. Categories of the PCOS Guideline recommendations: CCR, Clinical Consensus Recommendation; CCP, Clinical Practice Point; EBR, Evidence-based recommendation.

Table 10.4 Recommendations: behavioral strategies

CCR   Lifestyle interventions could include behavioral strategies such as goal-setting, self-monitoring, stimulus control, problem-solving, assertiveness training, slower eating, reinforcing changes and relapse prevention, to optimize weight management, healthy lifestyle and emotional well-being in women with PCOS.

CPP   Comprehensive health behavioral or cognitive behavioral interventions could be considered to increase support, engagement, retention, adherence and maintenance to a healthy lifestyle and improving health outcomes in women with PCOS.

capacities (aerobic fitness, maximal strength) when compared to minimal or no treatment. Other studies show that vigorous and sustained exercise is associated with better health outcomes and reduces the risk of the onset of chronic disease.

In the general population, evidence shows physical activity and structured exercise deliver clear health benefits. It is assumed these benefits apply to women with PCOS. Conversely, sedentary behaviors have been shown to be detrimental in the general population and are likely to exacerbate IR in women with PCOS. Other exercise studies conducted in a non-PCOS population reported physical activity, including formal exercise (aerobic and muscle-strengthening), improves body composition and clinical features compared to little or no exercise.[22] Specific exercise recommendations for adult women with PCOS are:

- For women wanting to maintain weight: 150 or more minutes per week of moderate exercise or 75 or more minutes per week of vigorous exercise – including weight-training activities.

- For women wanting to lose weight: 250 or more minutes per week of moderate exercise or 150 or more minutes per week of vigorous exercise – including two weight-training activities per week.

Unfortunately, despite the benefits of exercise in girls and women with PCOS, affected women report difficulty in accessing support and information that address their particular needs, such as unique barriers to exercising.[15] As women with PCOS may be focused on weight loss, it is important for health practitioners to stress the many benefits of exercise that may or may not include weight loss. The key points listed in the

Table 10.5 Recommendations: exercise intervention

CCR Health professionals should encourage and advise the following for prevention of weight gain and maintenance of health: in adults from 18 to 64 years, a minimum of 150 minutes/week of moderate-intensity physical activity or 75 minutes/week of vigorous intensity or an equivalent combination of both, including muscle-strengthening activities on 2 nonconsecutive days/week; in adolescents, at least 60 minutes of moderate to vigorous intensity physical activity/day, including activities that strengthen muscle and bone at least 3 times weekly – activity should be performed in at least 10-minute bouts or around 1 000 steps, aiming to achieve at least 30 minutes daily on most days.

CCR Health professionals should encourage and advise the following for modest weight loss, prevention of weight-regain and greater health benefits: a minimum of 250 minutes/week of moderate-intensity physical activity or 150 minutes/week of vigorous intensity activity or an equivalent combination of both, as well as muscle-strengthening activities involving major muscle groups on 2 non-consecutive days/week and minimizing sedentary, screen or sitting time.

CPP Physical activity includes leisure-time physical activity, transportation such as walking or cycling, occupational work, household chores, games, sports or planned exercise, in the context of daily, family and community activities. Daily, 10000 steps is ideal, including activities of daily living, and 30 minutes of structured physical activity or around 3000 steps. Structuring of recommended activities needs to consider women's and family routines as well as cultural preferences.

CPP Realistic physical activity SMART (Specific, Measurable, Achievable, Relevant and Timely) goals could include 10-minute bouts, progressively increasing physical activity by 5% weekly, up to and above recommendations.

CPP Self-monitoring, including with fitness tracking devices and technologies for step counts and exercise intensity, could be used as an adjunct to support and promote active lifestyles and minimize sedentary behaviors.

following section provide a range of key messages that may motivate girls and women to commence and sustain an exercise regime (see also Table 10.5).[1]

---

[1] See the PCOS and Lifestyle factsheet (Figure 10.1), which is also freely available as part of Monash's "Resources for Women with PCOS": www.monash.edu/medicine/sphpm/mchri/pcos/resources/resources-for-women-with-pcos.

Key Messages to Women and Girls with PCOS

Key messages for girls and women with PCOS that address identified motivators and barriers to commencing and sustaining an exercise regime are:

- Any physical activity is better than no activity.
- Start at a pace that you are comfortable with and slowly increase.
- Regular exercise improves PCOS symptoms and can improve your mood.
- If you have health concerns, talk to your doctor before commencing an exercise regime.
- Take control of you exercise plan and make adjustments in consultation with health professionals.
- Sitting and/or being inactive for long periods of time can worsen symptoms.
- Regular, moderate-intensity exercise is likely to result in a range of health benefits.
- To maintain your weight, do 150 or more minutes per week of moderate exercise or 75 or more minutes per week of vigorous exercise – include weight-training activities.
- To lose weight, do 250 or more minutes per week of moderate exercise or 150 or more minutes per week of vigorous exercise – include 2 weight-training activities per week.
- Get the support of an exercise physiologist or fitness expert for guidance and encouragement.
- Exercise will help you maintain your weight and prevent weight gain.
- Keep an exercise diary that includes changes in symptoms, energy and mood.

Health Literacy and PCOS

Health literacy is associated with obesity, poorer dietary intake and reduced physical activity.[24] It is "the cognitive and social skills which determine the motivation and ability of individuals to gain access to, understand and use information in ways which promote and maintain good health."[25] Women and girls with PCOS are at higher risk of being overweight and obese, which may be an outcome of both physiological and psychological factors.

Health literacy is also a determinant of health outcomes and is strongly linked to empowerment and self-efficacy.[26] These concepts are highly relevant to women with PCOS who need to manage their condition across the lifespan. Increased

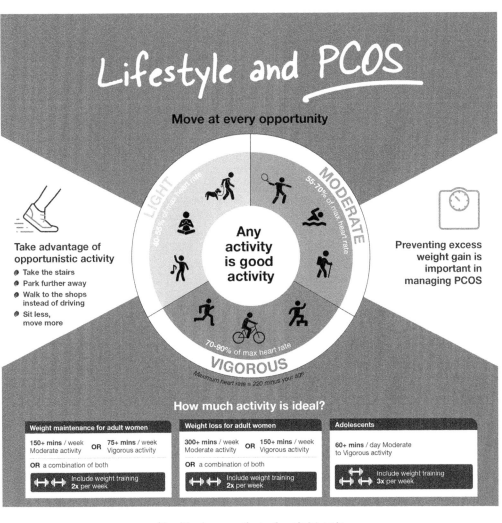

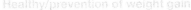

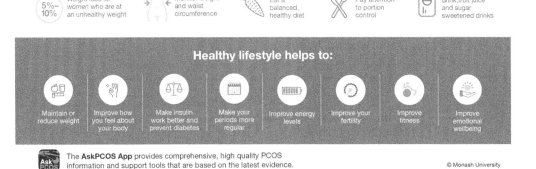

Figure 10.1 Lifestyle and PCOS
Source. Reprinted with permission from the copyright holder Monash University and the Monash Centre for Health Research and Implementation.

levels of health literacy in girls and women with PCOS are likely to result in stronger engagement with a range of health professionals and lead to better health outcomes. Also, it is important to understand that health literacy is context-dependent, so girls and women with high levels of health literacy may still struggle to manage a long-term condition such as PCOS and will require targeted and individualized support.[27]

Health literacy is enhanced through access to targeted, relevant and accessible information. Women and girls with PCOS report difficulty finding high-quality, accessible PCOS information. Health practitioners can enhance the health literacy of their patients by directing them to evidence-based PCOS resources and use of the teach-back method to check patients' knowledge and understanding. [27] In addition, tools such as a "question prompt list," [28] or an evidence-based PCOS app,[29] can increase health literacy and enhance self-care.[2]

The Role of Support Groups

Where possible girls and women with PCOS should be directed to peer-to-peer or facilitated PCOS support groups. Evidence shows that women exchange information and derive desired emotional and social support from support groups. They also report a range of benefits such as confidence in managing their condition and having greater agency in their healthcare.[30] Peer support is also useful for the self-management of chronic conditions by providing time, rehearsal and problem-solving around key health behaviors, as well as emotional and social support and encouragement.[31] Ideally, support groups should have partnerships with healthcare providers to ensure accuracy in the information being shared. There are a number of online support groups and face-to-face groups. Women should ensure these groups are guided by the best available evidence.

Conclusion

PCOS is a common and complex endocrine condition. Its heterogeneous expression creates diagnostic, treatment and management challenges for both health professionals and affected women. Despite the significant health burden of PCOS, women report delayed diagnosis and unsatisfactory information and support provision. In particular, they report difficulties in accessing clear guidance and ongoing support on necessary lifestyle changes.

More high-quality evidence is needed to fully understand the spectrum of health benefits of an optimized lifestyle in girls and women with PCOS. Encouragingly, current studies indicate a range of health benefits such as weight management, improved reproductive and metabolic health, optimized hormonal outcomes, improved emotional well-being and enhanced quality of life.

Health practitioners play a critical role in the provision of evidence-based, targeted and individualized information and support to optimize healthy lifestyle behaviors across the lifespan. Best practice models of care indicate that an integrated, multidisciplinary team approach provides optimal care outcomes. Lifestyle interventions are central to effective PCOS management, with a focus on weight management (weight-gain prevention, modest weight loss where required and weight maintenance) and sustained healthy lifestyle (diet and physical activity) behaviors.

References

1 Bozdag, G., Mumusoglu, S., Zengin, D., Karabulut, E. and Yildiz, B. O. The prevalence and phenotypic features of polycystic ovary syndrome: A systematic review and meta-analysis. *Hum Reprod* 2016; 31(12): 2841.

2 Stepto, N. K., Moreno-Asso, A., McIlvenna, L. C., Walters, K. A. and Rodgers, R. J. Molecular mechanisms of insulin resistance in polycystic ovary syndrome: Unraveling the conundrum in skeletal muscle? *J Clin Endocrinol Metab* 2019; 104(11): 5372.

3 Azziz, R., Kintziger, K., Li, R. et al. Recommendations for epidemiologic and phenotypic research in polycystic ovary syndrome: An androgen excess and PCOS society resource. *Hum Reprod* 2019; 34(11): 2254–2265.

4 Gibson-Helm, M., Teede, H., Dunaif, A. and Dokras, A. Delayed diagnosis and a lack of information associated with dissatisfaction in women with polycystic ovary syndrome. *J Clin Endocrinol Metab* 2017; 102(2): 604–612.

5 Teede, H., Misso, M., Costello, M. et al. *International Evidence-Based Guideline for the Assessment and Management of Polycystic Ovary Syndrome (PCOS)*. Melbourne: Monash University, 2018.

6 Tay, C., Moran, L., Wijeyaratne, C. et al. Integrated model of care for polycystic ovary syndrome. *Semin Reprod Med* 2018; 36(1): 86–94.

---

[2] High-quality PCOS resources are freely available as part of Monash's "Resources for Women with PCOS" toolkit: www.monash.edu/medicine/sphpm/mchri/pcos/resources/resources-for-women-with-pcos.

7   Teede, H. J. et al. Longitudinal weight gain in women identified with polycystic ovary syndrome: Results of an observational study in young women. *Obesity*. 2013; 21(8): 1526–1532.

8   Cassar, S., Misso, M. L., Hopkins, W. G., Shaw, C. S., Teede, H. J. and Stepto, N. K. Insulin resistance in polycystic ovary syndrome: A systematic review and meta-analysis of euglycaemic–hyperinsulinaemic clamp studies. *Hum Reprod* 2016; 31(11): 2619–2631.

9   National Health and Medical Research Council. *Australian Dietary Guidelines*. Canberra: National Health and Medical Research Council, 2013.

10 Geier, L. M., Bekx, M. T. and Connor, E. L. Factors contributing to initial weight loss among adolescents with polycystic ovary syndrome. *J Pediatr Adolesc Gynecol* 2012; 25(6): 367–370.

11 Kakoly, N. S., Earnest, A., Moran, L. J., Teede, H. J. and Joham, A. E. Group-based developmental BMI trajectories, polycystic ovary syndrome, and gestational diabetes: A community-based longitudinal study. *BMC Med* 2017; 15(1): 195.

12 Lim, S. S., Norman, R. J., Davies, M. J. and Moran, L. J. The effect of obesity on polycystic ovary syndrome: A systematic review and meta-analysis. *Obes Rev* 2013; 14(2): 95–109.

13 Tay, C. T., Teede, H. J., Hill, B., Loxton, D. and Joham, A. E. Increased prevalence of eating disorders, low self-esteem, and psychological distress in women with polycystic ovary syndrome: A community-based cohort study. *Fertil Steril* 2019; 112(2): 353–361.

14 Durrer Schutz, D., Busetto, L., Dicker, D. et al. European practical and patient-centred guidelines for adult obesity management in primary care. *Obes Facts* 2019; 12(1): 40–66.

15 Banting, L. K., Gibson-Helm, M., Polman, R., Teede, H. J. and Stepto, N. K. Physical activity and mental health in women with polycystic ovary syndrome. *BMC Women's Health* 2014; 14(1): 51.

16 Beauchamp, A., Batterham, R. W., Dodson, S. et al. Systematic development and implementation of interventions to OPtimise HEalth LIteracy and Access (Ophelia). *BMC Public Health*. 2017; 17(1): 230.

17 Teede, H., Deeks, A, L. M. Polycystic ovary syndrome: A complex condition with psychological, reproductive and metabolic manifestations that impacts on health across the lifespan. *BMC Med* 2010; 8(1): 41.

18 Damone, A. L., Joham, A. E., Loxton, D., Earnest, A., Teede, H. J. and Moran, L. J. Depression, anxiety and perceived stress in women with and without PCOS: A community-based study. *Psychol Med* 2019; 49(9): 1510.

19 Shaw, K., et al. Psychological interventions for overweight or obesity. *Cochrane Database of Syst Rev* 2005; (2).

20 Stepto, N., Patten, R. K., Tassone, E. C. et al. Exercise recommendations for women with Polycystic Ovary Syndrome: Is the evidence enough? *Sports Med* 2019; 49(8): 1143–1157.

21 Haqq, L., McFarlane, J., Dieberg, G. and Smart, N. Effect of lifestyle intervention on the reproductive endocrine profile in women with polycystic ovarian syndrome: A systematic review and meta-analysis. *Endocr Connect* 2014; 3(1): 36–46.

22 Haqq, L., McFarlane, J., Dieberg, G. and Smart, N. The effect of lifestyle intervention on body composition, glycemic control, and cardiorespiratory fitness in polycystic ovarian syndrome: A systematic review and meta-analysis. *Int J Sport Nutr Exerc Metab* 2015; 25(6): 533–540.

23 Harrison, C. L., Lombard, C. B., Moran, L. J. and Teede, H. J. Exercise therapy in polycystic ovary syndrome: A systematic review. *Hum Reprod Update*. 2011; 17(2): 171–183.

24 Garad, R., McPhee, C., Chai, T. L., Moran, L., O'Reilly, S. and Lim, S. The role of health literacy in postpartum weight, diet, and physical activity. *J Clin Med*. 2020; 9(8).

25 WHO (World Health Organization). *Health Promotion Glossary*. Geneva: WHO, 1998.

26 Osborne, R. H., Beauchamp, A. and Batterham, R. Health literacy: A concept with potential to greatly impact the infectious diseases field. *Int J Infect* 2016; 43: 101–102.

27 Yen, P. H. and Leasure, A. R. Use and effectiveness of the teach-back method in patient education and health outcomes. *Fed Pract* 2019; 36(6): 284–289.

28 Khan, N. N., Vincent, A., Boyle, J. A. et al Development of a question prompt list for women with polycystic ovary syndrome. *Fertil Steril* 2018; 110(3): 514–522.

29 Xie, J., Burstein, F., Garad, R., Teede, H. and Boyle, J. Personalized mobile tool AskPCOS delivering evidence-based quality information about polycystic ovary syndrome. *Semin Reprod Med* 2018; 36(1): 66–72.

30 Avery, J., Ottey, S., Morman, R., Cree-Green, M. and Gibson-Helm, M. Polycystic ovary syndrome support groups and their role in awareness, advocacy and peer support: A systematic search and narrative review. *Curr Opinion Endocr Metab Res* 2020; 12: 98–104.

31 Duggan, M., Chislett, W. and Calder, R. The *State of Self-Care in Australia*. Melbourne: Australian Health Policy Collaboration (AHPC), 2017.

Ovulation Induction in Polycystic Ovary Syndrome

Evert J. P. van Santbrink

Introduction

Chronic oligo- or anovulation is a major problem for women seeking pregnancy. This is reflected by the fact that about 20% of patients visiting a fertility clinic present with anovulation. The majority (about 80%) of these patients will meet the criteria for polycystic ovary syndrome (PCOS), as captured and agreed in the international Rotterdam consensus conference and modified in 2003 (see also Chapter 5).[1] Altogether, this results in PCOS being the most common hormonal disorder in women.

When the diagnosis PCOS is determined after ruling out other causes of anovulation like hyperprolactinemia, hypo- or hyperthyroidism or adrenal pathology (Cushing's syndrome and congenital adrenal hyperplasia), this may be followed by treatment, which, in case of a wish to conceive, in the first place should be restoration of normal physiology, that is, selection and growth of a single dominant follicle resulting in mono-ovulation. This description meets the definition of *ovulation induction* and should not be confused with alternative ovarian-stimulation protocols pursuing a different goal such as "controlled ovarian hyperstimulation" as used for in vitro fertilization (IVF).

The PCOS patient group is a very heterogeneous population in which, next to anovulation, obesity, biochemical or clinical hyperandrogenism (alopecia, acne or hirsutism) and insulin resistance may also play an important role. The Rotterdam PCOS consensus criteria even broadened the definition compared to the National Institutes of Health (NIH) criteria: patients with anovulation and polycystic ovary morphology but without hyperandrogenism are included. As hyperandrogenism is considered by some as one of the main characteristics of PCOS, it is not surprising that this resulted in an extensive and ongoing debate, which may only be concluded when it is possible to add a descriptive genotype to the definition of PCOS (see also Chapter 2). This heterogeneity of the PCOS population may explain the various effective treatment approaches possible for ovulation induction, which are discussed in this chapter.

Interventions

The clinical manifestation of anovulation is oligomenorrhea (intermenstrual period > 35 days) or amenorrhea (intermenstrual period > 6 months). Although ovulation may occur in oligomenorrhea, the longer the time period between menstruation, the smaller the chance of that cycle being ovulatory. The primary aim of treatment in PCOS patients trying to conceive is restoration of a regular mono-ovulatory menstrual cycle.

Lifestyle Interventions

The first intervention offered to the individual or couple who present with anovulatory infertility should be optimization of health and lifestyle (as discussed in Chapters 10 and 16). This counseling could encompass advice on diet, exercise, smoking cessation and other patient-specific risk factors. Moreover, a substantial number of PCOS patients struggle with obesity, which at least promotes the PCOS phenotype. Optimization of lifestyle and weight could improve the endocrine profile, the likelihood of ovulation occurring both naturally and in response to ovulation induction agents as well as the chance of having a healthy pregnancy. In addition, attention should be given to possible decreased emotional well-being and psychosexual function, as women with PCOS and subfertility may be more prone to this (see also Chapter 17).

Pharmacological Interventions

The general goal of all pharmacological interventions is to increase the action of follicle-stimulating hormone (FSH) at the receptor site. This may be done either by increasing the serum FSH concentration or by optimizing the FSH sensitivity of the ovaries. The most commonly used interventions are discussed in this section.

Aromatase Inhibitors

Third-generation aromatase inhibitors, such as letrozole and anastrozole, result in inhibition of aromatase activity by competitive binding to the heme of the cytochrome p450 subunit of the aromatase enzyme. Thus, it blocks the production of estrogen from the androgen precursor not only in the ovarian granulosa cells but also in other tissues. The lack of negative feedback of estrogen on the hypothalamic–pituitary level increases the pituitary release of gonadotropins and results in ovarian stimulation. A secondary working mechanism of aromatase inhibitors as an ovulation induction agent may be that they increase the availability of androgens in the ovary by inhibiting conversion of androgen to estrogen and thus improving sensitivity of the FSH receptor. The half-life of letrozole is approximately two days and considerably shorter compared to clomiphene citrate (CC) as discussed in the section "Anti-estrogens."

Aromatase inhibitors were initially used in a continuous protocol for breast cancer therapy and until now that has been their only registered indication. Despite that, the aromatase inhibitor letrozole has been used for ovulation induction since 2001 in a similar protocol as is used for CC: starting treatment on day 3 after a spontaneous or progesterone-induced withdrawal bleeding and continued for 5 days with a dose of 2.5 mg/day. In the case of persistent anovulation, the dose may be increased in two steps to a maximum of 7.5 mg/day. After 6–12 ovulatory treatment cycles without conception, usually second-line treatment is initiated.

After initial positive results with the use of letrozole for ovulation induction, the publication of a study on potential fetal toxicity in a comparison to CC resulted in a warning by the pharmaceutical company (Novartis Pharmaceuticals) not to use letrozole for this indication.[2] In follow-up studies (multiple case series, multicenter randomized controlled trials [RCTs] and a recent systematic review), this possible increased risk of

congenital anomalies could not be reproduced and the risk of letrozole was even lower or at least comparable to the reported risk of CC and the general population (5–8%).[3]

The reported risk for multiple pregnancy, abortion and ovarian hyperstimulation syndrome (OHSS) was no different for letrozole or CC (see Table 11.1). Side effects reported during use of aromatase inhibitors include gastrointestinal disturbances, hot flushes, headaches and back pain but are seldom a reason for discontinuation of treatment. The results of ovulation induction with letrozole as a first-line treatment in a PCOS population are a 75% ovulation rate, 36% clinical pregnancy rate and 31% cumulative live birth rate.[4]

In conclusion, letrozole is an effective first-line treatment intervention for ovulation induction in PCOS patients. With regard to safety, there seems to be no increased potential fetal toxicity with letrozole compared to CC or the general population. In many countries, letrozole is not registered for use as an ovulation induction agent (off-label use) so patients should be informed and should consent before prescription.

Anti-estrogens

Anti-estrogens, like CC and tamoxifen, act as nonselective estrogen receptor blockers thus interfering with the negative feedback of estrogens at the hypothalamic–pituitary level. This results in a rise in the pituitary release of gonadotropins, especially FSH, and thereby increased ovarian stimulation. The half-life of CC can vary between five days and three weeks, depending on the chosen clomiphene isomer predominance (clomiphene is a racemic mixture of enclomiphene and zuclomiphene). As CC occupies its receptor for such a prolonged period, this may have a negative effect of estrogen action on cervical mucus and the endometrium and cause decreased sperm penetration and survival during this period.[5] Treatment protocol, results and complications of CC and tamoxifen are comparable, but tamoxifen is rarely used for ovulation induction and consequently will not be further discussed in this chapter.

Like aromatase inhibitors, CC was initially used for breast cancer therapy but even its use for ovulation induction goes back to the early 1960s. Since then, it has been a first-line treatment choice for patients with chronic anovulation because it is effective, safe, patient-friendly,

103

cheap and is registered for ovulation induction in most countries.

As discussed, CC is generally started on day 3 after a spontaneous or progesterone-induced withdrawal bleeding and continued for 5 days with a dose of 50 mg/day. In the case of persistent anovulation, the dose may be increased in two steps to a maximum of 150 mg/day. Several studies reported an effect of the chosen starting day: when CC treatment was started on day 5 rather than day 3, this resulted in a decreased ovulation and pregnancy rate. In general, the use of CC for longer than 12 months is not recommended because there may be a possible increased risk for ovarian cancer,[6] and the chance of pregnancy decreases substantially after 12 ovulatory menstrual cycles without pregnancy.

Reported side effects are hot flushes and nausea especially on the days CC is used. This may sometimes be a reason to change treatment compound. Development of multiple follicles has been reported, often resulting in a multiple pregnancy rate of between 5% and 10%. Severe OHSS has not been reported following CC treatment. Treatment results with CC as a first-line treatment modality in PCOS patients are a 73% ovulation rate, 36% clinical pregnancy rate and a 29% live birth rate after 6 months of treatment.[7]

In conclusion, CC is an effective first-line treatment compound for ovulation induction in PCOS patients. It has been registered for this indication, is cheap, safe and has been used as such for a very long time. However, for some time now there has been debate on whether letrozole or CC should be the first-line choice in anovulation treatment of PCOS patients.[4]

Insulin Sensitizers

Insulin sensitizers used for ovulation induction in PCOS patients may not all have the same mechanism of action but they do have a common end point in improving serum glucose regulation. Metformin (a biguanide) reduces hepatic gluconeogenesis and insulin concentrations, while pioglitazone and rosiglitazone (thiazolidinediones) enhance glucose uptake in adipose and muscle tissue and decrease hepatic glucose output. Inositol (hydroxyl-cyclohexaan) is a nutritional supplement that increases the insulin signal in the intracellular milieu. Their common aim is to restore the endocrine milieu: decreasing insulin resistance and hyperandrogenism and normalizing ovarian FSH responsiveness and thereby promoting the restoration of ovulatory cycles.

Although insulin sensitizers were developed at first to treat patients with diabetes, as insulin resistance also plays an important role in the pathogenesis of PCOS, there is particular interest for their use in this patient group. Concomitant hyperandrogenism in PCOS patients may be explained by the fact that hyperinsulinemia increases ovarian androgen production and decreases sex hormone-binding globulin (SHBG) serum concentrations, resulting in an increased bioavailability of androgens. Moreover, hyperinsulinemia promotes estrogen hyper-responsiveness on ovarian FSH stimulation that induces FSH to drop (too) early. This may cause FSH-dependent follicle growth arrest in the early follicular phase and the classic polycystic morphology image of the ovaries on ultrasound.[8]

It may be no surprise that the most prominent benefit of insulin sensitizers for ovulation induction is reported in obese patients. This also stresses the role of weight reduction through lifestyle modification as a possible primary solution for this problem (see Chapters 10 and 16).

Of the insulin-sensitizing compounds used for ovulation induction, only metformin has been widely used and investigated since 1994 and therefore has the most reassuring safety profile. Alternative insulin sensitizers such as pioglitazone, rosiglitazone and inositol (myo-inositol or D-chiro-inositol) currently are reported in too few publications and thus there is too little evidence to draw any conclusions regarding their effectiveness for this indication.[9]

The treatment schedule of metformin is started as a daily dose of 2–3 × 500 mg to a maximum daily dose of 2 000 mg/day. It may take up to three months until the maximal effect has been reached. There is no reported benefit of metformin alone or in combination with CC compared to CC alone as a first-line treatment compound for ovulation induction in PCOS patients, but there may be a reported benefit for the addition of metformin to CC in patients remaining anovulatory during CC first-line treatment.[9] This effect will increase in a more obese population.[10]

Common side effects while using insulin sensitizers are gastrointestinal complaints: nausea, vomiting and diarrhea. These are ameliorated in most subjects when used over a longer period.

A very rare but more serious complication is lactic acidosis, which is only reported in patients with comorbidity (renal insufficiency, liver disease or congestive heart failure). Metformin may reduce the risk of gestational diabetes and it may be safe for use during pregnancy,[11] but convincing evidence is lacking.

In conclusion, no recommendation can be made for the use of metformin as a first-line treatment modality for ovulation induction in PCOS patients. In the case of persistent anovulation after the highest dose of CC, adding metformin is reported to improve treatment outcome.

Gonadotropins

In the ovarian theca cell, luteinizing hormone (LH) promotes conversion of cholesterol to androstenedione and testosterone, while subsequently FSH induces aromatization of these androgens in the ovarian granulosa cells to estrone and estradiol. Although in general both hormones are required for adequate follicle growth, in PCOS patients the amount of endogenous LH is sufficient to facilitate normal follicle growth and concomitant estrogen production while using exogenous FSH alone for ovarian stimulation.

The pituitary gonadotropins LH and FSH have been available for ovulation induction since the early 1960s. Back then, they were extracted from urine collected by postmenopausal women (human menopausal gonadotropin). Subsequently, purification was performed to remove nonactive proteins, resulting in highly purified urinary gonadotropin preparations. To assure the continuous availability of FSH, since the 1990s, recombinant DNA technology can be used to produce human recombinant FSH in Chinese hamster ovary cell lines. Nowadays, recombinant instead of urinary gonadotropins are preferably used for ovulation induction, although treatment results comparing urinary and recombinant FSH are not different.[12]

There are mainly two approaches in treatment regimens of ovulation induction using gonadotropins, of which the "step-up" protocol is most widely accepted. In the "step-up" protocol, the initial low FSH dose (37.5–50.0 IU/day) is increased by small increments (37.5–50.0 IU/day) until finally the FSH threshold for ongoing follicle growth and ovulation is surpassed. In contrast, the "step-down" protocol has a starting dose of FSH that equals the "FSH response dose" and will thereby instantly cause ongoing follicle growth.[13] From that point, the daily FSH dose may be decreased (37.5–50.0 IU) every three days, resulting in the development of a single dominant follicle.

While the step-down protocol mimics the physiologic serum FSH profile more closely, and establishes dominant follicle growth more quickly, the step-up protocol results in a lower risk for ovarian hyper-response and subsequent cancellation of stimulation.[14] To solve this dilemma, and to determine the individual "FSH response dose," a dose-finding step-up cycle can be used and consecutive treatment cycles may be performed according to the step-down protocol, unless the starting dose equals the response dose. In that case, a fixed-dose regimen may be used.[15] Urinary or recombinant hCG can be used to trigger ovulation when at least one follicle with a minimal diameter of 16–18 mm is present. Stimulation may be cancelled when more than three follicles > 12 mm in diameter are present.

While reported multiple pregnancy rates after gonadotropin ovulation induction are about 5%, the contribution of ovulation induction to higher-order multiple pregnancies is substantial. The chances of OHSS and multiple pregnancy after gonadotropin ovulation induction are largely related to frequent monitoring by experienced practitioners and strict cancellation criteria.[16] Reported treatment results with gonadotropins are about 70% mono-ovulatory cycles, 20% pregnancy rate per cycle and cumulative single live birth rate of 43% after 6–12 months of treatment.[17]

In conclusion, gonadotropin use for ovulation induction is safe and highly effective as a second-line treatment, while frequent monitoring by experienced practitioners and strict cancellation criteria restrain the risk of complications.

Clinical Practice and Treatment Outcome

Parental health and nutrition play an important role in conception, pregnancy and healthy aging of the future child. It is recommended that the first step to reduce risks for the mother and child would be individualized advice and preconception lifestyle optimization, including a healthy weight.

Table 11.1 Comparison of ovulation induction treatment results with letrozole and clomiphene, both as first-line ovulation induction agent in WHO2 anovulation

	Clomiphene citrate	Letrozole	OR
Cumulative ovulation %	77	75	NS
Clinical pregnancy rate %	26.4	35.9	1.56 (1.37–1.78)
Live birth rate %	21.4	31.4	1.68 (1.42–1.99)
Miscarriage %	20	19	0.94 (0.43–1.24)
Multiple birth %	1.7	1.3	0.73 (0.43–1.24)

Source. Franik et al. Aromatase inhibitors (letrozole) for subfertile women with polycystic ovary syndrome. *Cochrane Database Syst Rev* 2018; 5(5): CD010287.

First-Line Treatment

The anti-estrogen CC offers a reliable, effective, safe and cheap treatment modality for ovulation induction in PCOS patients and also is registered for this indication in most countries. Therefore, it has been a first-line treatment choice for decades and CC was generally accepted as the most adequate first-line treatment in PCOS patients. However, more recent reports state that the aromatase inhibitor letrozole when used as first-line ovulation induction modality in PCOS patients generates better treatment results in comparison to CC (see Table 11.1), while multiple pregnancy and miscarriage rates were comparable.

Recommendation from the 2018 international evidence-based guideline on PCOS proposes that letrozole be considered as a first-line treatment because significant higher ovulation, pregnancy and live birth rates were reported compared to CC.[18] In comparison to clomiphene citrate, aromatase inhibitors have the potential advantage of the lack of anti-estrogenic effect on target organs such as the endometrium and cervical mucus. This may explain the better treatment outcomes.

An important note from the authors of the guideline is that this recommendation is based solely on the clinical fact that most treatment populations are not therapy-naïve, because, if that was taken as selection criterion for comparing treatment results, there would have been no difference between the two interventions for any outcome. Another important point to consider is that most studies included in the analysis have been performed in US populations that have specific characteristics (e.g. morbid obesity) and therefore may not be comparable to treatment populations and outcomes in other countries.

Although letrozole (in certain treatment populations) may have benefits in efficacy over CC as an ovulation induction agent, there still may be uncertainty about its safety and off-label use in most countries. This results in the conclusion that the primary recommendation for first-line ovulation induction in PCOS patients may be letrozole as well as CC, which still may be considered as an effective, safe and reliable alternative choice.

Second-Line Treatment

After first-line ovulation induction treatment has failed, due to the persistent absence of ovulatory cycles or despite 6–12 ovulatory cycles without conception, second-line treatment may be initiated. Exogenous gonadotropins are traditionally utilized for second-line ovulation induction treatment. As treatment with gonadotropins requires daily injections and multiple visits for ultrasound monitoring, most patients experience it to be more intensive and stressful compared to first-line treatment modalities. Adverse hormonal effects reported are in general less profound compared to CC or letrozole.

If the classic ovulation induction sequence is followed of using CC as the first-line treatment and then second-line gonadotropin treatment is evaluated, this turns out to be a rather successful approach (Figure 11.1). A cumulative pregnancy rate of 71% resulting in singleton live birth after 24 months of follow-up was reported in a therapy-naïve PCOS population of 240 patients.[19]

Compared to any alternative second-line treatment choice, gonadotropin ovulation induction has a superior treatment outcome, but it also has relatively high complication risks because the ovarian response to gonadotropin stimulation is hard to predict. Although this is due to large

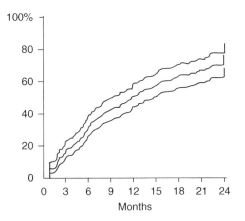

Figure 11.1 Cumulative singleton live birth rate of 71% with a 95% confidence interval after a 24-month follow-up period in the classical ovulation induction algorithm (CC followed by exogenous FSH in case of treatment failure) in 240 therapy-naïve PCOS patients
Source. Adapted from Eijkemans et al. High singleton live birth rate following classical ovulation induction in normogonadotrophic anovulatory infertility (WHO 2). *Hum Reprod* 2003; 18: 2357–2362.

inter- and intra-individual variation, frequent monitoring and strict cancellation criteria are capable of limiting this risk.[18]

While the traditional treatment modalities used for ovulation induction in PCOS patients are focused on increasing the FSH serum concentration in order to "surpass the FSH threshold" for dominant follicle growth (antiestrogens, aromatase inhibitors, exogenous FSH), more recent attention has been given to improvement of the endocrine ovarian milieu, resulting in enhanced FSH responsiveness of the ovaries (lifestyle modification, insulin sensitizers, and laparoscopic electrocautery of the ovaries; see Chapter 12). This favorable endocrine milieu may also benefit implantation and embryo development. A combination of both strategies could be used to individualize treatment in a patient-tailored way: for every patient, an optimal effective treatment plan is devised based on specific individual characteristics.[15] Unfortunately, subgroups of patients who may benefit from certain strategies are difficult to identify clearly. Until recently, attempts to identify these subgroups were performed based on specific patient characteristics. Future knowledge and availability of the genetic profiles involved in ovulation induction may be helpful in accelerating the identification process and will improve the differentiation for individual patients.

First-line treatment modality for ovulation induction with metformin alone or in combination with CC reported no better treatment outcome than with CC alone. On the other hand, for second-line intervention, after persistent anovulation with the first-line treatment, the addition of metformin to CC results in increased ovulation and pregnancy rates, especially in women who are more overweight. Moreover, the addition of metformin to gonadotropin ovulation induction may also have comparable benefits: improved ovulation, pregnancy and live birth rates compared to gonadotropin treatment alone.[20] It can be concluded that the addition of metformin to CC and gonadotropins may be able to optimize ovarian response to stimulation and thus may be considered as a second-line co-treatment for ovulation induction in PCOS patients, especially in patients with obesity.[10]

Although the exact mechanism of action is unknown, laparoscopic electrocautery of the ovaries (LEO) may be an alternative treatment strategy in PCOS patients remaining anovulatory after first-line treatment for ovulation induction (see also Chapter 12). Although limited damage to the ovaries is done during LEO, and it requires an invasive surgical intervention under general anesthesia, it may be a favorable alternative compared to starting daily gonadotropin injections with intensive ultrasound monitoring. Moreover, when regular monofollicular ovulations return after LEO this may increase natural pregnancy chances for a longer period without an increased risk for multiple gestation in comparison to ovulation induction using gonadotropins. While a higher bodyweight is predictive for failure of LEO treatment [21], this modality may be considered especially for PCOS patients with a lower weight (BMI < 28 kg/m^2).

Complications

The most important complications resulting from ovulation induction are caused by the limited control of follicular development. This may result in ovarian hyperstimulation and multiple pregnancy. Although the chances of pregnancy will increase with multi-follicular development and ovulation, multiple pregnancies result in increased perinatal morbidity and mortality but may also result in postnatal stress for the parents who have to take care of multiple neonates.

With antiestrogen treatment, multi-follicular development is regularly reported but multiple pregnancy rate is low at 2–13%. Severe OHSS has not been reported following CC treatment. [7] In FSH ovulation induction, the extended half-life of FSH makes it hard to predict how many follicles are actually reaching the dominant status and sometimes daily ovarian ultrasound monitoring is required to adjust the treatment dosage before multi-follicular development is a fact. This may result in daily hospital visits and increased patient inconvenience.[16]

An alternative way besides ultrasound to monitor follicle development could be the measurement of circulating estradiol during ovarian stimulation. In a large retrospective analysis of intrauterine insemination (IUI) treatment cycles in combination with gonadotropin stimulation, a significant association was reported between multiple pregnancy rates and E_2 serum concentration on the day of hCG administration. The odds of having a multiple gestation significantly increased when the E_2 level exceeded 400 pg/mL (OR 8.24; $p < 0.01$), and these odds increased even further when the E_2 level exceeded 650 pg/mL (OR 11.11; $p < 0.01$). Interestingly, the E_2 serum concentration had no impact on clinical pregnancy rate, which remained at approximately 13% despite the E_2 level.[22]

It may be concluded that, in ovulation induction, all follicles with a diameter greater than 12 mm should be considered prone for ovulation. Stimulation should be cancelled when more than three follicles > 12 mm in diameter are present or E_2 serum levels exceed 400 pg/mL. Monitoring ovarian stimulation should be performed using ultrasound and may be extended with E_2 serum measurements to prevent multiple gestation. To minimize the risk for multiple pregnancy and OHSS, frequent monitoring by experienced practitioners and strict cancellation criteria are mandatory to prevent complications.

Conclusions

Patients presenting with a wish to conceive and chronic anovulation due to PCOS should be offered ovulation induction after optimization of lifestyle and health. First-line ovulation induction treatment in PCOS patients may be initiated using the antiestrogen CC or aromatase inhibitor letrozole. In the case of persistent anovulation or

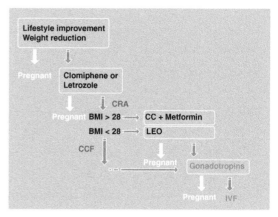

Figure 11.2 Ovulation induction treatment algorithm for PCOS patients with chronic anovulation and a wish to conceive

absence of pregnancy after 6–12 ovulatory months, second-line treatment may be started using gonadotropins. Alternatively, when first-line treatment does not result in regular ovulatory cycles, second-line treatment may be continued with the addition of metformin to CC in patients who are significantly overweight (BMI > 28 kg/m^2) or with LEO in leaner patients (BMI < 28 kg/m^2). If the latter strategy proves not to be effective, this still offers the opportunity to start gonadotropin ovulation induction. When 6–12 ovulatory cycles of gonadotropin ovulation induction have passed without pregnancy, assisted reproduction (IVF) should be offered.

Complications resulting from ovulation induction are mainly caused by the limited control of ovarian reaction to stimulation. Follicle development during ovarian stimulation should therefore be carefully monitored by experienced practitioners and strict cancellation criteria are imperative to limit this risk.

Ovulation induction in PCOS patients may be laborious but also quite effective (Figure 11.2). Because the problem of anovulation is a clear obstruction to conception, treatment to reversing this may turn out to be very rewarding.

References

1   The Rotterdam ESHRE/ASRM-Sponsored PCOS Consensus Workshop Group. Revised 2003 consensus on diagnostic criteria and long-term health risks related to polycystic ovary syndrome (PCOS). *Hum Reprod* 2004; 19(1): 41–47.

2   Mitwally, M. F., Biljan, M. M. and Casper, R. F. Pregnancy outcome after the use of an aromatase inhibitor for ovarian stimulation. *Am J Obstet Gynecol* 2005; 192(2): 381–386.

3   Tatsumi, T., Jwa, S. C., Kuwahara, A. et al. No increased risk of major congenital anomalies or adverse pregnancy or neonatal outcomes following letrozole use in ART. *Hum Reprod* 2017; 32(1): 125–132.

4   Franik, S., Eltrop, S. M., Kremer, J. A. M. et al. Aromatase inhibitors (letrozole) for subfertile women with polycystic ovary syndrome. *Cochrane Database Syst Rev.* 2018; 5(5): CD010287.

5   Caspar, R. F. and Mitwally, M. F. M. Aromatase inhibitors for ovulation induction. *J Clin Endocrinol Metab* 2006; 91(3): 760–771.

6   Rossing, M. A., Daling, J. R., Weiss, N. S., Moore, D. E. and Self, S. G. Ovarian tumors in a cohort of infertile women. *N Engl J Med* 1994; 331(12): 771–776.

7   Homburg, R. Clomiphene citrate – end of an era? A mini-review. *Hum Reprod* 2005; 20(8): 2043–2051.

8   Coffler, M. S., Patel, K., Dahan, M. H. et al. Enhanced granulosa cell responsiveness to follicle-stimulating hormone during insulin infusion in women with polycystic ovary syndrome treated with pioglitazone. *J Clin Endocrinol Metab* 2003; 88(12): 5624–5631.

9   Morley, L. C., Tang, T., Yasmin, E. et al. Insulin-sensitizing drugs (metformin, rosiglitazone, pioglitazone, D-inositol) for women with PCOS, oligo amenorrhoea and subfertility. *Cochrane Database Syst Rev* 2017; 11(11): CD003053.

10 Rausch, M. E., Legro, R .S., Barnhart, H. X. et al. Predictors of pregnancy in women with polycystic ovary syndrome. *J Clin Endocrinol Metab* 2009; 94(9): 3458–3466.

11 Glueck, C. J., Goldenberg, N., Pranikoff, J. et al. Height, weight, and motor-social development during the first 18 months of life in 126 infants born to 109 mothers with polycystic ovary syndrome who conceived on and continued metformin through pregnancy. *Hum Reprod* 2004; 19(6): 1323–1330.

12 Weiss, N. S., Kostova, E., Nahuis, M. et al. Gonadotrophins for ovulation induction in women with polycystic ovary syndrome. *Cochrane Database Syst Rev* 2019; 1(1): CD010290.

13 van Santbrink, E. J. and Fauser, B. C. Urinary follicle-stimulating hormone for normogonadotropic clomiphene-resistant anovulatory infertility: Prospective, randomized comparison between low dose step-up and step-down dose regimens. *J Clin Endocrinol Metab* 1997; 82(11): 3597–3602.

14 Christin-Maitre, S. and Hugues, J. N. Recombinant FSH Study Group: A comparative randomized multicentric study comparing the step-up versus step-down protocol in polycystic ovary syndrome. *Hum Reprod* 2003; 18(8): 1626–1631.

15 van Santbrink, E. J., Eijkemans, M. J., Laven, J. S. and Fauser, B. C. Patient-tailored conventional ovulation induction algorithms in anovulatory infertility. *Trends Endocrinol Metab* 2005; 16(8): 381–389.

16 Balen, A. H., Morley, L. C., Misso, M. et al. The management of anovulatory infertility in women with polycystic ovary syndrome: An analysis of the evidence to support the development of global WHO guidance. *Hum Reprod Update* 2016; 22(6): 687–708.

17 Mulders, A. G., Eijkemans, M. J., Imani, B. et al. Prediction of chances for success or complications in gonadotrophin ovulation induction in normogonadotrophic anovulatory infertility. *Reprod BioMed Online* 2003; 7(2): 170–178.

18 Teede, H. J., Misso, M. L., Costello, M. F. et al. Recommendations from the international evidence-based guideline for the assessment and management of polycystic ovary syndrome. *Fertil Steril* 2018; 110(3): 364–379.

19 Eijkemans, M. J., Imani, B., Mulders, A. G., Habbema, J. D. and Fauser, B. C. High singleton live birth rate following classical ovulation induction in normogonadotrophic anovulatory infertility (WHO 2). *Hum Reprod* 2003; 18(11): 2357–2362.

20 Bordewijk, E. M., Nahuis, M., Costello, M. F. et al. Metformin during ovulation induction with gonadotrophins followed by timed intercourse or intrauterine insemination for subfertility associated with polycystic ovary syndrome. *Cochrane Database Syst Rev* 2017; 1(1): CD009090.

21 Amer, S. A., Li, T. C., Ledger, W. L. Ovulation induction using laparoscopic ovarian drilling in women with polycystic ovarian syndrome: Predictors of success. *Hum Reprod* 2004; 19(8): 1719–1724.

22 Goldman, R. H., Batsis, M., Petrozza, J. C. and Souter, I. Patient-specific predictions of outcome after gonadotropin ovulation induction/ intrauterine insemination. *Fertil Steril* 2014; 101(6): 1649–1655.

Chapter 12

Ovarian Surgery for Ovulation Induction

Gabor T. Kovacs

History

Although the history of polycystic ovary syndrome (PCOS) was discussed in detail in Chapter 1, a brief review here is warranted. Stein and Leventhal were not only the first to describe the condition in 1934/5;[1] they also reported on a surgical treatment for anovulation, which resulted in two pregnancies. By 1964, Stein reported on a successful series of 108 anovulatory PCOS women treated by bilateral ovarian wedge resection (BOWR).[2]

Until the availability of oral and injectable ovulation induction agents, BOWR was the only treatment for anovulatory infertility in women with PCOS. However, the treatment required laparotomy and often resulted in periovarian/peritubal scarring, which had its own negative effect on fertility. In 1976, Toaff and colleagues reported that all seven patients who underwent laparoscopy subsequent to BOWR had extensive periovarian and peritubal adhesions.[3] They concluded: "our observations support the plea to relegate the surgical approach to a minor position in patients with Stein-Leventhal syndrome." Consequently, wedge resection was only performed in conjunction with another surgical procedure that already required laparotomy.

The development of laparoscopy opened up an opportunity to revisit a surgical approach to treat anovulatory infertility. As laparoscopy became a part of gynecology, and with the development of forceps for grasping the ovary, combined with diathermy, it was possible to carry out ovarian surgery with minimally invasive techniques. The first pregnancies after ovarian biopsy and electro-cautery were described by Palmer and Cohen in 1972.[4] By 1972, Jean Cohen and colleagues in Paris had reported 21 pregnancies from 57 successive ovarian biopsies and electrocautery.[5] Several French gynecologists applied the technique to treating their PCOS patients by ovarian biopsy.[6]

The modern resurgence of ovarian surgery to induce ovulation in anovulatory PCOS women was inspired by Gjönnaess,[7] who in 1984 described an ovulation rate of 92% in a series of 62 women who were treated by laparoscopic ovarian unipolar diathermy. Other reports followed and the first 17 published reports of these case series are summarized in Table 12.1.[6]

Methods of Ovarian Surgery

Unipolar Diathermy

The original reports from France described biopsying the ovary and using unipolar diathermy resulting in ovulation. Gjönnaess also used unipolar ovarian cautery; and, as it was readily available and can be performed by any laparoscopically trained operating gynecologist, it was the most popular method used. Semm forceps were used for grasping the ovary while burning. However, it is difficult to grasp the enlarged ovary with forceps with a narrow jaw opening, something that could be compared to trying to grasp a football with ice tongs. The technique was significantly improved with the development of an insulated needle (Corson needle). This enabled the ovarian capsule to be pierced and the cortex to be burned. The ovary needed to be grasped to give counterpressure to the penetrating needle, but the conventional forceps can easily damage the fragile veins in the ovarian pedicle. To overcome this, atraumatic forceps have been designed.

Unipolar diathermy does have the danger of flash burns, and bipolar diathermy is safer as the current only passes between the two jaws of the forceps. Although bipolar forceps were developed, it is difficult to use for ovarian cautery because, again, the opening and separation of the two jaws is limited and they were not widely used.

Table 12.1 Laparoscopic ovarian biopsy and drilling: initial reports

Author	Year	Technique	Number of women	Spontaneous ovulation (%)	Pregnancies (%)
Cohen et al. [5]	1972	Biopsy	51		41
Gjönnaess [7]	1984	Cautery	62	92	84
Greenblatt and Casper	1987	Cautery	6	71	56
Huber et al.	1988	Laser	8	42	
Cohen	1989	Cautery	778		32
Daniell and Miller	1989	Laser	85	84	67
Gadir et al.	1990	Cautery	29	26	44
Tasaka et al.	1990	Cautery	11	91	36
Utsonomiya et al.	1990	Biopsy	16	94	50
Gurgan et al.	1991	Cautery	40	71	57
Kovacs et al.	1991	Cautery	10	70	20
Gurgan et al.	1992	Laser	40	70	50
Ostrzenski	1992	Laser	12	92	92
Pellicer and Remohi	1992	Cautery	131	67	53
Armar and Lachelin	1993	Cautery	50	86	66
Campo et al.	1993	Resection	23	56	56
Gjönnaess	1994	Cautery	252	92	84

Source. Modified after J. Cohen, Laparoscopic surgical treatment of infertility related to PCOS revisited. In G. T. Kovacs and R. Norman, eds. *Polycystic Ovary Syndrome*. Cambridge: Cambridge University Press, 2007, 159–176, with permission of Cambridge University Press.

Laser

Laser technology was adapted for use in laparoscopic surgery in the 1980s and 1990s, and laser ovarian drilling was then applied to ovarian cautery. The use of a CO_2 laser in PCOS was first described by Daniell and Miller.[8] They used a 25 W continuous-mode laser to destroy some of the subcapsular cysts, recommending 25–40 vaporization sites in each ovary. It was postulated that fewer adhesions resulted from laser vaporization than unipolar diathermy. Support for this came from a study on sheep by Petrucco.[9] However, this was negated by a report from Keckstein who found adhesion in three of seven women treated by CO_2 laser ovarian drilling.[10]

The use of the Holmium:YAG (Ho:YAG) laser was reported by Asada and colleagues,[11] who reported on eight women with PCOS-related anovulation who did not respond to clomiphene citrate (CC) and who were treated with laparoscopic ovarian drilling (LOD) using the Ho:YAG laser at the Saiseikai Kanagawaken Hospital, Yokohama. The Ho:YAG laser has a wavelength of 2.14 microns and is approximately 100 times more highly absorbed in water than the Nd:YAG laser. Ho:YAG laser energy is transmitted by a standard quartz fiberoptic light guide and achieves a controlled penetration depth in tissue of around 0.5 mm. Ho:YAG energy produces a consistent zone of thermal necrosis of less than 1.0 mm, and the thermal damage is independent of pigmentation. Ovulation occurred spontaneously in all the patients, with a cumulative probability of conception at 13 months after surgery of 87.5%. They concluded that LOD using the Ho:YAG laser could be an effective treatment of anovulatory women with PCOS who did not respond to CC.

Various other laser types, argon, KTP and Nd:YAG, have all been used.[12, 13] The initial Cochrane Review of ovarian drilling for anovulatory PCOS concluded that "None of the studied modalities of drilling technique had any obvious advantages."[14] We can conclude that the use of laser is far more restricted, more expensive and can be performed by fewer clinicians without any demonstrated benefits.

Unilateral or Bilateral

Stein and Leventhal removed about a quarter of each ovary to achieve ovulation. Gjönnaess inflicted about 10–12 punctures to each ovary, but the minimum number of lesions needed to induce ovulation was not known. A novel modification of the technique was reported by Balen and Jacobs. They demonstrated no difference in efficacy whether they undertook cautery of only one ovary at four sites or carried out the more radical method of multiple cautery to both ovaries.[15]

Supportive evidence for such a conservative unilateral approach came from several other units. Abu Hashim and colleagues published a meta-analysis of 8 studies involving 484 women comparing unilateral (ULOD) and bilateral laparoscopic ovarian drilling (BLOD).[16] As far as effectiveness was concerned, there was no difference in ovulation or clinical pregnancy and live birth rates between ULOD and BLOD. As far as effect on ovarian reserve, there was no difference in anti-Müllerian hormone (AMH) levels, but a significantly higher antral follicle count (AFC) at six-month follow-up was found with ULOD (MD 2.20; 95% CI 1.01 to 3.39). They concluded that clinicians should utilize ULOD concordant with the *primum non nocere* principle if LOD is used.

Transvaginal Hydrolaparoscopy

An alternate way to visualize the ovaries is to use a transvaginal telescope using saline solution (hydrolaparoscopy), which was first described by Gordts and colleagues in 1998.[17] Transvaginal hydrolaparoscopy (TVHL) was then applied to ovarian drilling in PCOS when Gordts and colleagues reported on drilling of the ovarian capsule using THL with a 5-Fr bipolar needle (Karl Storz, Tuttlingen, Germany) and creating 10–15 holes to a depth of 1–2 mm +/−0.20 mm in each ovary.[18] Of 39 clomiphene-resistant PCOS patients who underwent THL and ovarian drilling, a total of 25 out of 33 patients (76%) (6 lost to follow-up) became pregnant. They recommended that THL for ovarian capsule drilling offered a valuable and less invasive alternative to the standard laparoscopic procedure. Supportive evidence came from France from a series of 80 women with CC-resistant PCOS who underwent operative "transvaginal fertiloscopy" with a coaxial bipolar electrode.[19] The cumulative pregnancy rate was 39.7% (29/73). No complications occurred.

Although THL has had limited uptake by gynecologists, by 2018 Giampaolino and colleagues reported on 117 CC-resistant PCOS patients who underwent THL ovarian drilling.[20] Ovulation rate was 64.1% one month after treatment, 79.5% after three months and 82.9% after six months. Pregnancy rate was 70.1%. However, a randomized controlled trial (RCT) of TVHL drilling compared to treatment with follicle-stimulating hormone (FSH) was stopped after the screening of 40 patients (when results were available for 34) because the pregnancy rate was significantly higher in the medical group 8/16 versus 3/18 in the surgical group ($p = 0.04$).[21] As THL is only practiced by a minority of gynecologists, its use for ovarian drilling has been limited.

Ultrasound-Guided Transvaginal Ovarian Needle Drilling

An alternate technique of ovarian drilling was described by Badawy and colleagues who reported using transvaginal ultrasound guidance to drill the ovaries as an alternative to the traditional laparoscopic electrosurgical drilling.[22] In a randomized, controlled, prospective trial of 163 women with CC-resistant PCOS randomized to treatment with either ultrasound-guided transvaginal needle ovarian drilling (UTND; $n = 82$) or laparoscopic electrosurgical ovarian drilling ($n = 81$), there were no significant differences between the two groups with regard to resumption of normal menstruation, ovulation, pregnancy, hirsutism or acne. UTND has the advantage that it can be adopted as an outpatient office procedure with reduced costs and rapid recovery.

Zhu and colleagues modified UTND by applying laser energy.[23] They suggested minimizing damage to the ovarian surface by intra-ovarian coagulation, which created a spot 10 mm in diameter, at least 5 mm from the surface. Api had a number of reservations about this technique.[24] While he agreed that interstitial laser treatment would prevent ovarian surface damage, and thus have a theoretical advantage of preventing postoperative adhesion formation over LOD, he postulated that it might damage intraovarian vessels as the blood supply enters the ovary from the hilum. He also pointed out that, as the fiberoptic cable is 400 μm in diameter, it is not easily visualized using ultrasound. Because the technique is not under direct visualization, he was also concerned about the risk of unrecognized inadvertent hemorrhage from the ovary and adjacent pelvic organ damage. Furthermore, any unintentional movement of the patient during the procedure may cause inadvertent needle movements inside the ovary, with catastrophic consequences if the fiberoptic cable tip reaches beyond the ovarian surface when the laser energy is activated. Also, as there is no direct visualization of the pelvic organs, it is not possible to assess the tubo-ovarian relationship, tubal patency or the presence of adhesions and endometriosis. Api concluded that this novel treatment method has not yet been investigated thoroughly.

Laparoscopic Ovarian Multi-Needle Intervention

To refine the technique of ovarian drilling a specially designed laparoscopic device and technique was described by Kaya and colleagues.[25] Kaya designed a laparoscopic instrument (Kaya laparoscopic drilling device; Aygun Medical Devices Limited Company, Samsun, Turkey), which is inserted through the 5 mm ancillary port. It is 37 cm long with a distal grasper-like tip containing two prongs. Each prong is 25 mm by 4 mm in area and consists of 10 needle-like teeth, which are 2 mm in length and 0.4 mm in diameter. The ovary is grasped between the jaws of the instrument and squeezed by applying some force. This is repeated again and again until the entire ovarian surface is treated and is then repeated for the other ovary. Thirty-five infertile CC-resistant women with PCOS were treated: 17 by laparoscopic ovarian multi-needle intervention (LOMNI) and 18 by ovulation induction. There was no significant difference in outcomes, but the cost of LOMNI was significantly ($p < 0.001$) lower than the ovulation induction treatment. They concluded that LOMNI may be a safe and effective procedure for the treatment of CC-resistant infertility in patients with PCOS, without the unwanted effects (such as adhesion formation) of LOD.

Table 12.2 Complications of surgical laparoscopy/ovarian drilling

Anesthetic Complications
Associated with Insertion of Verres Needle or Laparoscopic Trochar
• Laparoscopic injury at insertion
• Gas complication – CO_2 embolism
• Mis-insufflation into tissues
• Trauma to viscus or vessel
Associated with the Actual Operation
• Heat damage at time of drilling
• Bowel, bladder or vessel damage during procedure, especially bleeding from ovarian pedicle where grasped

Possible Complications of Ovarian Cautery/Drilling

Complications of ovarian cautery or drilling are summarized in Table 12.2. While there are no accurate figures from large studies for the incidence of operative complications after ovarian cautery or laser drilling, their frequency can be deduced from complications experienced after operative laparoscopy. Complications of laparoscopy can be divided into those associated with the insufflation and insertion of the Veres needle or trochars (air embolism, damage to a blood vessel or damage to viscera) and those associated with the procedure itself (intraoperative bleeding or damage to an organ – bowel, ureter or bladder). A study of 25764 gynecological laparoscopies from Holland in 1994 reported 145 complications (5.7/1000 in all types of operations).[26] A national study from Finland from 1995/6, reporting on 32205 gynecological laparoscopies, reported a complication rate for operative laparoscopies of 12.6/1000.[27] This is probably the best estimate for the complication rate after ovarian cautery/laser.

Postoperative – Delayed

The complications specific to ovarian drilling with possible effects on future fertility include the risk of ovarian adhesions and possible reduction of ovarian reserve.

Periovarian and Tubal Adhesions

It became obvious that BOWR often resulted in significant adhesions, which led to a plea to abandon it as a treatment for anovulation.[3] It was hoped that the less destructive laparoscopic approach would not result in significant adhesions. On reviewing the literature,[6] ovarian adhesions between 0% and 100% have been reported after laparoscopic drilling.

As early as 1993, Nather and Fisher reported on a "second look" in 62 PCOS patients who had undergone LOD and found an adhesion rate of 19.3%.[28] They also reported that, in women who had a post-cautery lavage, the incidence decreased to 16.6%. Mercorio and colleagues reported on 96 women who underwent laparoscopic drilling followed by a short-term, second-look minilaparoscopy.[29] They detected adhesion formation in 54 of the 90 women (60%) and in 83 of the 180 (46%) ovaries treated. They concluded that there was a significant incidence of adhesions after LOD and that the extent and severity of adhesions were not influenced by the number of ovarian punctures. They also noted that the left ovary appeared more prone to develop severe adhesions than the right one. A study by Giampaolino and colleagues in 2016 found that 73 of 123 patients who underwent LOD showed the presence of ovarian adhesion. [30] This was compared to 123 women who underwent TVHL with an adhesion rate of 15.5%. This difference was highly significant with a p-value < 0.0001 and a relative risk of 0.22 (95% IC 0.133 to 0.350). They suggested that TVHL may have a lower rate of postoperative adhesions than LOD.

Despite the findings that LOD does seem to sometimes result in adhesion formation, postoperative pregnancy rates appear comparable to those obtained by ovulation induction.

Premature Ovarian Failure

There is a theoretical concern that cautery/laser energy to the ovary may result in the destruction of ovarian follicles or damage to the blood supply and thus result in decreased ovarian reserve.

In 2009, Api reviewed the available literature on whether LOD is harmful to the ovarian reserve markers and found four articles that specifically reported on the ovarian reserve tests before and after surgery.[31] He found in some reports that there were statistically significant differences between day 3 FSH, inhibin B levels, ovarian volume and AFC. Although the post-LOD values

were found to be lower than the pre-LOD values, they were still higher when compared with women without PCOS. He concluded that most of the changes in the ovarian reserve markers observed after LOD could be interpreted as normalization of ovarian function rather than as a reduction of ovarian reserve.

Weerakiet and colleagues compared ovarian reserve assessed by AMH levels and day 3 FSH, AFC and inhibin B in 21 PCOS women undergoing LOD to women who did not undergo LOD (the PCOS group) and normal ovulatory women (the control group).[32] The PCOS women both with and without LOD had significantly greater ovarian reserve than the age-matched controls. Only inhibin B levels seemed to be lower in the LOD than in the non-operated PCOS group.

Hendriks and colleagues carried out experimental comparisons of damage from CO_2 laser, monopolar electrocoagulation and bipolar electrocoagulation on bovine ovaries.[33] They found that bipolar electrocoagulation resulted in significantly more destruction per burn than the CO_2 laser and monopolar electrocoagulation (287.6 mm^3 vs. 24.0 mm^3 and 70.0 mm^3, respectively). Given the same clinical effectiveness of the various procedures, they recommended that the least destructive method should be used and that the first choice should be CO_2 laser or monopolar electrocoagulation.

To assess whether ovarian damage is through impairment of blood supply, a study was carried out by Vizer and colleagues.[34] They used a 3D color power angiography (CPA) to evaluate and quantify intraovarian blood flow before and after LOD. They found that ovarian volume decreased and 3D CPA showed increased intraovarian flow intensity after laparoscopic electrocautery. They also compared hormone levels of serum luteinizing hormone (LH) and testosterone (T) levels in 10 women and found that 5-alpha-reductase enzyme activity and androgen to cortisol metabolites decreased; serum FSH levels increased one week after laparoscopy and correlated well with changes in 3D sonographic features. They concluded that 3D ultrasonography may be a useful adjunct and noninvasive method for correlating clinical parameters with the blood flow alterations in PCOS patients.

Reassurance comes from a 15–25-year follow-up of 150 patients who underwent the more destructive procedure of BOWR,[35] which in

88% of women showed regular menstrual patterns lasting up to 25 years after the surgery.

Cost Analysis

There are limited data on the cost-benefit equation of LOD against ovulation induction with gonadotropins. My colleagues and I compared the cost of LOD using electrocautery with the cost of ovulation induction using injectable FSH in the Australian private health system.[36] The cost of LOD using unipolar diathermy was 84% of the cost of one cycle of ovulation induction using FSH (including the cost of hormones, biochemistry, medical costs and ultrasound).

Farquhar also compared the costs of LOD with gonadotropins.[37] The total cost of treatment in the Netherlands for the ovarian drilling group was 4664 euros and for the gonadotropins group was 5418 euros. In New Zealand, the costs of a live birth were a third lower in the group that underwent laparoscopic ovarian diathermy compared with those women who received gonadotropins (NZ$19640 and NZ$29836, respectively).

An opposing cost assessment was published by DeFrene and colleagues from Ghent, Belgium, in 2015.[38] They carried out a retrospective health economic evaluation in 43 women who had human menopausal gonadotropin (hMG) therapy compared with 35 women who had LOD followed by ovulation induction with CC and/or hMG if spontaneous ovulation did not occur within 2 months. Data were collected until the patients were pregnant. The cost per patient, up to an ongoing pregnancy, was significantly higher after LOD than in the hMG group (adjusted mean difference 1073 euros; 95% CI 180 to 1967). Consequently, each clinician must calculate the relative costs in 1803 their health economic environment.

Mechanism of Action

How wedge resection of the ovaries worked was never understood, although Stein and Leventhal postulated a decrease in crowding of the cortex, thus enabling the growth of normal follicles to the surface. With LOD, Gjönnaess suggested that the benefit of drilling was either nonspecific stromal destruction or the discharge of the contents of subcapsular cysts.[7] Daniell and Miller hypothesized that laser energy was effective by opening the follicular capsules by laser energy – follicular fluid

containing androgens was released, thus removing the block to ovulation.[8]

There have been a number of studies on changes in reproductive hormones after LOD. Campo reviewed data regarding anovulatory PCOS patients, 679 of them treated by classical ovarian resection after laparotomy, 720 by laparoscopic electrocauterization, 322 by laparoscopic laser vaporization and 82 by laparoscopic multiple biopsies.[39] He found that hormone variations after surgery consisted of a remarkable fall in serum androgen levels (androstenedione and T), an FSH increase, reduced biological activity and reduced amplitude of LH pulses, and an LH:FSH ratio trending toward normal levels. My colleagues and I reported in agreement with Campo that there was a significant and persistent fall in serum T levels; and we were able to measure inhibin levels, which showed a transient fall with subsequent rise.[36] However, a study by Amer and colleagues of 50 anovulatory women with PCOS who underwent LOD found no statistically significant change in inhibin B after LOD.[40] They concluded that it was unlikely that inhibin had any role to play in the mechanism of action of LOD.

In support of the reduction of androgen theory, Seow and colleagues confirmed that the reduction of serum androgen level is the likely mechanism behind LOD in improving spontaneous ovulation and promoting fertility in women with PCOS.[41]

Vizer and colleagues,[34] in addition to their study of intraovarian blood flow with 3D CPA histogram analysis before and after laparoscopic ovarian electrocautery, also compared the hormonal effects of surgery with 3D sonographic findings. They also found that serum LH and T levels, ratios of urinary steroids reflecting 5-alpha-reductase enzyme activity and androgen and cortisol metabolites decreased; serum FSH levels increased one week after laparoscopy and correlated well with changes in 3D sonographic features.

Further confirmation for a decrease in LH and androgen concentrations after LOD, and four possible mechanisms for this, came from S. L. Tan's unit in Montreal in 2000.[42] First, they postulated that this might be due to the destruction of the androgen-producing ovarian stroma and drainage of the follicles, which have high androgen levels, by decreasing the amount of substrate available for peripheral aromatization to estrogens. This restores the feedback mechanism to the hypothalamus and the pituitary gland, allowing appropriate gonadotropin stimulation for follicular development and ovulation. Secondly, at the ovarian level, the elevated intra-follicular androgen levels may inhibit granulosa cell function and follicular growth. Reduction in intraovarian androgen after surgery allows follicular development. A third mechanism is a reduction in the circulating levels of inhibin after surgery, which results in the secondary rise in serum FSH in combination with the reduction of local androgen, which may facilitate follicular growth. Fourthly, surgery may also provoke an increased blood flow to the ovary, allowing increased delivery of gonadotropin.

Efficacy Compared with Alternative Methods of Ovulation Induction

Consensus Expert Opinion

A group of international experts gathered in Thessaloniki in Greece in 2007 to draft some consensus statements on various aspects of the management of PCOS.[43] With respect to laparoscopic ovarian surgery (LOS), they concluded that:

- LOS can achieve uni-follicular ovulation with no risk of ovarian hyperstimulation syndrome (OHSS) or high-order multiples.
- Intensive monitoring of follicular development is not required after LOS.
- LOS is an alternative to gonadotropin therapy for CC-resistant anovulatory PCOS.
- This treatment is best suited to those for whom frequent ultrasound monitoring is impractical.
- LOS is a single treatment using existing equipment.
- The risks of surgery are minimal but include the risk of the laparoscopy, adhesion formation and destruction of normal ovarian tissue. Minimal damage should be caused to the ovaries. Irrigation with an adhesion barrier may be useful, but there is no evidence of efficacy from prospective studies.
- Surgery should be performed by appropriately trained personnel.
- LOS should not be offered for non-fertility indications.

Evidence-Based "Meta-analyses"

Six Cochrane Reviews of ovarian drilling have been undertaken, with the most recent carried out in 2020.[44] Although the first review in 2000 concluded that the value of LOD was undetermined, by the 2005 review they concluded that there was no difference in live birth rates when CC-resistant PCOS patients were treated by LOD or by gonadotropins. In all the reviews, they highlighted the lack of multiple pregnancies after LOD.

In 2018 an international evidence-based guideline was produced on the assessment and management of women with PCOS.[45] The guideline recommended that LOS could be a second-line therapy for women with PCOS who are CC-resistant and with anovulatory infertility and no other infertility factors. The 2018 international consensus statement compares outcomes for LOS against a number of medical treatment alternatives.[45] These include LOS versus metformin; LOS versus CC; LOS versus CC plus metformin; LOS versus aromatase inhibitors; and LOS versus gonadotropins.

Laparoscopic Ovarian Surgery vs. Metformin

Two medium-quality RCTs compared LOS to metformin and found that there were conflicting results in the two studies, thus there was insufficient evidence to make a recommendation about LOS compared to metformin for live birth rate per patient, ovulation rate per cycle, pregnancy rate per cycle, pregnancy rate per patient, multiple pregnancies and miscarriage rate per pregnancy.[46, 47]

Laparoscopic Ovarian Surgery vs. Clomiphene Citrate

Two high-quality RCTs (level II) with a low risk of bias compared LOS to CC and found that there was no difference between LOS and CC for live birth rate per patient and pregnancy rate per patient, ovulation rate per patient and miscarriage rate per pregnancy.[48, 49] These results are today less relevant because few would advocate LOS as a first-line treatment, and letrozole (off license) is now the recommended first-line treatment rather than CC.

Laparoscopic Ovarian Surgery vs. Clomiphene Citrate plus Metformin

The 2018 guideline quoted the same three studies included in the 2012 Cochrane Review.[50] The conclusion was that there was insufficient evidence to support or refute the use of LOS over CC plus metformin for ovulation rate per patient.

Laparoscopic Ovarian Surgery vs. Aromatase Inhibitors

The Cochrane Review of 2012 combined these studies in a meta-analysis of pregnancy rate per patient, multiple pregnancy rate per pregnancy and miscarriage rate per pregnancy and there was no statistical difference between the two interventions. Thus there was insufficient evidence of a difference between the two options.

Laparoscopic Ovarian Surgery vs. Gonadotropins

Again, with reference to the 2012 Cochrane Review,[50] the 2018 guideline quoted one high-quality RCT and found no difference in any of the success factors, but a better (lower) multiple pregnancy rate (OR 0.13; 95% CI 0.03 to 0.59) for 4 studies with 303 participants was noted.

The sixth updated review includes 38 trials (3326 women). The studies were predominantly from Egypt (12 studies) while four studies were included each from India, Iran, Italy and the UK, two from Turkey, and one each from France, Jordan, New Zealand, Saudi Arabia and Yugoslavia. There is little additional data between the 2018 guideline [45] and this 2020 Cochrane Review. Its weakness is that the quality of the reported studies varied from "very low- to moderate-quality." The main limitations were due to poor reporting of study methods, with downgrading for risks of bias (randomization and allocation concealment) and lack of blinding, thus there being a danger of "rubbish in – rubbish out," meaning that, even by pooling data, it is hard to draw firm conclusions. Although pooled results suggest LOD may decrease live birth slightly when compared with medical ovulation induction alone (OR 0.71; 95% CI 0.54 to 0.92; 9 studies, 1015 women; $I^2 =$ 0%; low-quality evidence), when studies restricted to only RCTs with low risk of selection bias are considered (4 studies, 415 women), they suggested that there is no difference in outcomes between medical or surgical treatment (OR 0.90; 95% CI 0.59 to 1.36). This would suggest that LOD is not inferior to medical treatments.

The authors also conclude that "LOD probably reduces multiple pregnancy rates" (Peto OR 0.34; 95% CI 0.18 to 0.66; 14 studies, 1161 women; $I^2 = 2$%; moderate-quality evidence). However, as LOD restores spontaneous ovulation, it is obvious that the risk of ovarian hyperstimulation and consequent multiple pregnancy using LOD will be similar to that with natural conception. We do not need an RCT to conclude this. Similarly, the authors' conclusion states "LOD *may* result in less OHSS," which again is obvious and does not need an RCT. I would put this in the same category as requiring an RCT of "jumping out of an airplane with and without a parachute" to prove that parachutes are useful. The quality of evidence is insufficient to justify a conclusion on live birth, clinical pregnancy or miscarriage rate for the analysis of unilateral LOD versus bilateral LOD.

In summary, the four recommendations from the international guideline with respect to the role of LOS are:[45]

1. LOS could be a second-line therapy for women with PCOS who are CC-resistant (as well as letrozole-resistant – my words) with anovulatory infertility and no other infertility factors.
2. LOS could potentially be offered as a first-line treatment if laparoscopy is indicated for another reason than infertility and no other infertility factors.
3. The risk of laparoscopic surgery should be clearly explained to women considering LOS.
4. For each clinician, laparoscopic surgery consideration should be given to:
   - the comparative costs of medical versus LOS
   - the expertise required for each approach
   - especially in obese women, the operative and postoperative risks
   - a small risk of lower ovarian reserve after surgery
   - the risk of postoperative adhesions.

In conclusion, LOS seems to produce similar pregnancy results to ovulation induction with gonadotropins, without the need for extensive monitoring (because of mono-ovulation) and with only a background risk of multiple pregnancy.

However, it is an invasive surgical intervention with infrequent but possible complications, and there is a small risk of reduced ovarian reserve or loss of ovarian function as well as possible adhesion formation. In my practice, it is the preferred second-line therapy in anovulatory PCOS after failed clomiphene/letrozole treatment.

References

1   Stein, I. F. and Leventhal, M. L. Amenorrhoea associated with bilateral polycystic ovaries. *Am J Obstet Gynecol* 1935; 29(2): 181–191.

2   Stein, I. F. Duration of fertility following ovarian wedge resection: Stein-Leventhal syndrome. *West J Surg Obstet Gynecol* 1964; 72: 237–242.

3   Toaff, R., Toaff, M. E. and Peyser, M. R. Infertility following wedge resection of the ovaries. *Am J Obstet Gynecol* 1976; 124(1): 92–96.

4   Palmer, R. and Cohen, J. Biopsies percoelioscopiques. *Minerva Gynaecol* 1965; 17: 238–239.

5   Cohen, J., Audebert, A., de Brux, J. and Giorgi, H. Sterility due to dysovulation: Prognostic and therapeutic role of ovarian biopsy during calioscopy. *J Gynecol Obstet Biol Reprod (Paris)* 1972; 1: 657–671.

6   Cohen, J. Laparoscopic surgical treatment of infertility related to PCOS revisited. In G. T. Kovacs and R. Norman, eds. *Polycystic Ovary Syndrome*. Cambridge: Cambridge University Press, 2007, 159–176.

7   Gjönnaess, H. Polycystic ovarian syndrome treated by ovarian electrocautery through the laparoscope. *Fertil Steril* 1984; 41: 20–25.

8   Daniell, J. F. and Miller, W. Polycystic ovaries treated by laparoscopic laser vaporization. *Fertil Steril* 1989; 51: 232–236.

9   Petrucco, O. M. Laparoscopic CO_2 laser drilling of sheep ovaries: Interval assessment of histological changes and adhesion formation. Abstracts of the Seventh Annual Scientific Meeting of The Fertility Society of Australia, Newcastle; 1988: 21.

10 Keckstein, J. Laparoscopic treatment of polycystic ovarian syndrome. *Bailliere Clin Obstet Gynaecol* 1989; 3(3): 563–581.

11 Asada, H., Kishi, I., Kaseda, S. et al. Laparoscopic treatment of polycystic ovaries with the holmium: YAG laser. *Fertil Steril* 2002; 77: 852–853.

12 Gürgan, T., Yarali, H. and Urman, B. Laparoscopic treatment of polycystic ovarian disease. *Hum Reprod* 1994; 9: 573–577.

13 Heylen, S. M., Puttemans, P. J. and Brosens, I. A. Polycystic ovarian disease treated by laparoscopic argon laser capsule drilling: Comparison of vaporization versus perforation technique. *Hum Reprod* 1994; 9: 1038–1042.

14 Farquhar, C., Vandekerckhove, P., Arnot, M. and Lilford, R. Laparoscopic "drilling" by diathermy or laser for ovulation induction in anovulatory polycystic ovary syndrome. *Cochrane Database Syst Rev* 2000; 2: CD001122.

15 Balen, A. H. and Jacobs, H. S. A prospective study comparing unilateral and bilateral laparoscopic ovarian diathermy in women with the polycystic ovary syndrome. *Fertil Steril* 1994; 62: 921–925.

16 Abu Hashim, H., Foda, O. and El Rakhawy, M. Unilateral or bilateral laparoscopic ovarian drilling in polycystic ovary syndrome: A meta-analysis of randomized trials. *Arch Gynecol Obstet* 2018; 297 (4): 859–87.

17 Gordts, S., Campo, R., Rombauts, L. and Brosens, I. Transvaginal hydrolaparoscopy as an outpatient procedure for infertility investigation. *Hum Reprod* 1998; 13: 99–103.

18 Gordts, S., Gordts, S., Puttemans, P. et al. Transvaginal hydrolaparoscopy in the treatment of polycystic ovary syndrome. *Fertil Steril* 2009; 91: 2520–2526.

19 Fernandez, H., Watrelot, A., Alby, J. et al. Fertility after ovarian drilling by transvaginal fertiloscopy for treatment of polycystic ovary syndrome *J Am Assoc Gynecol Laparosc* 2004; 11(3): 374–378.

20 Giampaolino, P., deRosa, N., Della Corte, L. et al. Operative transvaginal hydrolaparoscopy improve ovulation rate after clomiphene failure in polycystic ovary syndrome. *Gynecol Endocrinol* 2018; 34(1): 32–35.

21 Fernandez, H., Cedrin-Durnerin, I., Gallot, V. et al. Using an ovarian drilling by hydrolaparoscopy or recombinant follicle stimulating hormone plus metformin to treat polycystic ovary syndrome: Why a randomized controlled trial fail? *J Gynecol Obstet Biol Reprod (Paris)* 2015; 44(8): 692–698.

22 Badawy, A., Khiary, M., Ragab, A., Hassan, M. and Sherief, L. Ultrasound-guided transvaginal ovarian needle drilling (UTND) for treatment of polycystic ovary syndrome: A randomized controlled trial. *Fertil Steril* 2009; 91: 1164–1167.

23 Zhu, W., Fu, Z., Chen, X. et al. Transvaginal ultrasound-guided ovarian interstitial laser treatment in anovulatory women with polycystic ovary syndrome: A randomized clinical trial on the effect of laser dose used on the outcome. *Fertil Steril* 2010; 94: 268–275.

24 Api, M. Could transvaginal, ultrasound-guided ovarian interstitial laser treatment replace laparoscopic ovarian drilling in women with polycystic ovary syndrome resistant to clomiphene citrate. *Fertil Steril* 2009; 6: 2039–2040.

25 Kaya, H., Sezik, M. and Ozkaya, O. Evaluation of a new surgical approach for the treatment of clomiphene citrate-resistant infertility in polycystic ovary syndrome: laparoscopic ovarian multi-needle intervention. *J Minim Invasive Gynecol* 2005; 12: 355–358.

26 Jansen, F. W., Kapiteyn, K., Trimbos-Kemper, T., Hermans, J. and Trimbos, J. B. Complications of laparoscopy: A prospective multicentre observational study. *Br J Obstet Gynaecol* 1997; 104(5): 595–600.

27 Harkki-Siren, P., Sjoberg, J. and Kurki, T. Major complications of laparoscopy: A follow-up Finnish study. *Obstet Gynecol* 1999; 94(1): 94–98.

28 Fisher, R. and Naether, O. G. Adhesion formation after laparoscopic electrocoagulation of the ovarian surface in polycystic ovary patients. *Fertil Steril* 1993; 60(1): 95–98.

29 Mercorio, F., Mercorio, A., Di Spiezio Sardo, A., Barba, G. V., Pellicano, M. and Nappi, C. Evaluation of ovarian adhesion formation after laparoscopic ovarian drilling by second-look minilaparoscopy. *Fertil Steril* 2007; 88: 894–899.

30 Giampaolino, P. , Morra, I. , Tommaselli, G. A., di Carlo, C., Nappi, C. and Bifulco, G. Post-operative ovarian adhesion formation after ovarian drilling: A randomized study comparing conventional laparoscopy and transvaginal hydrolaparoscopy. *Arch Gynecol Obstet* 2016; 294(4): 791–796.

31 Api, M. Is ovarian reserve diminished after laparoscopic ovarian drilling? *Gynecol Endocrinol* 2009; 25: 159–165.

32 Weerakiet, S., Lertvikool, S., Tingthanatikul, Y., Wansumrith, S., Leelaphiwat, S. and Jultanmas, R. Ovarian reserve in women with polycystic ovary syndrome who underwent laparoscopic ovarian drilling. *Gynecol Endocrinol* 2007; 2: 1–6.

33 Hendriks, M.-L., van der Valk, P., Lambalk, C. B. et al. Extensive tissue damage of bovine ovaries after bipolar ovarian drilling compared to monopolar electrocoagulation or carbon dioxide laser. *Fertil Steril* 2010; 93: 969–975.

34 Vizer, M., Kiesel, L., Szabó, I. et al. Assessment of three-dimensional sonographic features of polycystic ovaries after laparoscopic ovarian electrocautery. *Fertil Steril* 2007; 88: 894–899.

35 Lunde, O., Djoselend, O. and Grottum, P. Polycystic ovarian syndrome: A follow-up study on fertility and menstrual pattern in 149 patients 15–25 years after ovarian wedge resection. *Hum Reprod* 2001; 16: 1479–1485.

36 Kovacs, G., Buckler, H., Bangah, M. et al. Treatment of anovulation due to polycystic ovarian syndrome by laparoscopic ovarian electrocautery. *Br J Obstet Gynaecol* 1991; 98: 30–35.

37 Farquhar, C. M. An economic evaluation of laparoscopic ovarian diathermy versus gonadotrophin therapy for women with clomiphene citrate-resistant polycystic ovarian syndrome *Curr Opin Obstet Gynecol* 2005; 17(4): 347–353.

38 DeFrene, V., Gerris, J., Weyers, S. et al. Gonadotropin therapy versus laparoscopic ovarian drilling in clomiphene citrate-resistant polycystic ovary syndrome patients: A retrospective cost-effectiveness analysis. *Gynecol Obstet Invest* 2015; 80(3): 164–169.

39 Campo, S. Ovulatory cycles, pregnancy outcome and complications after surgical treatment of polycystic ovary syndrome. *Obstet Gynecol Surv* 1998; 53: 297–308.

40 Amer, S. A., Laird, S., Ledger, W. L. and Li, T. C. Effect of laparoscopic ovarian diathermy on circulating inhibin B in women with anovulatory polycystic ovary syndrome. *Hum Reprod* 2007; 22: 389–394.

41 Seow, K. M., Juan, C. C., Hwang, J. L. and Ho, L. T. Laparoscopic surgery in polycystic ovary syndrome: Reproductive and metabolic effects. *Semin Reprod Med* 2008; 26: 101–110.

42 Felemban, A., Tan, S. L. and Tulandi, T. Laparoscopic treatment of polycystic ovaries with insulated needle cautery: A reappraisal. *Fertil Steril* 2000; 73(2): 266–269.

43 Thessaloniki ESHRE/ASRM-sponsored PCOS Consensus Workshop Group. Consensus on infertility treatment related to polycystic ovary syndrome. *Hum Reprod* 2008; 23: 462–477.

44 Bordewijk, E. M., Ng, K. Y. B., Rakic, L. et al. Laparoscopic ovarian drilling for ovulation induction in women with anovulatory polycystic ovary syndrome. *Cochrane Database Syst Rev.* 2020; 2(2): CD001122.

45 Teede, H., Misso, M. , Costello, M. et al. *International Evidence-Based Guideline for the Assessment and Management of Polycystic Ovary Syndrome.* Melbourne: Monash University and NHMRC, Centre for Research Excellence in PCOS and the Australian PCOS Alliance, 2018.

46 Hamed, H. O., Hasan, A. F., Ahmed, O. G. and Ahmed, M. A. Metformin versus laparoscopic ovarian drilling in clomiphene- and insulin-resistant women with polycystic ovary syndrome. *Int J Gynaecol Obstet* 2010; 108(2): 143–147.

47 Palomba, S., Orio, F., Jr., Nardo, L. G. et al. Metformin administration versus laparoscopic ovarian diathermy in clomiphene citrate-resistant women with polycystic ovary syndrome: A prospective parallel randomized double-blind placebo-controlled trial. *J Clin Endocrinol Metab* 2004; 89(10): 4801–4809.

48 Abu Hashim, H., Foda, O., Ghayaty, E. and Elawa, A. Laparoscopic ovarian diathermy after clomiphene failure in polycystic ovary

syndrome: Is it worthwhile? A randomized controlled trial. *Arch Gynecol Obstet* 2011; 284(5): 1303–1309.

49 Amer, S. A., Li, T. C., Metwally, M., Emarh, M. and Ledger, W. L. Randomized controlled trial comparing laparoscopic ovarian diathermy with clomiphene citrate as a first-line method of ovulation induction in women with polycystic ovary syndrome. *Hum Reprod* 2009; 24(1): 219–225.

50 Farquhar, C. , Brown, J. and Marjoribanks, J. Laparoscopic drilling by diathermy or laser for ovulation induction in anovulatory polycystic ovary syndrome. *Cochrane Database Syst Rev* 2012; 6: CD001122.

Chapter 13

In Vitro Fertilization and Assisted Reproductive Technologies in Polycystic Ovary Syndrome

Susie Jacob and Adam Balen

Introduction

In vitro fertilization (IVF) should be viewed as a third-line treatment for those with polycystic ovary syndrome (PCOS). In the absence of known causative factors of infertility, such as tubal or sperm abnormalities, a methodical approach to treatment should first include lifestyle modification and an efficacious trial of ovulation induction (OI). Cumulative pregnancy rates of 62% within four treatment cycles have been shown with letrozole, an aromatase inhibitor [1] – now widely accepted as the first-line OI agent in PCOS.[2, 3] For those who remain refractory to different regimens of OI, the move to IVF, with the associated risk of ovarian hyperstimulation syndrome (OHSS), becomes justified. The presence of polycystic ovaries is a major risk factor for OHSS, necessitating careful planning of gonadotropin stimulation.

Diagnosis and Prevalence

PCOS is a heterogenous condition whose pathophysiology appears to be multifactorial and polygenic. Although the definition has been much debated, the Rotterdam international consensus definition remains the most widely recognized and accepted version.[4] Two of the following are required:

1. Oligo- and/or anovulation
2. Clinical and/or biochemical signs of hyperandrogenism
3. Polycystic ovary morphology (PCOM) on ultrasound

Other causes of androgen excess or menstrual disturbance must be excluded. Improved ultrasound technology has led to an increased follicle requirement to confirm PCOM. Previously > 12 peripherally placed follicles on a single ovary were pathognomonic of PCOM,[5] but now with modern transvaginal transducers with a frequency band width that includes 8 MHz, the threshold has increased to 20 and/or ovarian volume $\geq$ 10 mL ensuring no corpora lutea, cysts or dominant follicles are present.[3]

The prevalence of PCOS is determined by the diagnostic criteria used, ethnic origin and the population of women studied. PCOS remains the most common endocrinopathy affecting reproductive-aged women, with a prevalence of 8–13%.[3] The finding of PCOM is common and can be seen in upwards of 20% of reproductive-aged women. The prevalence of PCOS is higher in South Asian women compared with Caucasian women, and those from South Asia have increased insulin resistance and symptom severity.[6] Ethnicity also impacts on clinical outcome following assisted reproductive technologies (ART). The literature suggests that South Asian or Black Afro-Caribbean women have inferior outcomes following fresh transfer cycles but not with frozen cycles.[7] Underlying ovarian features including effects of insulin resistance and hyperandrogenemia appear to play an important part in these differences.

Hyperandrogenemia and Oocyte Competence

Hyperandrogenism, in conjunction with hyperinsulinemia, is a fundamental feature of PCOS. The hormonal interplay between key hormones in PCOS adds to perturbed folliculogenesis and oocyte competence.[8] Hyperandrogenism influences the hypothalamic–pituitary–ovarian axis in a number of ways. Furthermore, there are additional mechanisms that lead to increased GnRH pulsatility, hypersecretion of luteinizing hormone (LH), premature granulosa cell luteinization and abnormal oocyte maturation. Through direct and indirect mechanisms, hyperandrogenism impairs oocyte competence including causing premature oocyte maturation and activated proapoptotic signaling pathways in oocytes.[9] Teissier and colleagues showed that follicular testosterone levels were significantly elevated in PCOS, especially in meiotically incompetent oocytes. High androgen levels are likely to contribute to the reduced fertilization seen in oocytes from those with PCOS.[10] Anti-Müllerian hormone (AMH) is elevated in women with PCOS. High levels of AMH exert an inhibitory effect on follicle-stimulating hormone (FSH) induced aromatase activity. Failed conversion of androgen to estrogen leads to chronic hyperandrogenism, interrupting the follicles' ability to undergo cyclic recruitment among selectable follicles.[11]

Oxidative stress is caused by an imbalance between pro-oxidant molecules and antioxidants, culminating in increased concentrations of reactive oxygen species (ROS). Low levels of ROS in follicular fluid promote oocyte maturation and contribute to the release of a competent oocyte at the time of ovulation. Elevated ROS levels induce DNA damage and can interfere with oocyte competence. A hyperandrogenic ovarian milieu promotes oxidative stress, interfering with oxygen attainment and oxidative metabolism required for oocyte development.[8]

Serum androgen levels rise during ovarian stimulation and are higher in women with PCOS. Increased levels are thought to negatively impact on pregnancy outcome. Markers of endometrial receptivity include glycodelin, a secretory protein in the endometrium. A positive correlation exists between successful conception cycles following IVF and glycodelin. Increased androgen levels have been found to reduce glycodelin in women with PCOS and recurrent miscarriage.[12]

Hyperandrogenemia has been shown to contribute to altered gene expression associated with chromosome alignment and segregation.[13] Furthermore, there is altered metabolism in oocytes from women with PCOS, leading to premature separation of sister chromatids. Exposure to excess androgens in utero can have far-reaching effects, including epigenetic programming, particularly on genes regulating reproduction and metabolism.[14–16]

Reproductive Health in PCOS

A recent large retrospective study provides one of the largest datasets to date, reviewing the incidence of metabolic complications of pregnancy in PCOS women (PCOS $n = 14882$; "normal" $n = 9081906$).[17] At baseline, more pregnant women with PCOS were obese (22.3% vs. 3.5%, $p < 0.001$), had pregestational diabetes (4.1% vs. 0.9%, $p < 0.001$), had chronic hypertension (8.4% vs. 1.8%, $p < 0.001$) and had treated thyroid disease (12.6% vs. 2.4%, $p < 0.001$). Women with PCOS were more likely to have undergone IVF treatment (2.4% vs. 0.1%, $p < 0.001$) and have multi-gestation pregnancies (5.9% vs. 1.5%, $p < 0.001$). In all pregnancies, women with PCOS were more likely to develop gestational diabetes (adjusted odds ratio (aOR) 2.19; 95% CI 2.02 to 2.37), pregnancy-associated hypertension (aOR 1.38; 95% CI 1.27 to 1.50, $p < 0.001$) and preeclampsia (aOR 1.29; 95% CI 1.14 to 1.45).[17] This is in agreement with an earlier study, which also found an increased risk of preterm birth (OR 1.75; 95% CI 1.16 to 2.62). Babies born to mothers with PCOS had a significantly increased risk of admission to a neonatal intensive care unit (OR 2.31; 95% CI 1.25 to 4.26) and a higher perinatal mortality (OR 3.07; 95% CI 1.03 to 9.21) unrelated to multiple birth.[18] Obesity, a common occurrence in PCOS, is independently associated with adverse pregnancy outcomes, including miscarriage, preeclampsia, gestational diabetes and congenital abnormalities.

Lifestyle modification and health optimization prior to treatment and pregnancy are of paramount importance. A recent Cochrane Review addressed lifestyle changes in women with PCOS and concluded that intervention may improve endocrine profile, reproductive outcome and body mass index (BMI), although no studies assessed live birth or miscarriage rates.[19] Long-term health optimization is key for women with PCOS, both for reproductive health and for long-term overall health. The approach should ideally be long-term and sustained, as "quick fix" weight-loss programs prior to commencing ART are unlikely to substantially alter the ability to achieve a successful pregnancy through IVF.[20]

Obesity

Obesity is a major factor that influences all outcomes for women with PCOS. Between 38% and 66% of women with PCOS are overweight or obese, with BMI correlating with the severity of phenotypic features. Clinical pregnancy rates are significantly lower in the obese in either natural or ART cycles. This reduction in pregnancy rate is seen in both fresh and frozen transfer cycles. Women with PCOS undergoing IVF who have a very high BMI of greater than 40 kg/m² have been shown to have a significantly reduced clinical pregnancy rate (32% vs. 72%, relative risk (RR) 0.44).[21] Cycles were further complicated by increased gonadotropin requirement, difficult oocyte retrievals, fewer oocytes retrieved and impaired fertilization. Embryo quality was reduced with a greater degree of fragmentation. Similar findings are seen in freeze-only cycles. Qiu and colleagues showed a clear reduction in live birth rate (LBR) (aRR = 0.66; 95% CI 0.48 to 0.92) and increased miscarriage rate (aRR = 1.68; 95% CI 1.01 to 3.09) in those with a BMI > 30 kg/m² undergoing a frozen cycle.[22] This implies that obesity influences oocyte quality perhaps more than endometrial receptivity, both of which are considered key factors in obese patients with PCOS. If weight loss can be achieved, then one could logically expect an improved outcome. A recent large Swedish study of obese infertile women compared a strict calorie-controlled diet for 12 weeks and a period of weight stabilization prior to IVF with those who went straight to IVF.[23] While there was an improved chance of natural conception in those who achieved weight loss prior to IVF, in a subgroup analysis of those with PCOS who reduced weight by either 5 BMI points or to a BMI of less than 25, there was no difference in LBR following IVF. Therefore, short-term weight reduction may not always rectify the outcome for those who are overweight, and it may well be more important to focus on long-term lifestyle modification in order to alter the disordered hormonal and metabolic environment within which the oocyte develops and matures.

Conception alone should not be the only focus for those who are overweight. Maternal health is paramount both to improve the long-term outcome for the baby and to reduce any risks during pregnancy. In the most recent triennial report (2015–2017) into maternal death, more than 34% of women who died were obese and a further 24% were overweight.[24] Both obesity and PCOS increase the risk of developing gestational diabetes, preeclampsia and preterm birth. An increased need for operative delivery predisposes obese women to wound infection and thromboembolism. Preconceptional health advice and support are essential in order to reduce the spiraling effects of the obesity epidemic on fertility and childbirth. Obesity and PCOS are considered in detail in Chapter 16.

Ovarian Hyperstimulation Syndrome

Ovarian hyperstimulation syndrome (OHSS) is the most serious complication of superovulation in ART treatment. Ovarian stimulation leads to increased vascular permeability following release of vasoactive mediators from stimulated ovaries. Vascular endothelial growth factor (VEGF), a potent angiogenic mitogen, is a key mediator of ovarian folliculogenesis and therefore OHSS. The growth factor acts via two endothelial tyrosine kinase receptors, which either transduce or prevent signal transduction. The combined effect of these differing forms mediates the angiogenic properties of VEGF.[25] The process of OHSS culminates in fluid shifts from the vascular compartment into the third space, resulting in intravascular dehydration. Symptoms can rapidly progress from mild abdominal distension and nausea to oliguria, ascites and hematological disturbance. Severe manifestations of OHSS include hepatorenal disturbance, thrombosis, adult respiratory distress syndrome and even death.[26] The true incidence of OHSS remains unknown, but hospitalization for severe manifestations is low (0.5–2% of IVF cycles). Clinically significant moderate to severe OHSS affects up to 10% of IVF cycles, while milder forms may affect up to a third of cycles.[27]

Women with PCOS have an increased incidence of OHSS because of the increased recruitment of gonadotropin-responsive small antral follicles from the primordial pool. This is reflected in the increased levels of anti-Müllerian hormone (AMH) produced by the many antral follicles of the polycystic ovary. Although the initial response to gonadotropin stimulation may be slow, once the threshold is reached, the resultant follicular development may be exuberant. Further evidence for this was observed in women undergoing their first cycle of IVF in whom the incidence of severe OHSS was 2.7% in those with normal ovaries, 12.6% in those with PCOM and 15.4% in those with full-blown PCOS.[28] An increased expression of VEGF is seen in women with PCOS,[29]

123

with a concurrent reduction in the circulating signal transduction "preventing" receptor, leading to its increased bioavailability. Furthermore, insulin has been demonstrated to augment VEGF secretion, with hyperinsulinemia being a fundamental feature of many with PCOS.

Superovulation Strategies

GnRH Antagonist vs. Agonist Protocols

When considering the best protocol for superovulation in women with polycystic ovaries undergoing IVF the aim is to maximize synchronous follicular growth with oocyte maturation. Historically, the gonadotropin-releasing hormone (GnRH) agonist protocol brought significant benefit for women with PCOS,[30] although with improved oocyte yield and pregnancy rate came a sixfold increased incidence of OHSS. This was due in part to the longer duration and total dose of gonadotropin required for ovarian stimulation. [31] This fact is particularly pertinent for those with PCOS, who can have an explosive response when the effects of pituitary suppression are overcome. The agonist may interfere with the follicle selection process, preventing atresia of small antral follicles and allowing more mid-sized follicles to develop. Furthermore, following down-regulation, the low-basal levels of FSH may be sufficient to support growth of multiple small follicles up to the 2 mm gonadotropin-dependent stage. Indeed, OHSS is usually associated with a large number of small-to-moderate sized follicles (< 14 mm) rather than with larger, more mature follicles.

The use of GnRH agonists has now been superseded by the GnRH antagonist protocols with equivalent live birth rates but significantly reduced risks of OHSS.[32] The most recent Cochrane Review has found no difference in live birth rate between the antagonist or the long GnRH agonist protocol (OR 1.02; 95% CI 0.85 to 1.23; 12 RCTs, n = 2303, I^2 = 27%; moderate-quality evidence).[33] There is a significant reduction in the incidence of any grade of OHSS (OR 0.61; 95% C 0.51 to 0.72; 36 RCTs, n = 7944, I^2 = 31%; moderate-quality evidence) and a reduction in cycle cancellation for over-response (OR 0.47; 95% CI 0.32 to 0.69; 19 RCTs, n = 4256). It should be recognized that, while over-response is reduced, there may be increased cycle cancellation

for poor response with the antagonist cycle (OR 1.32; 95% CI 1.06 to 1.65; 25 RCTs, n = 5 230, I^2 = 68%; moderate-quality evidence). There is no difference in miscarriage rate between agonist or antagonist cycles (OR 1.03; 95% CI 0.82 to 1.29; 34 RCTs, n = 7 082, I^2 = 0%; moderate-quality evidence).

Pretreatment strategies such as using the combined oral contraceptive pill (COCP) are often employed to time cycles for planning a clinic's workload. In high-responding women with PCOS, this may be detrimental as some studies have shown an increased duration of stimulation and a reduction in pregnancy rate. The most recent Cochrane Review for COCP use concludes that there is insufficient evidence regarding OHSS with or without the pill but a significant reduction in pregnancy rates in the antagonist cycle (OR 0.74; 95% CI 0.58 to 0.95; 6 RCTs; 1335 women; I^2 = 0%; moderate-quality evidence) when the pill is used which should influence treatment selection.[34]

Gonadotropin Selection

FSH exists in a number of different isoforms, dependent on the number of branching carbohydrate moieties found on the molecule. Within the menstrual cycle, the more acidic isoform predominates the early follicular cycle with a switch to the less-acidic form around ovulation. This switch is controlled by estradiol levels. In vivo acidic isoforms have a longer half-life with a more controlled steroidogenic response and selective follicle growth. Less-acidic isoforms induce exponential growth, in a less selective manner, which theoretically could exacerbate OHSS with rapidly rising estradiol levels. Although there has been interest in the ratio of FSH isoforms between gonadotropins, in practice no difference in clinical outcome has been shown between preparations. There is no difference in outcome between recombinant or urinary-derived gonadotropins, with respect to live birth rate (28 trials, 7339 couples, OR 0.97; 95% CI 0.87 to 1.08) or incidence of OHSS in all women undergoing IVF (32 trials, 7740 couples; OR 1.18; 95% CI 0.86 to 1.61).[35] With respect to those with PCOS, a more recent meta-analysis again confirms no difference in clinical outcome between the types of gonadotropin used.[36] The authors of both meta-analyses suggest that the gonadotropin used should be selected based on cost and convenience for the individual.

The dose of gonadotropin used per cycle is clearly important in a high-responder population. It is important to tailor the dose of stimulation for each individual based on her age and ovarian reserve tests in order to optimize outcome and reduce the risk of OHSS.[37]

Pre-ovulatory Trigger

When considering the "pre-ovulatory trigger," the key issue is the protocol used. If a long GnRH agonist protocol has been used then it is important to use a low dose of human chorionic gonadotropin (hCG) (5000 IU) to initiate oocyte maturation rather than a dose of 10000 IU, which many clinics use in routine practice. A significant advantage of the GnRH antagonist protocol is the opportunity to use a GnRH agonist in place of hCG to complete oocyte maturation. The antagonist competitively binds to the GnRH receptor, producing its effect within hours of administration. The agonist can then displace the antagonist from the pituitary receptor, resulting in the release of native LH. While the released LH initiates oocyte nuclear maturation, there is a substantial reduction in surge duration compared with the use of hCG.[38] An adequate background of LH is required to ensure that optimal luteinization occurs. It has been shown that there are similar numbers of mature oocytes retrieved and embryo quality whether an agonist or hCG is used as the trigger.[39] Early use of the agonist trigger was associated with disappointing pregnancy rates despite a reduction in OHSS. Furthermore, standard luteal phase support was insufficient to overcome the severe luteal deficiency observed. The pathophysiology of luteal phase insufficiency was secondary to low-level endogenous LH and the shorter half-life of LH. Consequently, the corpus luteum degenerated leaving insufficient progesterone to support early pregnancy development.[40] Modified luteal phase support with either a small dose (1500 IU) of supplementary hCG at the time of oocyte retrieval and/or estradiol and progesterone overcomes this deficit to a certain extent. Haahr and colleagues performed a recent meta-analysis to qualify this point.[40] The results showed a nonsignificant difference in LBR favoring an hCG trigger (OR 0.84; 95% CI 0.62 to 1.14). OHSS was reported in a total of 4/413 cases in the GnRHa group compared with 7/413 in the hCG group (OR 0.48; 95% CI 0.15 to 1.60). The difference in LBR may be explained by a nonsignificant increase in miscarriage with the GnRH agonist triggered group compared with the hCG group (OR 1.85; 95% CI 0.97 to 3.54). This trend of inferiority has led some to question if further modification of luteal phase support can improve reproductive outcomes. Use of micro-dosing of hCG following the GnRH agonist trigger has been suggested to replace progesterone, although not yet proven in a high-responder PCOS population.[41]

Recombinant technology has allowed the production of recombinant LH, which has been tried as an alternative to hCG for final oocyte maturation. No difference in pregnancy rates or incidence of OHSS has been found and so this approach is no longer favored.[42]

Novel approaches for final oocyte maturation have been considered. Kisspeptins and the connected neuronal network of kisspeptin-neurokinin-B-dynorphon (KNDy) have provided insight into how upstream modulation of the GnRH signal can be harnessed to improve reproductive outcome. Following direct signaling to the GnRH neuron via the kisspeptin receptor, a pulsatile release of GnRH enters the portal circulation. In turn, this stimulates pituitary gonadotropin release, with a preferential secretion of LH and to a lesser extent FSH. By adopting a physiological approach using the hypothalamic endogenous GnRH reserve, a reduction in OHSS may be achieved. Kisspeptin has a half-life of only 28 minutes, in contrast to the extended effect of hCG or even a GnRH trigger. A study to address the optimum dose of kisspeptin, in a high-risk cohort for OHSS, resulted in high rates of oocyte maturation, high implantation rates and no cases of clinically significant OHSS.[43] Inclusion criteria were an AMH > 40 pmol/L or a total antral follicle count > 23 – a cohort likely to have PCOS but not defined as such. High pregnancy rates were seen throughout the study, with the greatest LBR of 62% following 9.6 nmol/kg kisspeptin-54. Mild OHSS was seen in only 4 out of the 60 women included. This suggests that kisspeptin is capable of inducing ovulation when there is a large cohort of follicles.[44]

Freeze-Only Strategy

A segmentation approach, with no fresh embryo transfer, but elective freezing of all suitable embryos and embryo transfer in frozen cycle only, has been advocated as a way to eliminate OHSS. A recent Cochrane Review compared fresh transfer versus a "freeze-all" approach.[45]. There was no clear difference in cumulative LBR (OR 1.09; 95% CI 0.91 to 1.31; 4 trials, 1892 women; I^2 = 0%; moderate-quality evidence). The prevalence of OHSS was lower (but interestingly not eliminated) in the freeze-all group (OR 0.24; 95% CI 0.15 to 0.38; 2 trials; 1633 women; I^2 = 0%; low-quality evidence); as was the risk of miscarriage (OR 0.67; 95% CI 0.52 to 0.86; 4 trials; 1892 women; I^2 = 0%; low-quality evidence). This latter point is presumed to be secondary to an improved endometrium without interference from ovarian hyperstimulation and lower circulating estradiol levels. Although this equivalence in pregnancy rate and reduction in OHSS may seem preferable, frozen cycles are associated with an increase in pregnancy complications (OR 1.44; 95% CI 1.08 to 1.92; 2 trials; 1633 women; low-quality evidence) and there is the inevitable increase in time to pregnancy. Indeed, segmentation and routine use of cryopreserved embryos may increase the incidence of macrosomia, placenta accreta and preeclampsia.[40] A study looking at fresh versus elective frozen cycles in a PCOS population only confirmed a significant increase in preeclampsia with frozen cycles compared with fresh transfer (4.4% vs. 1.4%; RR 3.12; 95% CI 1.26 to 7.73).[46] An important issue is an apparent increased incidence of still birth and neonatal death in the freeze-only group, secondary to prematurity. Further research is required to qualify the balance between safety, reproductive outcome and cost before a segmented-only approach should be adopted; nonetheless, most prefer this approach for those cycles with a high risk of OHSS.

Another strategy for reducing OHSS includes starting cabergoline around the time of hCG administration or oocyte pick-up.[27] Cabergoline, a dopamine agonist, inhibits phosphorylation of the VEGF receptor, thereby reducing its effects on vascular permeability.

Insulin Resistance and Metformin

Insulin resistance coupled with hyperandrogenemia are key factors in the pathophysiology of PCOS. Aberrant phosphorylation of tyrosine and serine residues on the insulin receptor increase insulin resistance and induce compensatory hyperinsulinemia. Insulin binds insulin-like growth factor 1 (IGF-1) receptors in the ovaries, augmenting the theca cell response to LH and resulting in excess androgen production. Hyperinsulinemia reduces hepatic synthesis of sex hormone-binding globulin (SHBG) and IGF-binding protein-1. In turn, this increases bioavailability of androgens IGF-1 and 2, which are important regulators of steroidogenesis and follicular maturation.

As hyperinsulinemia is well recognized in women with PCOS, a reasonable assumption would be that insulin-sensitizing drugs should improve many aspects of the syndrome, including reproductive outcome. Metformin, an oral biguanide, is the most widely researched agent in this category. Metformin reduces hepatic gluconeogenesis, increases peripheral utilization of glucose and mediates receptor kinase activity in thecal and granulosa cells.[47] A recent Cochrane Review evaluated metformin for OI.[48] This concluded that metformin may improve LBR compared with placebo (OR 1.59; 95% CI 1.0 to 2.51; 4 studies, 435 women; I^2 = 0%; low-quality evidence) but the evidence was inconclusive when compared with clomiphene. Interestingly, in subgroup analysis, obese patients may fare worse with respect to LBR on metformin compared with clomiphene (OR 0.30; 95% CI 0.17 to 0.52; 2 studies, 500 women). Many women were also found to have gastrointestinal side effects that may limit treatment.

A number of studies have investigated the effects of using insulin-sensitizing agents, mainly metformin, on women with PCOS undergoing IVF treatment. A Cochrane Review includes nine randomized controlled trials, all of which except one use a GnRH agonist protocol.[49] Dose and duration of metformin use were not uniform, ranging from 500 mg twice a day to 850 mg three times a day, for up to 16 weeks prior to hCG trigger. No clear difference in LBR was seen with additional metformin use (OR 1.39; 95% CI 0.81 to 2.40; 5 RCTs, 551 women; I^2 = 52%; low-quality evidence); but there was a significant reduction in the incidence of OHSS (OR 0.29; 95% CI 0.18 to 0.49; 8 RCTs, 798 women; moderate-quality evidence). Although a small study suggested promise in OHSS reduction in the antagonist cycle,[50] an adequately powered RCT did not confirm these findings.[51] There was no reduction in the incidence of moderate-to-severe OHSS (placebo (PLA) 12.2%, metformin (MET) = 16%; 95% CI −0.08 to 0.16, $p = 0.66$), total gonadotropin dose (PLA = 1200, MET = 1200; 95% CI −118.67 to 118.67, $p = 0.75$), oocytes retrieved (PLA = 15, MET = 14; 95% CI −2.37 to 4.37, $p = 0.66$) or fertilization rate (PLA = 60.7%, MET = 53.3%; 95% CI −0.96 to 14.94, $p = 0.07$). However, using metformin resulted in a reduced clinical pregnancy rate (CPR) per cycle started (PLA = 48.7%, MET = 28.6%; 95% CI 0.04 to 0.35, $p = 0.02$) and live birth rate (PLA = 51.6%, MET = 27.6%; 95% CI 0.05 to 0.40, $p = 0.02$). Furthermore, when ethnicity was taken into account there was a significant reduction in pregnancy outcome for the South Asian population irrespective of metformin or placebo use (CPR per cycle started, White Caucasian = 44.4%, South Asian = 19.4%; 95% CI 0.06 to 0.39, $p = 0.01$).

Although the agonist cycle has now been superseded by the antagonist cycle for high-responding women with PCOS,[3] if any women should require an agonist cycle, metformin should be added as an adjunct. For those on an antagonist cycle, metformin confers no advantage and may even be detrimental to the outcome.

In Vitro Maturation

In vitro maturation (IVM) of oocytes has been heralded as an OHSS elimination strategy. Oocytes are retrieved transvaginally from antral follicles in unstimulated or minimally stimulated ovaries. The oocyte then matures in vitro in a specially formulated medium for 24–48 hours, before undergoing fertilization with sperm via intra-cytoplasmic sperm injection. Despite promising results, there have not been high-quality trials confirming the viability of this method over standard IVF treatment.[52] Clinic and laboratory expertise are required for this method and it has not gained widespread popularity. With continued interest into the approach, reasonable pregnancy rates and confirmed safety of offspring,[53] there may yet be wider adoption of this method of assisted conception.

Conclusion

Women with PCOS undergoing IVF cycles respond differently to women with normal ovaries. Obesity further compounds differences in reproductive outcome. Weight loss and lifestyle modification should remain a pivotal feature before any move toward IVF, to improve success rates and reduce long-term sequelae for mother and child. The GnRH antagonist cycle has superseded the GnRH agonist in safety profile with equal live birth rates. Use of the GnRH agonist should be encouraged in high-responder patients with a modified luteal phase support to maintain an ongoing pregnancy. Metformin should continue to be used in GnRH agonist cycles to reduce OHSS but not in GnRH antagonist cycles. Segmentation of cycles with freezing of all embryos may become standard practice but the health of the mother through pregnancy should always be considered.

References

1 Amer, S. A., Smith, J., Mahran, A., Fox, P. and Fakis, A. Double-blind randomized controlled trial of letrozole versus clomiphene citrate in subfertile women with polycystic ovarian syndrome. *Hum Reprod* 2017; 32(8): 1631–1638.

2 Balen, A. H., Morley, L. C., Misso, M. et al. The management of anovulatory infertility in women with polycystic ovary syndrome: an analysis of the evidence to support the development of global WHO guidance. *Hum Reprod Update* 2016; 22(6): 687–708. https://doi.org/10.1093/humupd/dmw025

3 Teede, H. J., Misso, M. L., Costello, M. F. et al. Recommendations from the international evidence-based guideline for the assessment and management of polycystic ovary syndrome. *Fertil Steril* 2018; 110(3): 364–379.

4 The Rotterdam ESHRE/ASRM-Sponsored PCOS Consensus Workshop Group. Revised 2003 consensus on diagnostic criteria and long-term health risks related to polycystic ovary syndrome (PCOS). *Hum Reprod* 2004; 19: 41–47.

5 Balen, A. H., Laven, J. S. E., Tan, S. L. and Dewailly, D. Ultrasound assessment of the polycystic ovary: International consensus definitions. *Hum Reprod Update* 2003; 9: 505–514.

6 Wijeyaratne, C. N., Balen, A. H., Barth, J. H. and Belchetz, P. E. Clinical manifestations and insulin resistance (IR) in polycystic ovary syndrome (PCOS) among South Asians and Caucasians: Is there a difference? *Clin Endocrinol* 2002; 57(3): 343–350.

7 Mascarenhas, M. and Balen, A. H. Could ethnicity have a different effect on fresh and frozen embryo transfer outcomes: A retrospective study. *Reprod Biomed Online* 2019; 39(5): 764–769.

8 Palomba, S. and La Sala, G. B. Oocyte competence in women with PCOS. *Trends Endocrinol Metab* 2017; 28(3): 186–198.

9 Qiao, J. and Feng, H. L. Extra- and intra-ovarian factors in polycystic ovary syndrome: Impact on oocyte maturation and embryo developmental competence. *Hum Reprod Update* 2011; 17: 17–33.

10 Teissier, M. P., Chable, H., Paulhac, S. and Aubard, Y. Comparison of follicle steroidogenesis from normal and polycystic ovaries in women undergoing IVF: Relationship between steroid concentrations, follicle size, oocyte quality and fecundability. *Hum Reprod* 2000; 15(12): 2471–2477.

11 Dewailly, D., Robin, G., Peigne, M., Decanter, C., Pigny, P. and Catteau-Jonard, S. Interactions between androgens, FSH, anti-Müllerian hormone and estradiol during folliculogenesis in the human normal and polycystic ovary. *Hum Reprod Update* 2016; 22(6): 709–724. https://doi.org/10.1093/hu mupd/dmw027

12 Westergaard, L. G., Yding Andersen, C., Erb, K. et al. Placental protein 14 concentrations in circulation related to hormonal parameters and reproductive outcome in women undergoing IVF/ICSI. *Reprod Biomed Online* 2004; 8(1): 91–8.

13 Wood, J. R., Dumesic, D. A., Abbott, D. H. and Strauss, J. F., III. Molecular abnormalities in oocytes from women with polycystic ovary syndrome revealed by microarray analysis. *J Clin Endocrinol Metab* 2007; 92(2): 705–713.

14 Li, Z. and Huang, H. Epigenetic abnormality: A possible mechanism underlying the fetal origin of polycystic ovary syndrome. *Med Hypotheses* 2008; 70(3): 38–42.

15 Risal, S., Pei, Y., Lu, H. et al. Prenatal androgen exposure and transgenerational susceptibility to polycystic ovary syndrome. *Nature Medicine* 2019; 25(11).

16 Picton, H. M. and Balen, A. H. Transgenerational PCOS transmission. *Nat Med* 2019; 25(12): 1818–1820. https://doi.org/10.1038/s41591-019-06 78-x

17 Mills, G., Badeghiesh, A., Suarthana, E., Baghlaf, H. and Dahan, M. H. Polycystic ovary syndrome as an independent risk factor for gestational diabetes and hypertensive disorders of pregnancy: A population-based study on 9.1 million pregnancies. *Hum Reprod* 2020; 35(7): 1666–1674.

18 Boomsma, C. M., Eijkemans, M. J. C., Hughes, E. G., Visser, G. H. A., Fauser, B. C. J. M. and Macklon, N. S. A meta-analysis of pregnancy outcomes in women with polycystic ovary syndrome. *Hum Reprod Update* 2006; 12(6): 673–683.

19 Lim, S. S., Hutchison, S. K., Van Ryswyk, E., Norman, R. J., Teede, H. J. and Moran, L. J. Lifestyle changes in women with polycystic ovary syndrome. *Cochrane Database Syst Rev* 2019; 3: CD007506.

20 Norman, R. J. and Mol, B. W. J. Successful weight loss interventions before in vitro fertilization: Fat chance? *Fertil Steril* 2018; 110(4): 581–586.

21 Jungheim, E. S., Lanzendorf, S. E., Odem, R. R., Moley, K. H., Chang, A. S. and Ratts, V. S. Morbid obesity is associated with lower clinical pregnancy rates after in vitro fertilization in women with polycystic ovary syndrome. *Fertil Steril* 2009; 92(1): 256–261.

22 Qiu, M., Tao, Y., Kuang, Y. and Wang, Y. Effect of body mass index on pregnancy outcomes with the freeze-all strategy in women with polycystic ovarian syndrome. *Fertil Steril* 2019; 112(6): 1172–1179.

23 Einarsson, S., Bergh, C., Friberg, B. et al. Weight reduction intervention for obese infertile women prior to IVF: A randomized controlled trial. *Hum Reprod* 2017; 32(8): 1621–1630.

24 Knight, M., Bunch, K., Tuffnell, D. et al. (eds.). *Saving Lives, Improving Mothers' Care: Lessons Learned to Inform Maternity Care from the UK and Ireland Confidential Enquiries into Maternal Deaths and Morbidity 2016–18*. Oxford: National Perinatal Epidemiology Unit, University of Oxford and MBRACE-UK, 2020.

25 Holmes, D. I. and Zazhary, I. The vascular endothelial growth factor (VEGF) family: Angiogenic factors in health and disease. *Genome Biol* 2005; 6(2): 209.

26 Braat, D. D., Schutte, J. M., Bernadus, R. E., Mooij, T. M. and van Leeuwen, F. E. Maternal death related to IVF in the Netherlands 1984–2008. *Hum Reprod* 2010; 25(7): 1782–1786.

27 Mourad, S., Brown, J. and Farquhar, C. Interventions for the prevention of OHSS in ART cycles: An overview of Cochrane reviews. *Cochrane Database Syst Rev*. 2017; 23(1): CD012103.

28 Swanton, A., Storey, L., McVeigh, E. and Child, T. IVF outcome in women with PCOS, PCO and normal ovarian morphology. *Eur J Obstet Gynaecol Reprod Biol* 2010; 149(1): 68–71.

29 Peitsidis, P. and Agrawal, R. Role of vascular endothelial growth factor in women with PCO and PCOS: A systematic review. *Reprod Biomed Online* 2010; 20(4): 444–452.

30 Balen, A. H., Tan, S. L., MacDougall, J. and Jacobs, H. S. Miscarriage rates following in vitro fertilisation are increased in women with polycystic ovaries and reduced by pituitary desensitisation with buserelin. *Hum Reprod* 1993; 8: 959–964.

31 Tarlatzis, B. C. and Koblibianakis, E. M. GnRH agonists vs antagonists. *Best Pract Res Clin Obstet Gynaecol* 2007; 21(1): 57–65.

32 ESHRE Reproductive Endocrinology Guideline Group. *Ovarian Stimulation for IVF/ICSI: Guideline of the European Society of Human Reproduction and Embryology*. Grimbergen: ESHRE, 2019.

33 Al-Inany, H. G., Youssef, M. A., Ayeleke, R., Brown, J., Lam, W. and Broekmans, F. J. Gonadotrophin-releasing hormone antagonists for assisted reproductive technology. *Cochrane Database Syst Rev* 2016; 29(4): CD001750. https://doi.org/10.1002/14651858

34 Farquhar, C., Rombauts, L., Kremer, J. A. M., Lethaby, A. and Ayeleke, R. O. Oral contraceptive pill, progestogen or oestrogen pretreatment for ovarian stimulation protocols for women undergoing assisted reproductive techniques. *Cochrane Database Syst Rev* 2017; 5: CD006109.

35 van Wely, M., Kwan, I., Burt, A. L. et al. Recombinant versus urinary gonadotrophin for ovarian stimulation in assisted reproductive technology cycles. *Cochrane Database Syst Rev* 2011; 2: CD005354.

36 Weiss, N. S., Kostova, E., Nahuis, M., Mol, B. W. J., van der Veen, F., van Wely, M. Gonadotrophins for ovulation induction in women with polycystic ovary syndrome. *Cochrane Database Syst Rev* 2019; 1(1): CD010290.

37 Lensen, S. F., Wilkinson, J., Leijdekkers, J. A. et al. Individualised gonadotropin dose selection using markers of ovarian reserve for women undergoing in vitro fertilisation plus intracytoplasmic sperm injection (IVF/ICSI). *Cochrane Database Syst Rev* 2018; 2(2): CD012693.

38 Humaidan, P., Papanikolaou, E. G., Kyrou, D. et al. The luteal phase after GnRH-agonist triggering of ovulation: Present and future perspectives. *Reprod Biomed Online* 2012; 24(2): 134–141. https://doi.org/10.1016/j.rbmo.2011.11.00

39 Fauser, B. C., de Jong, D., Olivennes, F. et al. Endocrine profiles after triggering of final oocyte maturation with GnRH agonist after cotreatment with the GnRH antagonist ganirelix during ovarian hyperstimulation for in vitro fertilization. *J Clin Endocrinol Metab* 2002; 87(2): 709–715.

40 Haahr, T., Roque, M., Esteves, S. C. and Humaidan, P. GnRH agonist trigger and LH activity luteal phase support versus hCG trigger and conventional luteal phase support in fresh embryo transfer IVF/ICSI cycles: A systematic PRISMA review and meta-analysis. *Front Endocrinol (Lausanne)* 2017; 8: 116. https://doi.org/10.3389/fendo.2017.00116

41 Andersen, C. Y., Elbaek, H. O., Alsbjerg, B. et al. Daily low-dose hCG stimulation during the luteal phase combined with GnRHa triggered IVF cycles without exogenous progesterone: A proof of concept trial. *Hum Reprod* 2015; 30(10): 2387–2395. https://doi.org/10.1093/humrep/dev184

42 Youssef, M. A., Abou-Setta, A. M. and Lam, W. S. Recombinant versus urinary human chorionic gonadotrophin for final oocyte maturation triggering in IVF and ICSI cycles. *Cochrane Database Syst Rev* 2016; 4(4): CD003719.

43 Abbara, A, Jayasena, C. N., Christopoulos, G. et al. Efficacy of kisspeptin-54 to trigger oocyte maturation in women at high risk of ovarian hyperstimulation syndrome (OHSS) during in vitro fertilization (IVF) therapy. *J Clin Endocrinol Metab* 2015; 100(9): 3322–3331. https://doi.org/10.1210/jc.2015-2332

44 Jeon, Y. E., Lee, K. E., Jung, J. A. et al. Kisspeptin, leptin and retinol-binding protein 4 in women with PCOS. *Gynecol Obstet Invest* 2013; 75(4): 268–274. https://doi.org/10.1159/000350217

45 Wong, K. M., van Wely, M., Mol, F., Repping, S. and Mastenbroek, S. Fresh versus frozen embryo transfers in assisted reproduction. *Cochrane Database Syst Rev* 2017; 3: CD011184.

46 Chen, Z.-J., Shi, Y., Sun, Y. et al. Fresh versus frozen embryos for infertility in the polycystic ovary syndrome. *N Engl J Med* 2016; 375: 523–533.

47 Diamanti-Kandarakis, E., Christakou, C. D., Kandaraki, E. and Economou, F. N. Metformin: An old medication of new fashion: Evolving new molecular mechanisms and clinical implications in polycystic ovary syndrome. *Eur J Endocrinol* 2010; 162: 193–212.

48 Sharpe, A., Morley, L. C., Tang, T., Norman, R. J. and Balen, A. H. Metformin for ovulation induction (excluding gonadotrophins) in women with polycystic ovary syndrome. *Cochrane Database Syst Rev* 2019; 12: CD013505.

49 Tso, L. O., Costello, M. F., Albuquerque, L. E., Andriolo, R. B. and Macedo, C. R. Metformin treatment before and during IVF or ICSI in women with polycystic ovary syndrome. *Cochrane Database Syst Rev* 2014; 11: CD006105.

50 Doldi, N., Persico, P., Di Sebastiano, F., Marsiglio, E., Ferrari, A. Gonadotropin-releasing hormone antagonist and metformin for treatment of polycystic ovary syndrome patients undergoing in vitro fertilization-embryo transfer. *Gynecol Endocrinol* 2006; 22(5): 235–238.

51 Jacob, S. L., Brewer, C., Tang, T., Picton, H. M., Barth, J. H. and Balen, A. H. A short course of metformin does not reduce OHS in a GnRH

antagonist cycle for women with PCOS undergoing IVF: A randomised placebo-controlled trial. *Hum Reprod* 2016; 31(12): 2756–2764. https://doi.org/10.1093/humrep/dew268

52 Siristatidis, C. S., Maheshwari, A., Vaidakis, D. and Bhattacharya, S. In vitro maturation in subfertile women with polycystic ovarian syndrome undergoing assisted reproduction. *Cochrane Database of Syst Rev* 2018; 11: CD006606.

53 Mostinckx, L., Segers, I., Belva, F. et al. Obstetric and neonatal outcome of ART in patients with polycystic ovary syndrome: IVM of oocytes versus controlled ovarian stimulation. *Hum Reprod* 2019; 34(8): 1595–1607.

Pregnancy Complications and Children Outcomes in Patients with Polycystic Ovarian Syndrome

Femi Janse and Bart C. J. M. Fauser

Introduction

Polycystic ovary syndrome (PCOS) is a notoriously heterogeneous, common reproductive disorder associated with many coexisting conditions, including hyperandrogenemia, obesity, insulin resistance and other signs of metabolic dysfunction.[1, 2] PCOS itself along with these coexisting conditions may lead – next to anovulatory infertility – to adverse pregnancy outcomes as well as adverse long-term health outcomes of children born to women with PCOS (Figure 14.1).

The current chapter focuses on the implications of PCOS for the course of pregnancy and the health of offspring. This is especially important considering the "Barker hypothesis." This hypothesis suggests that fetal programming by the (endocrine) milieu in utero takes place at an early stage of pregnancy, thus affecting neuroendocrine systems that regulate body weight, dietary metabolism and glycemic control and thereby influencing long-term health in the offspring.[3] In addition, complex genomic abnormalities associated with PCOS,[4] and resulting metabolic dysfunction, may give rise to abnormalities in offspring. It remains unknown what the relative contributions of nature (genetics) and nurture (environment) are for suboptimal offspring health in PCOS. It seems crucial to make a clear distinction between these two phenomena, since only the environment during early pregnancy could be modified to improve perinatal outcomes, whereas genetics cannot.

Being able to identify risk factors for adverse pregnancy outcomes in women with PCOS will bring forward potential leads for intervention and secondary prevention. Moreover, this knowledge should encompass possibilities to treat the condition of PCOS in a transgenerational approach (Figure 14.2).

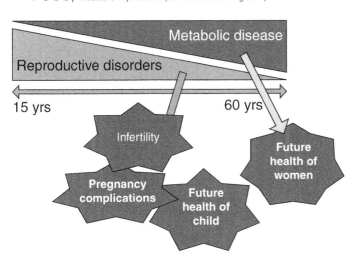

PCOS, *metabolic implications (both short- and long-term)*

Figure 14.1 Schematic representation concerning the major focus on reproductive dysfunction at young age and metabolic dysfunction at older age in women diagnosed with PCOS

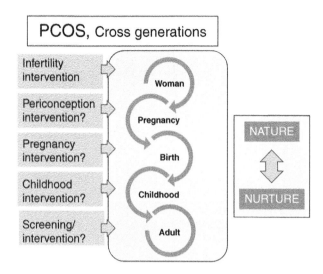

Figure 14.2 Schematic representation of cross-generational events in PCOS
It seems important to understand the natural cause of events in order to identify useful interventions during each stage of development.

PCOS and Infertility

PCOS is a common cause of anovulatory infertility. Although population studies demonstrate that a proportion of women with PCOS conceive spontaneously, the great majority require medical care (i.e. ovulation induction). Overall, prognosis of achieving a pregnancy is good. It is advised to first start with lifestyle modification and weight loss.[5] Pharmacologic treatment is commenced if cycles remain anovulatory. Classic ovulation induction is the first choice of treatment (see Chapters 11 and 12). In case aromatase inhibitors or clomiphene citrate are unsuccessful, this is usually followed by low-dose exogenous gonadotropins.[6] IVF treatment is recommended as a third-line, final treatment.

Repeatedly, the literature has shown that ovulation induction is successful in the majority of women with anovulation due to PCOS. The reported singleton birth rate is as high as 60% in one year and 78% in two years of conventional ovulation induction.[7, 8] When women with PCOS turn to IVF (see Chapter 13), there is no statistically significant difference in live birth, pregnancy and miscarriage rates compared to healthy controls.[9]

However, more recent data suggest that not all women with PCOS benefit from a "one-size-fits-all" infertility treatment strategy. It is important to identify those women who will experience prolonged time to pregnancy of more than two to three years. Multiple predictive models for couples with anovulatory infertility for predicting live birth

or pregnancy rate have been proposed. Owing to the significant heterogeneity of the phenotype of PCOS, it has proved difficult to achieve a prediction model with high validity and accuracy. However, repeatedly, the following predictors have been identified to be statistically significant: female age; duration of infertility; obesity or BMI; insulin concentrations; serum testosterone concentrations and free androgen index (FAI); serum sex hormone-binding globulin (SHBG) concentrations; and race. The identification of these predictors is valuable since it will aid in individualizing infertility treatment strategies in women with PCOS.[10] Keeping in mind the recommendations of the recent international PCOS guideline to initiate infertility treatment with aromatase inhibitors such as letrozole, future predictive studies should evaluate the effect of this new treatment on time to pregnancy and live birth rate.[6]

A point of concern is the risk of multiple pregnancy in infertility treatment. Multiple pregnancy itself is associated with many obstetric risks, such as hyperglycemia and gestational diabetes, hypertensive disorders and preterm birth. As will become more apparent in the next section, the condition of PCOS is also associated with these (and other) adverse obstetric factors. When infertility treatment is sought, women with PCOS should be counseled about these increased risks. Moreover, it is of the utmost importance to strive for singleton pregnancies in women with PCOS. When IVF is initiated, single embryo transfer should be advocated.[6, 11]

Table 14.1 Overview of adverse pregnancy outcomes in women with PCOS according to six published meta-analyses

Outcome	Boomsma, HRU 2006 [12]	Kjerulff, AJOG 2011 [13]	Qin, Reprod Biol Endocrinol 2013[14]	Yu, Medicine 2016[15]*	Bahri Khomami, Obes Rev 2018[16]	Sha, RBMO 2019[17]
Gestational diabetes	2.9 (1.7–5.1)	2.8 (1.9–4.1)	2.8 (2.0–4.0)	2.8 (2.3–3.4)	2.9 (2.4–3.5)	2.7 (1.4–5.0)
Preeclampsia	3.5 (2.0–6.2)	4.2 (2.8–6.5)	3.3 (2.1–5.2)	2.8 (2.3–3.4)	1.9 (1.6–2.3)	–
Preterm birth	1.8 (1.2–2.6)	2.2 (1.6–3.0)	1.3 (0.6–3.2)	1.5 (1.2–1.9)	–	1.6 (1.3–2.0)

Note. Data are odds ratios with associated 95% confidence intervals. * Data in the meta-analysis by Yu et al. are reported as relative risks with associated 95% confidence intervals.

PCOS and Pregnancy Complications

Extensive evidence suggests a negative impact of PCOS on the course of pregnancy and pregnancy outcome, even in singleton pregnancies.[2] Table 14.1 shows the odds ratios (ORs) with 95% confidence intervals (CIs) of the available meta-analyses for the most important pregnancy complications.[12–17]

Gestational diabetes mellitus. Longitudinal follow-up data suggest that as many as 16–42% of women with PCOS develop gestational diabetes mellitus (GDM).[18–20] Six meta-analyses demonstrated that women with PCOS have an almost threefold significantly higher chance of developing gestational diabetes compared with controls.[12–17]

There are multiple risk factors in women with PCOS that seem related to the increased incidence of gestational diabetes. Firstly, insulin metabolism is often disturbed preconceptionally. Preconceptionally measured insulin concentrations and homeostasis model assessment of insulin resistance (HOMA-IR) are statistically significant higher in women with PCOS who develop GDM compared with those who do not develop GDM. These risk factors remained significant even when adjusted for preconceptional BMI and body composition (i.e. waist circumference and waist-to-hip ratio).[21]

Secondly, different PCOS phenotypes play a role. In a recent prospective cohort study, it was shown that women with all three phenotype characteristics (hyperandrogenism + polycystic ovaries + cycle disturbances) experience a 30% higher chance of developing GDM compared to those women with only two phenotype characteristics (9 and 11%, $p = 0.05$).[22] In addition, another study showed that women with hyperandrogenic (defined as FAI > 4.5) PCOS significantly more often developed GDM compared with those with normoandrogenic PCOS (i.e. 45% vs. 24%, $p = 0.003$) (Figure 14.3).[20] Furthermore, preconceptionally measured lower sex hormone-binding globulin concentrations lead to increased incidence of GDM ($p < 0.001$). [18] Physiologically this can be explained because low levels of SHBG lead to an increase in circulating free androgens, thereby again highlighting the association of hyperandrogenism in PCOS and GDM.[23]

Thirdly, obesity is a known risk factor for developing gestational diabetes in general. In observational studies, women with PCOS often present with a significantly increased BMI. Therefore, some investigators mention that the higher BMI itself may be the main contributor to the increased incidence of GDM in women with PCOS. Others have identified that those women with PCOS who do develop GDM are generally more obese than those women with PCOS who do not develop GDM.[18] However, when prediction models for GDM in women with PCOS were constructed, the addition of body composition (i.e. waist circumference) leads to a nonsignificant contribution of BMI (OR 1.11; 95% CI 1.00 to 1.23), thereby indicating that BMI alone is not an independent risk factor for the development of GDM in women with PCOS.[18, 23, 24]

Hypertensive disorders of pregnancy. During normal, uncomplicated pregnancy, blood pressure rises with advancing gestation. This also

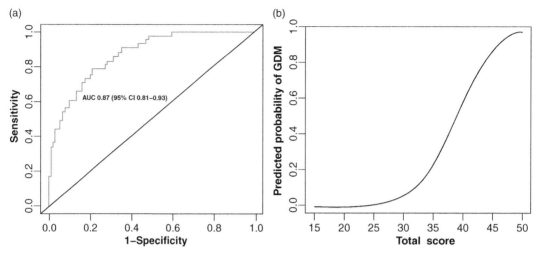

Figure 14.3 Prediction models for development of GDM in women with PCOS
Source. Reprinted from M. A. de Wilde et al. Preconception predictors of gestational diabetes: A multicentre prospective cohort study on the predominant complication of pregnancy in polycystic ovary syndrome. *Hum Reprod* 2014; 29: 1327–1336 with permission from Oxford University Press.
In a prospective cohort study of 326 women with PCOS a multivariate prediction model for the preconceptional identification of women with PCOS at increased risk for developing GDM was constructed.[19] Univariate and multivariate logistic regression of preconception patient characteristics were used. The area under the curve (AUC) of the receiver-operating characteristic was used to test the performance of the model (Figure 14.3(a)), and it was shown that the prediction model based on fasting glucose, fasting insulin, androstenedione, SHBG and first-degree relatives with type 2 diabetes performed well (AUC 0.87; 95% CI 0.81 to 0.93). Furthermore, the probability of developing GDM can be calculated by adding subscores for these five predictors (such as the levels of fasting glucose) and matching this total score with a probability of developing GDM, as is shown in Figure 14.3(b).

holds true for women with PCOS and does not seem to follow a different pattern. Furthermore, the incidence of pregnancy-induced hypertension is not significantly increased in women with PCOS compared to controls.[25, 26]

In contrast, preeclampsia (PE) is two to four times more frequently encountered in pregnant women with PCOS compared with controls (OR 1.9 to 4.2) (Table 14.1).[12–16] Similar to the incidence of GDM, the occurrence of PE in women with PCOS is dependent on PCOS phenotype. Hyperandrogenic forms of PCOS are associated with an increased risk for preeclampsia compared to normoandrogenic subtypes (OR 2.4; 95% CI 1.3 to 4.6; $p < 0.001$).[27] This increased risk remains statistically significant when controlling for a very common risk factor for PE, namely BMI. Another prospective follow-up study in a large cohort confirmed these results even when controlling for potential confounders such as preconceptionally measured markers of metabolic and cardiovascular disease: non-Caucasian ethnicity, family history of cardiovascular disease, smoking status, blood pressure, BMI, serum lipid levels, fasting insulin.[25] Importantly, women with normoandrogenic PCOS are not at increased risk for developing PE.[25, 27]

Preterm birth. The incidence of preterm birth is significantly increased in women with PCOS compared to healthy controls. The odds ratio (OR) varied between 1.3 and 2.2 in five of the abovementioned high-quality meta-analyses (Table 14.1).[11–15, 17] One could hypothesize that the increased preterm birth rate in women with PCOS could be due to increased induction of labor, for reasons such as placenta insufficiency associated with PE or GDM. However, data from large cohort studies show that the increased preterm birth rate is primarily due to spontaneous deliveries.[27, 28] The increased preterm birth rate is confined to late preterm birth and does not involve early preterm birth.[27]

As we have seen in GDM and PE, hyperandrogenism again plays a pivotal role in the high incidence of preterm birth in women with PCOS. It was shown that hyperandrogenic women with PCOS were almost three times more likely to deliver prematurely, while normoandrogenic women did not show a significantly increased risk compared to controls.[25, 27] No significant differences were seen between women with and women without oligomenorrhea or polycystic ovary morphology (PCOM) (Figure 14.4).

■ Feature present
▪ Feature absent

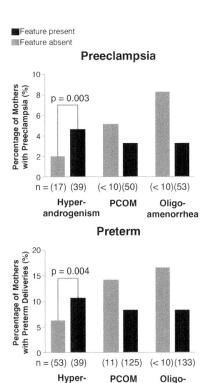

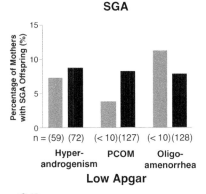

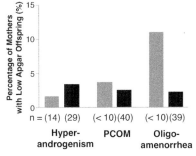

Figure 14.4 PCOS phenotype and pregnancy outcomes
Black bars represent women with the diagnostic feature, gray bars those without. Hyperandrogenism was identified as FAI ≥ 4.5 or Ferriman–Gallwey Score of ≥ 9.
Source. Reprinted from J. P. Christ et al. Pre-conception characteristics predict obstetrical and neonatal outcomes in women with polycystic ovary syndrome. *J Clin Endocrinol Metab* 2019;

Placental morphology. The placenta is suggested to play a key role in the development of pregnancy complications such as pregnancy-induced hypertension and preeclampsia. It is hypothesized that, in PCOS, early placentation is hampered because of detrimental contributors such as hyperandrogenemia and metabolic abnormalities like insulin resistance. Also obesity, which is encountered more often in women with PCOS, is associated with an increase in inflammatory response and pathologic lesions in the placenta.

Comparing placentas from women with PCOS to those of controls, more often chorioamnionitis (30 vs. 10%; $p = 0.001$), villitis (19 vs. 13%; $p = 0.045$), thrombosis (13 vs. 5%; $p = 0.02$), infarction (16 vs. 6%; $p = 0.01$) and villous immaturity (41 vs. 23%; $p = 0.009$) were identified. Subgroup analyses were performed to identify whether these differences could be explained by an increased incidence of pregnancy complications (such as GDM and PE); however, this was only the case for villitis and thrombosis. These findings suggest that PCOS by itself is associated with placenta abnormalities.[29] Increased placental inflammation has been related to pregnancy complications and maternal obesity, while thrombosis and infarction are signs of vascular damage and fetal hypoxia, both associated with PE and fetal growth restriction.

Animal models have shown that elevated androgen concentrations lead to an increase in the vascular tone of the uterine arteries, leading to decreased blood flow to the uterus. In addition, it has been shown that androgens reduce gene expression of proangiogenic factors, possible leading to impairment of spiral artery

Caption for Figure 14.4 (cont.)

104: 809–818 with permission from Oxford University Press. In a recent study data from 2768 well-phenotyped, prospectively followed-up women with PCOS were linked to data from a perinatal national registry. Women with PCOS were phenotyped preconceptionally, which involved BMI measurement, ultrasonography and extensive blood sampling, including androgens and lipids. The Dutch perinatal national registry included adverse pregnancy and neonatal outcome data such as preeclampsia, preterm birth, small for gestational age (SGA) and low Apgar scores. A significant increase in SGA risk by PCOS-specific features, such as preconceptionally increased FAI, could not be identified. Rather, the authors identified risk factors for SGA known in the general population, such as multiple gestation pregnancy, ethnicity, smoking and BMI. However, preeclampsia and preterm birth were significantly increased in women with a hyperandrogenic form of PCOS.

remodeling, which has been shown in women with PCOS also. In vitro studies have shown that insulin resistance, often encountered in women with PCOS, can impair IGF-1 signaling. IGF-1 is necessary for spiral artery remodeling by trophoblast invasion.[30]

PCOS and Offspring Health

Neonatal outcomes. Inevitably, pregnancy complications such as gestational diabetes and preeclampsia in PCOS mothers have a direct influence on neonatal outcomes. However, there is inconclusive evidence that PCOS alone is an independent risk factor for adverse obstetric and neonatal outcome.

Birth weight in children born to PCOS mothers is a much-debated topic. Four meta-analyses show inconsistent results with regard to risk for small for gestational age (SGA), large for gestational age (LGA) and macrosomia in these children (Table 14.2).[12, 13, 15, 17] Maternal obesity is a significant confounder for LGA and macrosomia. However, while some studies show that babies of obese PCOS mothers are at increased risk for LGA compared to obese non-PCOS mothers, others see an increase of SGA in obese women with PCOS.[23] Unfortunately, many studies published to date involve insufficiently large cohorts in which extensive phenotyping is lacking, which could lead to these conflicting findings. In recent years, however, two studies were published involving well-phenotyped women with PCOS. One study identified increased risk for SGA in women with PCOS (adjusted OR 3.3; 95% CI 1.3 to 8.4) compared to controls. Both studies also demonstrated that risk for SGA was even more pronounced in women with a hyperandrogenic form of PCOS (adjusted OR 5.3; 95% CI 2.0 to 13.8) (Table 14.3).[20] However, the other study involving well-phenotyped women with PCOS, and linking pregnancy outcomes with a perinatal national registry, could not identify a significant increase in SGA risk by PCOS-specific features, such as preconceptionally increased FAI. Rather, the authors identified risk factors for SGA known in the general population, such as multiple gestation pregnancy, ethnicity, smoking and BMI (Figure 14.4).[25]

Cesarean section rate is increased in women with PCOS (OR 1.5; 95% CI 1.4 to 1.6), even after controlling for obesity and pregnancy-associated hypertension. Congenital abnormalities appear to be at an almost twofold increase in PCOS offspring compared to controls. While it is known that first-trimester hyperglycemia and hyperinsulinemia are associated with increased risk for congenital abnormalities (cardiac, limb and neural tube defects), the finding persists after controlling for pregestational diabetes and GDM.[31]

Offspring follow-up. Long-term follow-up of the offspring of PCOS mothers is considered of great importance and is gaining increasing attention. Data derived from an American prospective

Table 14.2 Overview of adverse neonatal outcomes in women with PCOS according to four published meta-analyses

Outcome	Boomsma, HRU 2006 [12]	Kjerulff, AJOG 2011 [13]	Yu, Medicine 2016 [*15]	Sha, RBMO 2019 [17]
SGA	1.2 (0.3–5.1)	2.6 (1.4–5.1)	1.5 (0.96–2.20)	1.4 (0.8–2.3)
LGA	–	1.6 (0.9–2.6)	1.1 (0.9–1.4)	2.1 (1.01–4.4)
Macrosomia	1.1 (0.7–1.8)	–	–	–

Note. SGA = small for gestational age; LGA = large for gestational age. * Data in the meta-analysis by Yu et al are reported as relative risks with associated 95% confidence intervals.

In a study of 188 women with PCOS and 2889 healthy controls, women were prospectively followed-up during pregnancy for the identification of maternal and neonatal adverse outcomes. It was shown that women with the hyperandrogenic PCOS phenotype are especially at increased risk for any adverse pregnancy outcome (such as hypertensive disorders and GDM) (45%, adjusted OR 2.7; 95% CI 1.3 to 5.6) compared with those normoandrogenic PCOS (24%, adjusted OR 1.6; 95% CI 0.74 to 3.5) and controls (5%). Also a tendency for increased risk of any adverse neonatal outcome (such as preterm birth, LGA, SGA) was identified (adjusted OR 1.9; 95% CI 0.95 to 3.9), and adjusted OR 1.6 (95% CI 0.81 to 3.1), respectively. More specifically, SGA was significantly more frequently encountered in women with a hyperandrogenic form of PCOS (12%, adjusted OR 5.25; 95% CI 2.0 to 14) compared to women with normoandrogenic PCOS (8%, adjusted OR 3.3; 95% CI 1.3 to 8.4) and controls (6%).

Table 14.3 Univariate and multivariate logistic regression analysis of the pregnancy outcomes in women with hyperandrogenic PCOS (n = 76), women with normoandrogenic PCOS (n = 97) and the reference group (n = 2 889)

Outcome	OR (95% CI)			Adjusted OR (95% CI)a		
	Reference (n = 2889)	Normoandrogenic PCOS (n = 97)	Hyperandrogenic PCOS (n = 76)	Reference (n = 2889)	Normoandrogenic PCOS (n = 97)	Hyperandrogenic PCOS (n = 76)
Maternal complications						
Any maternal complicationb	Ref	2.24(1.37–3.65)	5.55(3.47–8.87)	Ref	1.60 (0.74–3.49)	2.67 (1.27–5.61)
Any hypertensive maternal complicationc	Ref	1.09 (0.52–2.27)	2.26(1.20–4.26)	Ref	1.50 (0.43–5.24)	1.77 (0.54–5.73)
Pregnancy-induced hypertension	Ref	0.94(0.41–2.18)	1.68(0.80–3.55)	Ref	1.26 (0.32–4.95)	1.20 (0.32–4.55)
Preeclampsia/HELLP	Ref	1.27(0.31–5.32)	3.36(1.18–9.57)	Ref	1.77 (0.13–24.2)	3.54 (0.46–27.3)
Gestational diabetes mellitus	Ref	3.91 (2.20–6.98)	11.1 (6.71–18.5)	Ref	3.17(1.28–7.84)	5.65 (2.49–12.8)
Neonatal complications						
Any neonatal complicationb	Ref	0.97 (0.59–1.59)	1.60 (0.98–2.61)	Ref	1.59 (0.81–3.11)	1.93 (0.95–3.91)
Spontaneous premature birth	Ref	1.82 (0.72–4.58)	2.35 (0.93–5.98)	Ref	1.06 (0.26–4.26)	0.62 (0.10–3.91)
Large for gestational age	Ref	0.57 (0.26–1.24)	0.73 (0.34–1.61)	Ref	0.88 (0.29–2.69)	0.64 (0.19–2.18)
Small for gestational age	Ref	1.35 (0.64–2.83)	2.00 (0.98–4.07)	Ref	3.26 (1.27–8.36)	5.25 (2.00–13.8)

Note. Hyperandrogenism was determined at initial screening before conception in the PCOS group. CI = confidence interval; HELLP = hemolysis elevated liver enzymes low platelets; OR = odds ratio; Ref = reference value.

a Odds ratio adjusted for body mass index, maternal age, parity, pregnancy after treatment (yes/no), and smoking during pregnancy;

b In some patients $\geq$ 1 complications occurred.

c Pregnancy-induced hypertension or preeclampsia/HELLP.

Source. M. A. de Wilde et al. Increased rates of complications in singleton pregnancies of women previously diagnosed with polycystic ovary syndrome predominantly in the hyperandrogenic phenotype. *Fertil Steril* 2017; 108: 333–340.

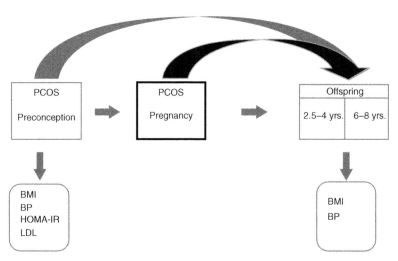

Figure 14.5 Offspring health of mothers with PCOS
BMI = body mass index; BP = blood pressure; HOMA-IR = homeostasis model assessment of insulin resistance; LDL = low-density lipoprotein-cholesterol. In blue: the investigated associations in this chapter; in gray: the potential role of pregnancy in mother–offspring associations.
Reprinted from M. N. Gunning et al. Associations of preconception body mass index in women with PCOS and BMI and blood pressure of their offspring. *Gynecol Endocrinol* 2019 ;35: 673–678 with permission from Taylor & Francis Ltd (www.tandfonline.com). A prospective follow-up study of preconceptionally well-phenotyped women with PCOS and their offspring reports on childhood BMI and blood pressure. In this study children were followed until age eight years. It was shown that preconceptional BMI of women with PCOS is positively associated with BMI in their offspring ($p = 0.01$), which is consistent with associations of BMI in offspring of the general population. No significant associations were identified between preconception systolic blood pressure, androgens, insulin resistance, and lipids, with offspring parameters.

birth cohort of 5000 children linked self-reported maternal PCOS phenotype data to infant growth. No differences were identified for height, weight and BMI between children born to women with PCOS ($n = 435$) compared to non-PCOS women, up until the age of three years. There was also no significant rapid weight gain in these children.[32]

A prospective follow-up study of preconceptionally well-phenotyped women with PCOS and their offspring also report on childhood BMI and blood pressure. In this study, children were followed until age eight years. It was shown that preconceptional BMI of women with PCOS is positively associated with BMI in their offspring ($p = 0.01$), which is consistent with associations of BMI in offspring of the general population. No significant associations were identified between preconception systolic blood pressure, androgens, insulin resistance and lipids with offspring parameters (Figure 14.5).[33]

Cardiovascular and metabolic health of the offspring of women with PCOS may be less favorable compared to controls. One study in children up to eight years of age, showed that young PCOS offspring have significantly higher arterial stiffness (measured by pulse pressure in the aorta),

significantly greater left ventricle diameter and significantly increased intima-media thickness of the carotids (a marker of preclinical atherosclerosis and stiffness). Also, LDL-cholesterol and triglyceride concentrations were significantly higher in offspring of women with PCOS compared with controls. These data suggest increased metabolic and cardiovascular risk in young children from mothers with PCOS. It remains to be elucidated to what extent this is related to (the combination of) the inherited predisposition, adverse intrauterine environment (hyperglycemia, hyperandrogenemia, preeclampsia) with epigenetic programming or lifestyle.[34]

Furthermore, neurodevelopmental development may be impaired in offspring of PCOS. A large population-based cohort study of a Finnish birth registry identified that maternal PCOS was associated with any psychiatric diagnosis (HR [hazard ratio] 1.32; 95% CI 1.27 to 1.38) in offspring. Specifically, sleeping disorders, attention-deficit/hyperactivity disorders, tic disorders, intellectual disabilities, autism spectrum, eating disorders and mood disorders were all significantly increased in offspring of women with PCOS. When adjusting for perinatal problems such as GDM, PCOS was still associated with increased incidence of impaired neurodevelopment. Children born to overweight PCOS women demonstrated the highest incidence of psychiatric illnesses.[35] These findings are supported by a recent meta-analysis. The offspring of women with PCOS were 66% more likely to be diagnosed with autism spectrum disorder compared with children of non-PCOS mothers, a finding that remained significant after correction for maternal age at birth, hypertension, obesity, diabetes mellitus, preterm birth or child gender. It was hypothesized that this increase could be due to previously known risk factors for development of autism spectrum disorders that are more prevalent in children of PCOS mothers: hyperandrogenic intrauterine environment, preeclampsia and birth through caesarean section. Whether the condition of PCOS itself is actually associated with autism remains unclear.[36]

Biomarkers. It is hypothesized that a maternal hyperandrogenic environment during pregnancy in women with PCOS may predispose the offspring to fetal hyperandrogenism and thereby potentially lead to long-term health consequences in offspring. Endocrine and cardiometabolic biomarkers have been studied in offspring of women with PCOS and compared with offspring of healthy controls. In one study, cord blood samples were drawn and estradiol, androstenedione, dehydroepiandrosterone sulfate (DHEAS), testosterone, SHBG, FAI, insulin, total cholesterol, low-density lipoprotein (LDL) cholesterol, high-density lipoprotein (HDL) cholesterol, triglycerides, c-reactive protein, adiponectin and leptin were measured. Only androstenedione proved to be statistically significantly increased in offspring of women with PCOS, after correction for maternal age, gestational age and birth weight. Preconceptional androgen levels of the PCOS mothers were not associated with differences in cord blood androgen measurements. [37] Another study could not identify the increase of any androgen concentration in cord blood from children born to women with PCOS.[38] Therefore, more research is needed to elucidate this topic.

Data from various studies focusing on specific cardiometabolic biomarkers in the offspring of women with PCOS have been studied together in a recently published individual participant data (IPD) meta-analysis. The IPD meta-analysis included data from 885 children, of whom nearly 300 children were born to women with PCOS, up to the age of 18 years. The data showed subtle but significant signs of altered cardiometabolic health in children of PCOS mothers, namely significantly lower HDL-cholesterol and lower birth weight in all PCOS offspring. Furthermore, in female offspring of PCOS women, higher insulin concentrations, higher HDL-cholesterol, lower LDL-cholesterol and lower total cholesterol were identified compared with female offspring of controls.[39] In addition, a small study on metabolic and inflammatory biomarkers in women with PCOS and their offspring also suggest increased chronic low-grade inflammation in PCOS offspring.[40] Together, these data suggest a potential detrimental effect of maternal PCOS on offspring cardiometabolic health, which may be gender-specific.

Conclusions

PCOS and associated coexisting conditions (i.e. hyperandrogenemia, obesity, insulin resistance and other signs of metabolic dysfunction) may lead – next to anovulatory infertility – to pregnancy complications, adverse perinatal outcomes and suboptimal long-term health of children born to women with PCOS. While pregnancy chances following infertility treatment in PCOS are favorable and chances for multiple pregnancies and associated complications have been reduced dramatically in recent years, there is no "one-size-fits-all" strategy and success rates are dependent on various factors such as female age, duration of infertility, BMI and serum insulin, testosterone and SHBG concentrations.

Convincing evidence demonstrates an increased risk for gestational diabetes (OR 2.7 to 2.9), hypertensive disorders of pregnancy (including preeclampsia, OR 1.9 to 4.2) and preterm birth (OR 1.5 to 2.2) in women with PCOS. Hyperandrogenemia plays an independent role in the occurrence of these pregnancy complications, while BMI or obesity alone is not an independent risk factor. Much uncertainty remains concerning the influence of PCOS on offspring health, especially regarding birth weight. However, measurements of cardiovascular health, metabolic risk factors and biomarkers point toward a less favorable profile in children born to women with PCOS, especially when a hyperandrogenic phenotype of PCOS is present. Future studies should focus on long-term follow-up of well-phenotyped PCOS offspring and specifically looking at cardiovascular and metabolic health.

References

1 The Rotterdam ESHRE/ASRM-Sponsored PCOS Consensus Workshop Group. Revised 2003 consensus on diagnostic criteria and long-term health risks related to polycystic ovary syndrome (PCOS). *Hum Reprod* 2004; 19(1): 41–47.

2 The Amsterdam ESHRE/ASRM-Sponsored 3rd PCOS Consensus Workshop Group. Consensus on women's health aspects of polycystic ovary syndrome (PCOS). *Hum Reprod* 2012; 27(1): 14–24.

3 Barker, D. J. Fetal programming of coronary heart disease. *Trends Endocrinol Metab* 2002; 13(9): 364–368.

4 Day, F., Karaderi, T., Jones, M. R. et al. Large-scale genome-wide meta-analysis of polycystic ovary syndrome suggests shared genetic architecture for different diagnosis criteria. *PLoS Genet* 2018; 14 (12): e1007813.

5 The Thessaloniki ESHRE/ASRM-Sponsored PCOS Consensus Workshop Group. Consensus on infertility treatment related to polycystic ovary syndrome. *Hum Reprod* 2008; 89(3): 505–522.

6 Teede, H. J., Misso, M. L., Costello, M. F. et al. Recommendations from the international evidence-based guideline for the assessment and management of polycystic ovary syndrome. *Hum Reprod* 2018; 33(9): 1602–1618.

7 Eijkemans, M. J., Imani, B., Mulders, A. G., Habbema, J. D. and Fauser, B.C. High singleton live birth rate following classical ovulation induction in normogonadotrophic anovulatory infertility (WHO 2). *Hum Reprod* 2003; 18(11): 2357–2362.

8 Veltman-Verhulst, S. M., Fauser, B. C. and Eijkemans, M. J. High singleton live birth rate confirmed after ovulation induction in women with anovulatory polycystic ovary syndrome: Validation of a prediction model for clinical practice. *Fertil Steril* 2012; 98(3): 761–768.

9 Heijnen, E. M., Eijkemans, M. J., Hughes, E. G., Laven, J. S., Macklon, N. S. and Fauser, B. C. A meta-analysis of outcomes of conventional IVF in women with polycystic ovary syndrome. *Hum Reprod Update* 2006; 12(1): 13–21.

10 Gunning, M. N., Christ, J., van Rijn, B. et al. Predicting pregnancy chances leading to term live birth within first year of treatment in women with Polycystic Ovary Syndrome (PCOS). Submitted 2020.

11 Fauser, B. C., Devroey, P. and Macklon, N. S. Multiple birth resulting from ovarian stimulation for subfertility treatment. *Lancet* 2005; 365(9473): 1807–1816.

12 Boomsma, C. M., Eijkemans, M. J., Hughes, E. G., Visser, G. H., Fauser, B. C. and Macklon, N. S. A meta-analysis of pregnancy outcomes in women with polycystic ovary syndrome. *Hum Reprod Update* 2006; 12(6): 673–683.

13 Kjerulff, L. E., Sanchez-Ramos, L. and Duffy, D. Pregnancy outcomes in women with polycystic ovary syndrome: A meta-analysis. *Am J Obstet Gynecol* 2011; 204(6): 558.e1–6.

14 Qin, J. Z., Pang, L. H., Li, M. J., Fan, X. J., Huang, R. D. and Chen, H. Y. Obstetric complications in women with polycystic ovary syndrome: A systematic review and meta-analysis. *Reprod Biol Endocrinol* 2013; 11(11): 56.

15 Yu, H., Chen, H., Rao, D.-P. and Gong, J. Association between polycystic ovary syndrome and the risk of pregnancy complications: A PRISMA-compliant systematic review and meta-analysis. *Medicine* 2016; 95(51): e4863.

16 Bahri Khomami, M., Joham, A. E., Boyle, J. A. et al. Increased maternal pregnancy complications in polycystic ovary syndrome appear to be independent of obesity: A systematic review, meta-analysis, and meta-regression. *Obes Rev* 2018; 20 (5): 659–674.

17 Sha, T., Wang, X., Cheng, W. and Yan, Y. A meta-analysis of pregnancy-related outcomes and complications in women with polycystic ovary syndrome undergoing IVF. *RBMO* 2019; 39(2): 281–293.

18 Veltman-Verhulst, S. M., van Haeften, T. W., Eijkemans, M. J., de Valk, H. W., Fauser, B. C. and Goverde, A. J. Sex hormone-binding globulin concentrations before conception as a predictor for gestational diabetes in women with polycystic ovary syndrome. *Hum Reprod* 2010; 25(12): 3123–3128.

19 de Wilde, M. A., Veltman-Verhulst, S. M., Goverde, A. J. et al. Preconception predictors of gestational diabetes: A multicentre prospective cohort study on the predominant complication of pregnancy in polycystic ovary syndrome. *Hum Reprod* 2014; 29(6): 1327–1336.

20 de Wilde, M. A., Lamain-de Ruiter, M., Veltman-Verhulst, S. M. et al. Increased rates of complications in singleton pregnancies of women previously diagnosed with polycystic ovary syndrome predominantly in the hyperandrogenic phenotype. *Fertil Steril* 2017; 108(2): 333–340.

21 de Wilde, M. A., Goverde, A. J., Veltman-Verhulst, S. M. et al. Insulin action in women with polycystic

ovary syndrome and its relation to gestational diabetes. *Hum Reprod* 2015; 30(6): 1447–1453.

22 Foroozanfard, F., Asemi, Z., Bazarganipour, F., Taghavi, S. A., Alland, H. and Aramesh, S. Comparing pregnancy, childbirth, and neonatal outcomes in women with different phenotypes of polycystic ovary syndrome and healthy women: A prospective cohort study. *Gynecol Endocrinol* 2020; 36(1): 61–65.

23 Palomba, S., de Wilde, M. A., Falbo, A., Koster, M. P., La Sala, G. B. and Fauser, B. C. Pregnancy complications in women with polycystic ovary syndrome. *Hum Reprod Update* 2015; 21(5): 575–592.

24 Palm, C. V. B, Glintborg, D., Boye Kyhl, H. et al. Polycystic ovary syndrome and hyperglycaemia in pregnancy: A narrative review and results from a prospective Danish cohort study. *Diabetes Res Clin Pract* 2018; 145: 167–177.

25 Christ, J.P., Gunning, M. N., Meun, C. et al. Pre-conception characteristics predict obstetrical and neonatal outcomes in women with polycystic ovary syndrome. *J Clin Endocrinol Metab* 2019; 104(3): 809–818.

26 Nielsen, J. N., Birukov, A., Jensen, R. C. et al. Blood pressure and hypertension during pregnancy in women with polycystic ovary syndrome: Odense Child Cohort. *Acta Obstet Gynecol Scand* 2020; 99 (10): 1354–1363.

27 Naver, K. V., Grinsted, J., Larsen, S. O. et al. Increased risk of preterm delivery and pre-eclampsia in women with polycystic ovary syndrome and hyperandrogenaemia. *BJOG* 2014; 121(5): 575–581.

28 Roos, N., Kieler, H., Sahlin, L., Ekman-Ordeberg, G., Falconer, H. and Stephansson, O. Risk of adverse pregnancy outcomes in women with polycystic ovary syndrome: Population-based cohort study. *Br Med J* 2011; 343: d6309.

29 Koster, M. P., de Wilde, M. A., Veltman-Verhulst, S. M. et al. Placental characteristics in women with polycystic ovary syndrome. *Hum Reprod* 2015; 30 (12): 2829–2837.

30 Kelley, A. S., Smith, Y. R. and Padmanabhan, V. A narrative review of placental contribution to adverse pregnancy outcomes in women with polycystic ovary syndrome. *J Clin Endocrinol Metab* 2019; 104(11): 5299–5315.

31 Mills, G., Badeghiesh, A., Suarthana, E., Baghlaf, H. and Dahan, M. H. Associations between polycystic ovary syndrome and adverse obstetric and neonatal outcomes: A population study of 9.1 million births. *Hum Reprod* 2020; 35(8): 1914–1921.

32 Bell, G. A., Sundaram, R., Mumford, S. L. et al. Maternal polycystic ovarian syndrome and offspring growth: The Upstate KIDS Study. *J Epidemiol Community Health* 2018; 72(9): 852–855.

33 Gunning, M. N., van Rijn, B. B., Bekker, M. N., de Wilde, M. A., Eijkemans, M. J. C. and Fauser, B. C. J. M. Associations of preconception body mass index in women with PCOS and BMI and blood pressure of their offspring. *Gynecol Endocrinol* 2019; 35(8): 673–678.

34 de Wilde, M. A., Eising, J. B., Gunning, M. N. et al. Cardiovascular and metabolic health of 74 children from women previously diagnosed with polycystic ovary syndrome in comparison with a population-based reference cohort. *Reprod Sci* 2018; 25(10): 1492–1500.

35 Chen, H. R., Kong, L., Piltonen, T., Gissler, M. and Lavebratt, C. Association of polycystic ovary syndrome or anovulatory infertility with offspring psychiatric and mild neurodevelopmental disorders: A Finnish population-based cohort study. *Hum Reprod* 2020; 35(10): 2336–2347.

36 Katsigianni, M., Karageorgiou, V., Lambrinoudaki, I. and Siristatidis, C. Maternal polycystic ovarian syndrome in autism spectrum disorder: A systematic review and meta-analysis. *Mol Psychiatry* 2019; 24(12): 1787–1797.

37 Daan, N. M., Koster, M. P., Steegers-Theunissen, R. P., Eijkemans, M. J. and Fauser, B. C. Endocrine and cardiometabolic cord blood characteristics of offspring born to mothers with and without polycystic ovary syndrome. *Fertil Steril* 2017; 107 (1): 261–268.e3.

38 Caanen, M. R., Kuijper, E. A., Hompes, P. G. et al. Mass spectrometry methods measured androgen and estrogen concentrations during pregnancy and in newborns of mothers with polycystic ovary syndrome. *Eur J Endocrinol* 2016; 174(1): 25–32.

39 Gunning, M. N., Petermann, T., Crisosto, N. et al. Cardiometabolic health in offspring of women with PCOS compared to healthy controls: A systematic review and individual participant data meta-analysis. *Hum Reprod Update* 2020; 26(1): 103–117.

40 Daan, N. M., Koster, M. P., de Wilde, M. A. et al. Biomarker profiles in women with PCOS and PCOS offspring: A pilot study. *PLoS One* 2016; 11 (11): e0165033.

The Role of In Vitro Maturation in Polycystic Ovary Syndrome

Roger J. Hart and Melanie Walls

Introduction

In vitro maturation (IVM) should be viewed as an alternative form of in vitro fertilization (IVF) treatment, whereby the patient receives little or no gonadotropin stimulation prior to oocyte retrieval, and the oocytes complete their final stages of maturation in the laboratory, as opposed to in vivo in a traditional IVF cycle. The proposed benefits of its use over the traditional IVF approach will be discussed in detail, but for women with polycystic ovary syndrome (PCOS), primarily they relate to the complete avoidance of the serious medical condition of ovarian hyperstimulation syndrome (OHSS), which is a particular risk.

IVM technology has been around for many years and was first described using an animal model in the 1930s.[1] The technique was later demonstrated to be feasible in humans in 1965, when oocytes aspirated from unstimulated follicles underwent spontaneous maturation.[2] The first live birth was recorded in 1991, after oocytes were collected and matured after ovarian biopsy, [3] and then in 1994 using transvaginal collection. [4] Subsequently, several centers around the world adopted and developed the IVM technology; however, the pregnancy rates achieved after IVM technology were low, due in part to poor embryo and endometrial development, and synchronization, with a fresh embryo transfer cycle. Consequently, this led to the technology not being widely accepted by the broader clinical infertility community and, for those sites persisting with the IVM technology, they adopted the approach of multiple embryo transfers to avoid the low implantation potential of each embryo. Essentially, it was not until the publication of the seminal paper by Junk and Yeap,[5] who were the pioneers of this technology in Western Australia, that there was a resurgence of international interest in IVM technology.

In Vivo Oocyte Maturation

In a normal menstrual cycle, the increasing serum concentration of estradiol produced by granulosa cells initiates a mid-cycle surge of pituitary gland secretion of luteinizing hormone (LH). This LH surge initiates several events that lead to in vivo oocyte maturation. The synchrony of nuclear and cytoplasmic maturation are two critical processes that are essential for oocyte competency and successful embryonic development. Nuclear maturation allows for the development and organization of the oocyte's nuclear material and arrests after the second meiotic division, metaphase II (MII). With the resumption of meiosis, subsequent to the LH surge, the germinal vesicle breaks down and the nuclear membrane disappears, chromatin condenses and the chromosomes align at the equatorial region of the meiotic spindle and spindle migration to the oocyte cortex occurs. The polar body is then extruded following homologous chromosome separation and the oocyte arrests at MII. Simultaneous with this maturation, cytoplasmic maturation occurs, which involves structural and functional modifications, changes that support oocyte activation, fertilization and embryo development. The oocyte gains the potential to undergo activation by concentrating cortical granules just below the oolemma. It is these cortical granules that are released in response to microinjection or sperm penetration.

Fertilization

It is the release of the cortical granules that initiates the hardening of the outer "shell" of the oocyte, the zona pellucida, which then acts as a functional block to further sperm penetration. Furthermore, cytoplasmic maturation is a prerequisite for successful sperm head decondensation and mitochondrial redistribution occurs, with the mitochondria relocating to the perinuclear region. Consequently, successful embryonic development relies on successful and synchronous cytoplasmic and nuclear maturation.[6]

In Vitro Maturation

To try to replicate the in vivo maturation of oocytes has been problematic and has led to refinements of specific culture conditions,[7] stimulation protocols,[8] patient selection[9] and fertilization techniques[10] to try to improve clinical outcomes. This chapter will discuss the current situation of IVM treatment offered in the particular centers with an interest in this field.

PCOS As an Indication for IVM Technology

In a natural menstrual cycle, the mid-cycle LH surge initiates the series of events that lead to follicle rupture that is ovulation. At the same time, inflammatory cytokines are released from the follicle into the vascular system. Consequently, as in standard IVF, the normal menstrual cycle is significantly amplified by gonadotropins to maximize the number of developing follicles. This ensures a patient will have several oocytes available for her treatment, hence a woman with many ovarian follicles will be at substantial risk of OHSS. OHSS describes the situation whereby inflammatory cytokines, released by the ovarian follicles, are disseminated into the vascular system and cause intravascular hemoconcentration and extravasation of fluid into the abdominal and pleural cavities, which lead to significant patient discomfort and the risk of a thrombotic event.[11] Consequently, a woman with multiple follicles, a typical ovarian polycystic appearance, is a very suitable patient for IVM technology because, with IVM treatment, there is no risk of OHSS.[12] The reason why there is no risk of OHSS is that the follicles are aspirated at a much smaller size (12 mm) than in a standard IVF treatment cycle and that, in most treatment protocols, no "trigger" injection is administered to initiate in vivo oocyte maturation with the release of inflammatory cytokines.[12] Consequently, the woman is spared the significant discomfort of OHSS and has a chance of conceiving that is similar to if she had embarked on a standard IVF cycle.[12] Our personal data suggest that a woman will end up with half the number of oocytes that she has follicles developing and that fertilization and blastocyst development are similar to standard IVF, without the discomfort. However, pregnancy rates using cryopreserved embryos have generally been much better than with the transfer of fresh embryos,[12] so this is our standard approach. Furthermore, we feel that to offer IVM to a woman of 37 years or older is not appropriate as the success rates of the treatment markedly diminish, perhaps as the older oocyte has a greater difficulty in synchronizing nuclear and cytoplasmic maturation, leading to compromised blastocyst development.[12, 13] However, it maybe that, with the use of refined culture conditions, the treatment can be extended to older women in the future.

It is also worth noting that another reason to advocate IVM treatment for a young woman with a good antral follicle count is her geographical location, as a woman who potentially is at risk of OHSS is obliged to stay in close proximity to her treating unit until the risk of OHSS subsides. This can be a significant impost on a woman who resides in a distant rural community. Hence it is perhaps not surprising that two centers with long track records of IVM treatment, Western Australia and Quebec,[12, 14] have large regional populations that have enabled them to develop their protocols and expertise.

Despite the very encouraging reports from centers with a special interest in IVM, there has been a limited take-up of this technology across the world. The reason for this may be due to the relatively recent introduction into traditional stimulation treatment protocols of multiple treatment strategies that minimize OHSS risk for susceptible patients. These therapies to minimize the risk of OHSS consist of the use of an agonist trigger in an antagonist cycle and adopting a "freeze-only" approach to the embryos, virtually eliminating the risk of OHSS for the majority of patients.[15] Furthermore, other well-established strategies consist of the concurrent use of metformin, the use of an antagonist for ovarian downregulation and cabergoline administered from the time of trigger, and the procedure of ovarian drilling.[16]

Other Potential Indications for the Use of IVM Technology

Perhaps the most rewarding alternative indication for the use of an IVM cycle is that it can be performed with either no or minimal ovarian stimulation at any stage of the menstrual cycle, over a short time frame. Hence, for an oncological patient with PCOS, it is possible to review a patient and immediately commence treatment and collect oocytes within a 3–5-day time frame, enabling a rapid progression to oncological management after successful oocyte verification as a method of fertility preservation. IVM also has its place as a method of fertility preservation for women with estrogen-sensitive tumors, such as breast or endometrial cancer, where these patients are understandably very concerned about any potential consequences of an elevated estradiol concentration during a stimulated IVF cycle on their malignancy. An alternative approach is to undergo IVM treatment, as generally follicles are aspirated at a maximal diameter of 12 mm, hence the serum estradiol concentrations generally approximate those found typically in mid-cycle for a woman in a spontaneous ovulatory cycle. A further potential use of IVM technology for a woman with PCOS who desires fertility preservation, who is undergoing oophorectomy as part of her treatment, is the possibility of aspirating follicles at the time of oophorectomy and maturing the oocytes in vitro. We have reported collecting 22 immature oocytes at the time of surgery, which, after 24 hours of culture, resulted in 15 MII oocytes and, after a further 24 hours of culture, 3 more oocytes matured, resulting in 18 oocytes vitrified for her future use.[17]

Stimulation Protocols

The development of protocols for IVM treatment have focused on ovarian stimulation and the need (or lack of) for a "trigger" injection. Various IVM stimulation protocols have been employed and documented and extensively debated in the literature.[18] Protocols differ with respect to the need for ovarian stimulation with follicle-stimulating hormone (FSH) prior to oocyte retrieval – namely, "ovarian priming," which ensures a cohort of follicles starts to develop until the lead follicle is approximately 12–14 mm in diameter at the time of follicular aspiration, versus the "natural cycle" approach, whereby follicular aspiration is performed without the use of FSH injections. Initial studies appeared to demonstrate that FSH priming in ovulatory women without a polycystic ovarian morphology did not improve oocyte numbers retrieved, their

maturation rate or the embryo cleavage rate or embryo development.[19] However, a further study by the same group showed that FSH priming improved the oocyte maturation potential and embryo implantation rates for women with PCOS.[20] In more recent years, the use of FSH priming to enable the development of larger and a greater cohort of follicles has become standard, as it led to the highest reported success rates.[5]

Additionally, there exists further debate as to the requirement to administer a "trigger" injection prior to follicular aspiration, mimicking the mid-cycle LH surge. While the use of the trigger is vigorously debated,[18] the only randomized controlled trial of the use, or not, of a trigger injection did not demonstrate any significant differences in embryological or clinical outcomes. [21] As protocols vary to a significant degree, each institution should audit their individual practice. A recent Chinese retrospective review of the use of human chorionic gonadotropin (hCG) priming in unstimulated IVM cycles, for women with PCOS, did not lead to any improvements in any clinical outcomes,[22] in line with the Cochrane Review published in 2016.[23]

It is our opinion that IVM means that oocyte maturation, from germinal vesicle breakdown to the development of a MII oocyte, should be completed in the laboratory. Our protocol involves the administration of ovarian stimulation for follicular priming, approximately 150 IU of FSH. No trigger injection is administered, follicles are aspirated at a maximum diameter of 12 mm and the maturation of the oocytes takes place in the laboratory with the interval transfer of a single blastocyst. This has led to clinical pregnancy rates approximating those of a standard IVF cycle.[12]

Oocyte Collection Procedure

Oocyte collection protocols for IVM vary widely, although they are very similar to the standard transvaginal oocyte aspiration procedure performed for IVF treatment, with slight modifications to collect oocytes from smaller follicles while minimizing the potential harm to the cumulus oocyte complexes. The collection procedure for IVM is important in order to maximize oocyte yield, as generally the number of oocytes collected is approximately half the number of follicles present.[12] For collection, a 16-guage needle is

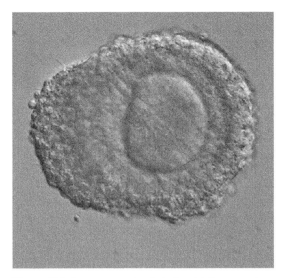

Figure 15.1 Immature oocyte displaying tightly compact corona radiata after IVM oocyte collection

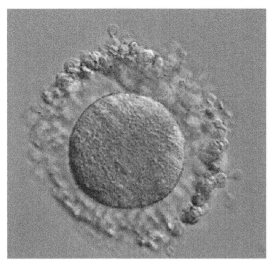

Figure 15.2 Immature oocyte displaying limited coronal cells and visible GV stage nucleus after IVM oocyte collection

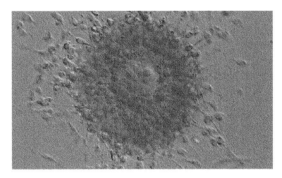

Figure 15.3 IVM oocyte displaying expanding and proliferating coronal cells after 24 hours in maturation culture

used, while maintaining the integrity of the oocyte. The oocyte retrieval procedure is more difficult than with a standard IVF collection, with aspiration pressures between 52.5 mmHg [9] and 200 mmHg.[24]

A comparison of single versus double lumen needles for IVM oocyte collection demonstrated no difference in the amount of oocytes collected. However, with the double lumen, there was a reduction in the amount of clots present in the collection fluid, making oocyte identification easier.[25] Variations in flushing solutions include Hartmann's [12] or Hepes [24] supplemented with heparin or no flushing at all,[8] and most centers use a mesh cell strainer to filter follicular aspirates.[8] Alternatively, this can be done by sight,[5, 12] which reduces the potential

harm from manipulation but does increase the length of the procedure, as the germinal vesicle (GV) stage oocytes do not have an expanded cumulus complex (Figures 15.1 and 15.2) and are therefore more difficult to identify than oocytes in standard IVF. All these protocol differences make a comparison of different techniques and approaches difficult.

Oocyte Maturation Culture

Culture Media
The oocyte and its cumulus complex must be maintained to prevent spontaneous oocyte maturation and to prevent asynchrony between the cytoplasm and the nucleus of the cell.[26] Commercial culture media are available, including Sage (Cooper Surgical, USA) and Medicult (Origio, Denmark), and have been shown to be equally effective.[27] Our protocol is to use blastocyst culture media,[5] which compares well with commercial IVM media.[28] Oocytes are maintained in maturation culture for at least 24 hours, [5] by which time expansion and proliferation of the coronal cells should be seen (Figures 15.3 and 15.4) as well as rates of maturation between 65% and 80%.

One of the only consistent methodologies for IVM treatment is the addition of gonadotropins to the culture media. FSH is the most common additive, aiding expansion of the cumulus oocyte

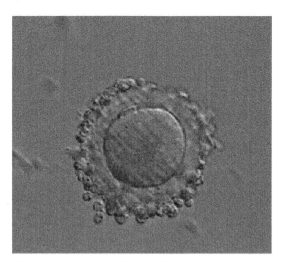

Figure 15.4 IVM oocyte displaying limited expanding and proliferating coronal cells after 24 hours in maturation culture with visible polar body

complex and oocyte maturation. In the literature, the most widely used concentration of FSH added to the media is reported as 0.075 IU/mL.[19, 29, 30] We use a concentration of 0.1 IU/mL.[5] Recombinant LH or hCG are necessary components of IVM media to aid the resumption of meiosis and the final stages of oocyte maturation, normally provided by the mid-cycle LH surge. The concentration of administered LH or hCG ranges from 0.1 IU/mL[30] to 0.75 IU/mL.[31]

A source of protein is currently essential in human IVM culture, with the most commonly used being maternal serum, human follicular fluid or, as is the case with commercial IVM media, human serum albumin. Serum contains complex components, including growth factors and amino acids that are essential for a maturing oocyte. However, serum also contains several elements that are not found in the normal follicular environment, which are potentially detrimental to oocyte and embryo development. Additionally, serum may lead to the generation of ammonia and subsequent mitochondrial disruption. Other culture media additives, including various growth factors, have shown promising results and are discussed later in this chapter, though these components are currently not widely used in clinical IVM programs.

Fertilization Methods

Insemination of IVM oocytes has predominantly been by intracytoplasmic sperm injection (ICSI),

owing to the perception that the extended time in culture may harden the zona pellucida. Another benefit of ICSI is that it allows for a more accurate assessment of nuclear maturation, by removing the coronal cells, and identification of the polar body. Following successful maturation, fertilization rates in IVM oocytes are generally similar to those seen with standard IVF and range from 62.9% to 90.7%. Insemination using IVF has demonstrated a significant reduction in fertilization of IVM oocytes compared to ICSI from retrospective data.[30] However, our data suggest that insemination using IVF is equally effective,[10] and this has been replicated recently by another group.[32]

Embryo Culture and Transfer

Following maturation culture and fertilization, embryo culture for IVM is no different from standard IVF. Embryo cleavage following IVM should demonstrate high rates of division upward of 90% in successful programs,[9] and blastocyst formation rates have also been reported at approaching 40%.[13] Use of time-lapse imaging suggest that IVM embryos may have difficulty transitioning from maternal to embryonic control of development due to high rates of early embryo arrest,[13] providing a potential explanation for the lower implantation rates in earlier IVM studies, where cleavage-stage transfer was commonplace.

An additional contributing factor to lower pregnancy rates reported in IVM may be the asynchrony between the embryo and the endometrium. In our practice, we found that embryos derived from IVM treatment show significantly greater live birth rates following frozen embryo transfers compared to fresh.[12]

Success Rates of IVM

In early studies, without the use of FSH priming but employing a trigger injection, the success rates of IVM programs were poor. However, much higher success rates can be achieved when utilizing a short FSH priming protocol, without a hCG trigger, for women with a polycystic ovarian morphology when using a freeze-only protocol. This is our standard approach, as it provides similar implantation and live birth rates to standard IVF, with a similar miscarriage rate.[12]

Neonatal and Childhood Outcomes

Children born from IVM treatment do not appear to have an increased risk of congenital malformations when compared to standard IVF,[12] although the number of births included in the studies was small. The largest longer-term follow-up study of children born resulting from IVM treatment studied the obstetric, neonatal and longer-term health outcomes of 184 children born from IVM treatment in comparison to 366 children born following standard IVF treatment. [33] The children were followed-up for a mean of 7.5 years, and no differences were found between the two groups with respect to obstetric or neonatal complications, congenital abnormalities, developmental delay, growth or hospital admissions.[33] The most recent study analyzed the growth and general health of 74 singleton children conceived in Belgium up to 2 years of age, and their findings, in comparison to children conceived from standard controlled ovarian stimulation, were very reassuring.[34] It is also interesting to note that the DNA methylation patterns and mRNA expression of imprinted genes within blastocysts derived from IVM treatment appear not to differ from standard controlled ovarian stimulation.[35] This is important, as the DNA methylation patterns within imprinted genes are being established in late follicular development and early in embryonic development,[35] and hence would be particularly susceptible to disruption during IVM.

Future Research

With a view to significantly improving the success of IVM programs, research has been directed toward improving the maturation of the oocyte in vitro. This has in part been accomplished by the integration of the oocyte-secreted paracrine factors (GDF9) and bone morphogenic protein 15 (BMP-15) as the heterodimer "Cumulin,"[36] with early human studies showing promise in improved embryo development.[36] Modulators of cAMP (IBMX), which prevents the dramatic drop in cAMP concentrations, after removal of the GV-stage oocyte from the in vivo follicular environment, have proven to be safe and effective in early human trials.[37] Further work involving the addition of Areg with FSH in the IVM culture media together with C-type natriuretic peptide (CNP) in pre-IVM-type systems has also demonstrated increased rates of embryo development.[38] Furthermore, recent research has suggested that supplementation with coenzyme Q10 may reduce postmeiotic aneuploidies in human IVM oocytes.[39] Hence, the incorporation of one, or a combination, of these factors into a commercially available culture media may in the future lead to improved success rates of IVM programs and lead to the widespread uptake of IVM. However, before IVM can be widely adopted as a successful assisted reproductive treatment for women with PCOS, it is essential that large randomized control trials comparing IVM treatment with standard IVF are performed. Hence, we await the results of a couple of trials that are currently underway.[40, 41]

References

1 Pincus, G. and Enzmann, E. V. The comparative behavior of mammalian eggs in vivo and in vitro. *J Exp Med* 1935; 62(5): 665–675.

2 Edwards, R. G. Maturation in vitro of mouse, sheep, cow, pig, rhesus monkey and human ovarian oocytes. *Nature* 1965; 208(5008): 349–351.

3 Cha, K. Y., Koo, J. J., Ko, J. J., Choi, D. H., Han, S. Y. and Yoon, T. K. Pregnancy after in vitro fertilization of human follicular oocytes collected from nonstimulated cycles, their culture in vitro and their transfer in a donor oocyte program. *Fertil Steril* 1991; 55(1): 109.

4 Trounson, A., Wood, C. and Kausche, A. In vitro maturation and the fertilization and developmental competence of oocytes recovered from untreated polycystic ovarian patients. *Fertil Steril* 1994; 62(2): 353.

5 Junk, S. M. and Yeap, D. Improved implantation and ongoing pregnancy rates after single-embryo transfer with an optimized protocol for in vitro oocyte maturation in women with polycystic ovaries and polycystic ovary syndrome. *Fertil Steril* 2012; 98 (4): 888–892.

6 Eppig, J. J. Coordination of nuclear and cytoplasmic oocyte maturation in eutherian mammals. *Reprod Fertil Dev* 1996; 8(4): 485–489.

7 Ben-Ami, I., Komsky, A., Bern, O., Kasterstein, E., Komarovsky, D. and Ron-El, R. In vitro maturation of human germinal vesicle-stage oocytes: Role of epidermal growth factor-like growth factors in the culture medium. *Hum Reprod* 2011; 26(1): 76–81.

8 Hreinsson, J., Rosenlund, B., Fridén, B. et al. Recombinant LH is equally effective as recombinant hCG in promoting oocyte maturation in a clinical in-vitro maturation programme: a randomized study. *Hum Reprod* 2003; 18(10): 2131–2136.

9   Child, T. J., Abdul-Jalil, A. K., Gulekli, B. and Lin Tan, S. In vitro maturation and fertilization of oocytes from unstimulated normal ovaries, polycystic ovaries, and women with polycystic ovary syndrome. *Fertil Steril* 2001; 76(5): 936–942.

10 Walls, M., Junk, S., Ryan, J. and Hart, R. IVF versus ICSI for the fertilization of in-vitro matured human oocytes. *Reprod Biomed Online* 2012; 25(6): 603–607.

11 Tang, H., Hunter, T., Hu, Y., Zhai, S. D., Sheng, X. and Hart, R. J. Cabergoline for preventing ovarian hyperstimulation syndrome. *Cochrane Database Syst Rev.* 2012; 2: CD008605.

12 Walls, M. L., Hunter, T., Ryan, J. P., Keelan, J. A., Nathan, E. and Hart, R. J. In vitro maturation as an alternative to standard in vitro fertilization for patients diagnosed with polycystic ovaries: A comparative analysis of fresh, frozen and cumulative cycle outcomes. *Hum Reprod* 2015; 30 (1): 88–96.

13 Walls, M. L., Ryan, J. P., Keelan, J. A. and Hart, R. In vitro maturation is associated with increased early embryo arrest without impairing morphokinetic development of useable embryos progressing to blastocysts. *Hum Reprod* 2015; 30 (8): 1842–1849.

14 Chian, R. C., Buckett, W. M., Too, L. L. and Tan, S. L. Pregnancies resulting from in vitro matured oocytes retrieved from patients with polycystic ovary syndrome after priming with human chorionic gonadotropin. *Fertil Steril* 1999; 72(4): 639–642.

15 Radesic, B. and Tremellen, K. Oocyte maturation employing a GnRH agonist in combination with low-dose hCG luteal rescue minimizes the severity of ovarian hyperstimulation syndrome while maintaining excellent pregnancy rates. *Hum Reprod* 2011; 26(12): 3437–3442.

16 Boothroyd, C., Karia, S., Andreadis, N. et al. Consensus statement on prevention and detection of ovarian hyperstimulation syndrome. *Aust N Z J Obstet Gynaecol* 2015; 55(6): 523–534.

17 Walls, M. L., Douglas, K., Ryan, J. P., Tan, J. and Hart, R. In-vitro maturation and cryopreservation of oocytes at the time of oophorectomy. *Gynecol Oncol Rep* 2015; 13: 79–81.

18 Dahan, M. H., Tan, S. L., Chung, J. and Son, W. Y. Clinical definition paper on in vitro maturation of human oocytes. *Hum Reprod* 2016; 31(7): 1383–1386.

19 Mikkelsen, A. L., Smith, S. D. and Lindenberg, S. In-vitro maturation of human oocytes from regularly menstruating women may be successful without follicle stimulating hormone priming. *Hum Reprod* 1999; 14(7): 1847–1851.

20 Mikkelsen, A. and Lindenberg, S. Benefit of FSH priming of women with PCOS to the in vitro maturation procedure and the outcome: A randomized prospective study. *Reproduction* 2001; 122(4): 587–92.

21 Zheng, X., Wang, L., Zhen, X., Lian, Y., Liu, P. and Qiao, J. Effect of hCG priming on embryonic development of immature oocytes collected from unstimulated women with polycystic ovarian syndrome. *Reprod Biol Endocrinol* 2012; 10: 40.

22 Lin, Y., Zheng, X., Ma, C. et al. Human chorionic gonadotropin priming does not improve pregnancy outcomes of PCOS-IVM cycles. *Front Endocrinol* 2020; 11: 279.

23 Reavey, J., Vincent, K., Child, T. and Granne, I. E. Human chorionic gonadotrophin priming for fertility treatment with in vitro maturation. *Cochrane Database Syst Rev.* 2016; 11: CD008720.

24 Yoon, H.-G., Yoon, S.-H., Son, W.-Y. et al. Clinical assisted reproduction: Pregnancies resulting from in vitro matured oocytes collected from women with regular menstrual cycle. *J Assist Reprod Genet* 2001;18(6):325–329.

25 Rose, B. I. and Laky, D. A comparison of the Cook single lumen immature ovum IVM needle to the Steiner-Tan pseudo double lumen flushing needle for oocyte retrieval for IVM. *J Assist Reprod Genet* 2013; 30(6): 855–860.

26 Sasseville, M., Gagnon, M. C., Guillemette, C., Sullivan, R., Gilchrist, R. B. and Richard, F. J. Regulation of gap junctions in porcine cumulus-oocyte complexes: Contributions of granulosa cell contact, gonadotropins, and lipid rafts. *Mol Endocrinol* 2009; 23(5): 700–710.

27 Pongsuthirak, P. and Vutyavanich, T. Comparison of Medicult and Sage media for in vitro maturation of immature oocytes obtained during cesarean deliveries. *JFIV Reprod Med Genet* 2015; 3: 136.

28 Pongsuthirak, P., Songveeratham, S. and Vutyavanich, T. Comparison of blastocyst and Sage media for in vitro maturation of human immature oocytes. *Reprod Sci* 2015; 22(3): 343–346.

29 Mikkelsen, A. L., Smith, S. and Lindenberg, S. Impact of oestradiol and inhibin A concentrations on pregnancy rate in in-vitro oocyte maturation. *Hum Reprod* 2000; 15(8): 1685–1690.

30 Söderström-Anttila, V., Mäkinen, S., Tuuri, T. and Suikkari, A.-M. Favourable pregnancy results with insemination of in vitro matured oocytes from unstimulated patients. *Hum Reprod* 2005; 20(6): 1534–1540.

31 Le Du, A., Kadoch, I. J., Bourcigaux, N. et al. In vitro oocyte maturation for the treatment of infertility associated with polycystic ovarian

syndrome: The French experience. *Hum Reprod* 2005; 20(2): 420–424.

32 Pongsuthirak, P. The effect of insemination methods on in vitro maturation outcomes. *Clin Exp Reprod Med* 2020; 47(2): 130–134.

33 Yu, E. J., Yoon, T. K., Lee, W. S. et al. Obstetrical, neonatal, and long-term outcomes of children conceived from in vitro matured oocytes. *Fertil Steril* 2019; 112(4): 691–699.

34 Belva, F., Roelants, M., Vermaning, S. et al. Growth and other health outcomes of 2-year-old singletons born after IVM versus controlled ovarian stimulation in mothers with polycystic ovary syndrome. *Hum Reprod Open* 2020; 1: hoz043.

35 Saenz-de-Juano, M. D., Ivanova, E., Romero, S. et al. DNA methylation and mRNA expression of imprinted genes in blastocysts derived from an improved in vitro maturation method for oocytes from small antral follicles in polycystic ovary syndrome patients. *Hum Reprod* 2019; 34(9): 1640–1649.

36 Mottershead, D. G., Sugimura, S., Al-Musawi, S. L. et al. Cumulin, an oocyte-secreted heterodimer of the transforming growth factor-beta family, is a potent activator of granulosa cells and improves oocyte quality. *J Biol Chem* 2015; 290(39): 24007–24020.

37 Spits, C., Guzman, L., Mertzanidou, A. et al. Chromosome constitution of human embryos generated after in vitro maturation including 3-isobutyl-1-methylxanthine in the oocyte collection medium. *Hum Reprod* 2015; 30(3): 653–663.

38 Sanchez, F., Lolicato, F., Romero, S. et al. An improved IVM method for cumulus-oocyte complexes from small follicles in polycystic ovary syndrome patients enhances oocyte competence and embryo yield. *Hum Reprod* 2017; 32(10): 2056–2068.

39 Ma, L., Cai, L., Hu, M. et al. Coenzyme Q10 supplementation of human oocyte in vitro maturation reduces postmeiotic aneuploidies. *Fertil Steril* 2020; 114(2): 331–337.

40 Zheng, X., Guo, W., Zeng, L. et al. Live birth after in vitro maturation versus standard in vitro fertilisation for women with polycystic ovary syndrome: Protocol for a non-inferiority randomised clinical trial. *BMJ Open* 2020; 10(4): e035334.

41 Vuong, L. N., Ho, V. N. A., Ho, T. M. et al. Effectiveness and safety of in vitro maturation of oocytes versus in vitro fertilisation in women with high antral follicle count: Study protocol for a randomised controlled trial. *BMJ Open* 2018; 8 (12): e023413.

The Treatment of Obesity in Polycystic Ovary Syndrome

Harry Frydenberg

Introduction

Obesity is an adiposity-based chronic disease that is becoming a global epidemic. The incidence of obesity in women of reproductive age diagnosed with PCOS has been estimated to be 30% and, when including the overweight group, is estimated to be 50% and thus the treatment of obesity plays a significant part in the management of this condition of polycystic ovary syndrome (PCOS).[1]

Obesity is defined as the abnormal excess of accumulated fat and as a disease when the accumulation is to the extent that health is impaired. The rise of obesity globally has been greater than 80% over the last 30 years,[2] with the increase being more in the "Westernized" countries compared to the Asian demographic group.[3] It has been shown that a small rise in body mass index (BMI) (weight/height^2) in the Asian demographic group is associated with a greater increase in comorbidities compared to the Caucasian demographic.[4] Obesity is most commonly defined by BMI and increased waist circumference, which, although not perfect, as it does not take into account the musculature and shape of the individual, does include central obesity in its waist measurement.

Obesity

Degrees of Obesity

The degree of obesity is expressed in BMI units, with 18.5–24.9 considered normal; 25–29.9 as overweight; 30–34.9 as Class 1 obesity (low risk); 35–39.9 as Class 2 obesity (moderate risk); 40 plus as Class 3 obesity (morbidly obese, high risk); and 50 plus as super-obese. Fat distribution follows two general patterns: android (central fat distribution) and gynoid (fat distribution around the hips). Android fat is more of a risk factor in coronary vascular disease (CVD) and type 2 diabetes, while gynoid distribution appears to be protective.[5]

The Causes of Obesity

To treat obesity, one must look at its causes. The genetic heritability of obesity has been put as between 40% and 70%,[5] with the obesity-related FTO gene situated on chromosome 16 occurring in 43% of people. There are more than 244 genes that affect adiposity, and they work by regulating food intake, regulating adipocyte differentiation and fat storage and regulating energy metabolism. The ALK gene has been described as and is thought to be the "thinness" gene, which has also been associated with cancers.[6] Other more general causes of obesity are physiological and psychosocial factors and gender, with male obesity being more prominent than female obesity. Society and lifestyle changes also contribute to increasing obesity.

Impact of Obesity

The impact of obesity is such that it causes disability, reduces quality of life and is a cause of premature death, increased medical costs and many other comorbidities, of which PCOS is one. Type 2 diabetes is a major comorbidity and is very closely associated with PCOS, whose other comorbidities include hypertension, hyperandrogenism and possibly some cancers. The mechanism of this impact is related to insulin resistance and various hormonal factors that will be described in the section "Polycystic Ovarian Syndrome." The incidence of type 2 diabetes associated with obesity (i.e. a BMI > 30) sits at 6.3% in the USA. In 2016, the World Health Organization (WHO) reported that, worldwide the incidence of overweight was 39% and obesity 13%.[7] According to the Centers for Disease Control and Prevention (CDC), in the USA, 75% of men and 60% of woman are overweight or obese and 8.1% morbidly obese. Globally, the incidence of PCOS is around 10% of all women of reproductive age,[8] and 30% of these are obese.[1] In the USA, however, the incidence of obesity with PCOS is 60%. In a study of morbidly obese women (BMI>40), 45.6% have PCOS.[9]

The Regulation of Obesity

The regulation of obesity is via three pathways: food intake, metabolism and energy expenditure. The set point is the range at which the body is programmed to function optimally. When one goes below the set point, both appetite and metabolism adjust to return one back to the "normal" set point. The physiological adaptation to changes in the set point occurs from the regulation of hormonal activity via adipose tissue, the stomach, the gut, the pancreas and muscle, with the hypothalamus as the regulatory organ, particularly the arcuate nucleus and the paravertebral nucleus, as well as the lateral hypothalamus with some input from the cortex (conscious will).

The regulation of hunger is via the "ghrelin" hormone, which is produced mainly in the fundus of the stomach to stimulate appetite via the hypothalamus.[10] The gut hormones cholecystokinin (CCK), oxyntomodulin, glucagon-like peptide-1 (GLP-1) and peptide YY (PYY) inhibit hunger via the hypothalamus.[11–13] The neurotransmitters neuropeptide Y (NPY) and agouti-related peptide (AGRP) are orexigenic and stimulate appetite, whereas proopiomelanocortin (POMC) and cocaine- and amphetamine-regulated transcript (CART) are anorexigenic (inhibit feeding).

Oxyntomodulin (OXM) is a product of post-translational processing of preproglucagon in the intestine and central nervous system (CNS). It acts like a GLP-1 receptor with anorectic action and reduced ghrelin levels in a human trial.[14] These act together to reduce food intake and increase resting energy expenditure. GLP-1 stimulates the anorexic system, reducing appetite, and advances glucose-induced insulin secretion as well as suppressing glucagon release. It also stimulates the beta cell and reduces beta cell apoptosis and in doing so influences changes in type 2 diabetes. It is produced mainly in the distal small bowel and the ileum.[15]

Leptin, which is mainly produced by adipose tissue, stimulates the anorexic system and inhibits hunger. It regulates fat storage in fat tissue via the hypothalamus and "increased circulating levels of leptin in obesity lead to hypothalamic leptin resistance, turning down anorexigenic and energy expenditure signals and further contributing to obesity."[16] Another fat-derived hormone, adiponectin stimulates glucose uptake and increases insulin sensitivity via the liver and skeletal muscle. It also acts via the vasculature and decreases levels of anti-inflammatory adipokines, such as adiponectin. In obesity, it produces a chronic state of low-grade inflammation, which promotes the development of insulin resistance and type 2 diabetes, hypertension and atherosclerosis.[17] Furthermore, pancreatic polypeptide (PP) is produced in the islets of Langerhans and is reported to reduce appetite in animals[18–21] and humans.[22]

Polycystic Ovarian Syndrome

PCOS is a hormonal disorder common among women of reproductive age. Women with PCOS may have infrequent or prolonged menstrual periods and excess male hormone (androgen) levels. The ovaries may develop numerous small collections of fluid (follicles) and fail to regularly release eggs. According to the Rotterdam criteria, polycystic ovarian syndrome is diagnosed in women presenting with at least two out of three of the following characteristics:

1. Clinical or biochemical hyperandrogenism
2. Ovulatory dysfunction
3. Polycystic ovarian morphology (PCOM)

Some definitions include all three.

The prevalence of PCOS is 6–20% in the literature and is the most common endocrine and metabolic disorder in women of reproductive age (Figure 16.1).[1, 23, 24] The incidence of obesity is estimated at 30% in women with PCOS,[1] whereas the incidence of PCOS in obese and overweight women is 28.3%.[25] The prevalence of PCOS did not increase with increasing grades of obesity and was independent of the presence or absence of metabolic syndrome.[26] "Insulin resistance is difficult to measure, but more than 50% of PCOS women, even as adolescents, have insulin resistance and they progress commonly to Metabolic Syndrome."[27–30] By the age of 50, 40% of PCOS women have diabetes,[31] and metabolic syndrome is prevalent in 40% of PCOS adolescents and 60% of obese PCOS adolescents.[32, 33]

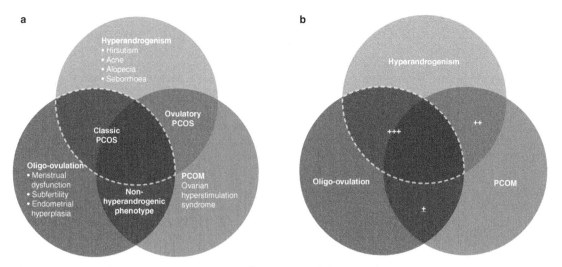

Figure 16.1 PCOS is a heterogeneous disorder in terms of phenotypes and clinical manifestations (part a) and in terms of metabolic consequences (part b).
Escobar-Morreale H.F (2018) Polycystic ovary syndrome: definition, aetiology, diagnosis and treatment Nat.Rev. Endocrinol

The etiology of PCOS is not certain but evidence suggests that it is a complex multigenic disorder with strong epigenetic and environment influences, which include diet and lifestyle factors. The genetic component of PCOS is approximately 10%.[34] It has been proposed by Hector Escobar-Morreale that "PCOS results from a vicious circle of androgen excess favoring abdominal adipose tissue deposition and visceral adiposity, by inducing insulin resistance and compensatory hyperinsulinemia, which further facilitates androgen secretion by the ovaries and adrenal glands in women with PCOS."[35]

As discussed, PCOS is commonly associated with obesity, particularly central obesity, insulin resistance and type 2 diabetes, and the treatment of obesity in PCOS is paramount in reversing the effects of this condition. "Obesity per se represents a condition of sex hormone imbalance in women,"[1] with levels of sex hormone-binding globulin (SHBG) decreasing with increased body fat, which leads to increased free androgens.[36]

Treatment of Obesity in PCOS

As outlined in the previous edition of this book, weight loss as a therapy is considered a mainstream approach to the treatment of PCOS, due to the association with central obesity, insulin resistance and hyperinsulinemia. The regulation of obesity previously outlined is instrumental in the success of weight-loss therapies. Both obesity and PCOS

have been shown to independently contribute to insulin resistance and hyperinsulinemia, which have been implicated in leading to hyperandrogenemia and anovulation.[37–40] Thus weight loss has shown improvements in both insulin resistance, fertility and the lowering of testosterone as well as increased SHBG in PCOS.[41] Moreover, the resultant reduction in serum insulin levels and leptin concentration produces improvement in ovulatory function and improvement in PCOS.[42]

Weight loss is also associated with the improvement of metabolic syndrome and the improvement in insulin-resistant type 2 diabetes, obstructive sleep apnea, hypertension and non-alcoholic steatohepatitis (NASH), all related to obesity, particularly central obesity in PCOS. As lifestyle changes in diet and exercise have been reported in Chapter 10, this chapter will look at the conservative aspects of the treatment of obesity, particularly pharmacotherapy.

Some of the older pharmacotherapeutic agents such as fenfluramine/sibutramine and Belviq (lorcaserin) have been withdrawn from the market because of cardiac or neoplastic concerns, whereas Duromine (an appetite suppressant) is still available. Qsymia, a combination of phentermine (an appetite suppressant) and topiramate (an anticonvulsant) is also used, but side effects such as numbness, tingling and suicidal thoughts have restricted its use. The newer medications available to achieve weight loss are Saxenda and Contrave.

Saxenda (liraglutide) is an injectable GLP-1 agonist medication,[43] which has shown to be effective in reducing appetite and reducing insulin resistance but needs to be maintained to keep on losing or maintaining weight. Side effects include nausea, headache and diarrhea. Weight loss results in a 16-week trial show 60% of participants lost > 5% TBW (total body weight) and 23% > 10% TBW.[44] In an observational study of overweight or obese women with PCOS treated with liraglutide over 27.8 weeks, 81.7% achieved weight loss of > 5% of TBW and 32.9% > 10% [43]. In an extension of this study, 64% of subjects lost > 5% TBW after one year and 85% of these maintained that weight loss after two years of treatment.[45]

Contrave is a new anorectic combination of Naltrexone Hcl (opioid antagonist) and bupropion Hcl (dopamine aminoketone antidepressant).[45] Side effects include nausea, constipation, headaches, suicidal thoughts, dizziness, insomnia and vomiting. The combination is theorized to work synergistically in the hypothalamus and mesolimbic dopamine circuit to promote satiety, reduce food intake and enhance energy expenditure.[46, 47] Weight loss results in a 56-week Contrave Obesity Research (COR) clinical trial [48] showed a 5.4% TBW loss compared to placebo, 1.3%, with 42% of participants (n = 538) losing > 5% and 21% losing > 10% TBW.[45]

Bariatric and Metabolic Surgery

Since the early 1970s, bariatric and metabolic surgery (often referred to as bariatric surgery) has undergone radical changes, with more than 90% of operations being carried out laparoscopically (keyhole) rather than as open procedures. The newer endoscopic procedures that have been done, such as endoscopic sleeve gastroplasty (ESG), have yet to prove their effectiveness and durability.

At the turn of the century, laparoscopic adjustable gastric banding (LAGB), vertical gastroplasty (VBG) and biliopancreatic bypass (BPD) were the main bariatric procedures, together with Roux-en-Y gastric pass. More recently, the sleeve gastrectomy has gained popularity and is currently the most commonly performed bariatric procedure around the world. Other procedures, including the one anastomosis gastric bypass

(OAGB), together with variants like the stomach intestinal preserving surgery (SIPS) and the single anastomosis duodeno-ileal bypass (SADI) approach, both being similar procedures, have found a place in the treatment of obesity and metabolic disorders including PCOS. Bariatric surgery has been shown to greatly improve metabolic disease and metabolic syndrome,[49] and bariatric surgery showed much better weight loss in the morbidly obese than conservative methods.[50]

Surgical Procedures

There are several bariatric procedures in current practice. The four listed below are the ones most commonly used in the bariatric surgical field:

Laparoscopic gastric banding, which attained peak popularity in the 1990s and the early 2000s, is substantially a restrictive procedure, although there have been studies that predict early satiety as being the means of achieving weight loss and that have been able to achieve > 50% of excess body weight loss.[51, 52]

Laparoscopic sleeve gastrectomy has become the most common, or popular, bariatric surgical procedure in the last 10 years, and it has achieved substantial weight loss and improvement in metabolic comorbidities. The technique requires removal of more than three-quarters of the stomach vertically to leave a long narrow gastric stomach remnant of approximately 100 cc, reducing one's capacity to consume food. Apart from the ability to limit intake, the removal of the fundus (the major site of ghrelin production) leads to reduction in appetite by reducing the amount of ghrelin, the appetite-stimulating hormone.

Roux-en-Y gastric bypass, the "gold standard of bariatric surgery for many years," does not remove any tissue but creates a small gastric pouch, which is attached to a "roux" loop to the pouch with an enteroenterostomy further down the tract. The biliopancreatic limb is usually around 50–100 cm and the elementary limb is around 130 cm, joined with an enteroenterostomy into the common limb where the bile and the digestive juices mix with the food from the alimentary limb.

Duodenal-jejunal diversion (DJB) is a variation of the BPD with the preservation of the pylorus.

The variations of this technique are SIPS and SADI, which are basically a sleeve gastrectomy with a single loop duodenal ileostomy or a roux loop to the first part of the duodenum beyond the pylorus, thus reducing or limiting any reflux of bile back into the stomach and more particularly into the esophagus to avoid the possibility of Barrett's esophagus, a precancerous condition. The length of the proximal and distal limbs regulates the degree of malabsorption and to some extent the degree of weight loss.

Modern techniques include the use of robotic instrumentation to assist in these procedures. The procedures are done laparoscopically but with the assistance of robotic arms, which can be manipulated remotely. Some surgeons attribute fewer complications because of the easier surgical ability of this approach; others see its benefits to limited types of cases only.

Risks Associated with Bariatric Surgery

Bariatric surgery presents with potential risks and effects, which are both physical and metabolic. The minimally invasive techniques have been associated with a reduction in morbidity and mortality. Laparoscopic gastric banding, where the major risk is band slippage and reflux, has a low mortality and morbidity but does have longer-term complications and a higher reoperation rate.

The risks associated with laparoscopic sleeve gastrectomy are mainly twofold. One is the risk of leak, which may lead to septicemia or even death and may be difficult to treat. The leak rate was originally around 2% but has reduced to 0.4–0.6% today. Reflux is a further complication of sleeve gastrectomy as there is a possibility of the development of Barrett's esophagus as a result of sleeve gastrectomy in the future.

As mentioned, Roux-en-Y gastric bypass is termed the "gold standard," but the risks are also those of leak, stomal stenosis, dumping syndrome, bowel obstruction and nutritional deficiencies and it can be associated with frequent bowel motions. The other procedures of SIPS, SADI and DJB also fall into this group, with dumping not usually a feature of these procedures as the pyloric integrity is preserved.

OAGB is a procedure that was introduced many years ago but which only more recently has been taken up in the bariatric field. It is a loop bypass similar to the Roux-en-Y gastric bypass but which reduces the number of anastomoses from two to one. It has been associated with gastric/bile reflux and there has been concern regarding the possible development of Barrett's esophagus, although this risk appears to be quite low.

Endoscopic Bariatric Surgical Techniques

Endoscopic procedures are the newer bariatric surgical technique developed over the last few years utilizing an endoscopic approach. The endoscopic sleeve gastroplasty (ESG) uses an endoscopic suturing device (Apollo OverStitch), suturing the internal aspects of the stomach from side to side starting at the fundus to the gastric antrum to form a vertical sleeve without gastric resection. The results are equivocal at present with not enough studies carried out.

Endoscopic balloons have been in place for more than 20 years, with the Garren bubble being the early prototype. Of the newer balloons, the most recent is the ORBERA gastric balloon. The balloon is inserted endoscopically and kept in for up to one year. Reported weight loss has been in the range of 12–26 kg after 6 months,[53, 54] with nausea being the most frequent side effect requiring early removal. A review of eight studies involving three intragastric balloons had a pooled weight loss of 9.7% total body weight loss (TBWL).[55] Other more novel techniques and devices are still being evaluated.

Weight loss owing to bariatric surgery is significant and, accordingly, results in improvements in metabolic syndrome and PCOS, as well as type 2 diabetes.

Bariatric Surgical Mechanism of Action

The mechanisms of action of bariatric procedures include a number of factors. Restrictive components reduce the capacity to eat, as occurs in gastric banding, gastric bypass and sleeve gastrectomy, where the stomach's capacity is reduced in some cases to < 150 mL. The bariatric procedures, which involve the removal of the fundus, do lead to a reduction in ghrelin (the anorectic hormone), which is produced mainly in the fundus of the stomach. The metabolic effects of the bypass procedures show improvement in diabetes, as well as hyperlipidemia, dyslipidemia and hypertension, and a reduction in insulin resistance and this is attributed to the increase in GLP-1, PYY and other gut hormones. Their action in this way can explain the improvement in PCOS following these surgical procedures.[56, 57]

There are two major theories postulated to explain these changes, the hindgut theory and the foregut theory. The hindgut theory states that the rapid delivery of food and nutrients to the distal ileum increases GLP-1 gut hormone, which results in improved glucose metabolism via stimulation of insulin secretion and glucagon suppression, as well as cerebral effects on appetite, [58] whereas the foregut theory states that exclusion of food to the proximal small bowel reduces the anti-incretin hormones with an improvement in glucose control.[59] These procedures also influence leptin, reducing levels to 50% post laparoscopic Roux-en-Y gastric bypass, which influences the fat metabolism and storage, as expressed in the section "The Regulation of Obesity."[51, 56, 60, 61]

A systematic review and meta-analysis by Buchwald and colleagues of 136 fully extracted studies, including 22 094 subjects, indicated the following % excess body weight loss (EBWL): 61.2% EBWL for all patients; for gastric banding, 47.7% EBWL; Roux-en-Y gastric bypass, 68.2 % EBWL; and for biliopancreatic diversion (BPD), 70.1% EBWL.[51] For the restrictive procedures, 30-day mortality was 0.1%; 0.5% for gastric bypass; and 1.1% for BPD. OAGB has shown 35.4% TBWL and 74.8% for EWBL at two years [62] and 72.9% EBWL at five years.[63]

Bariatric Surgery and Changes in PCOS

In a study by Escobar-Morreale and colleagues, [64, 65] which studied morbidly obese PCOS reproductive-aged women after bariatric surgery (either LAGB or BPD) followed prospectively for 26 months, most women (12/17) regained normal menstrual function and most returned to spontaneous ovulation (10/17), with an average weight loss of 41 kg. These patients showed improvement in hirsutism, androgen profiles and a 50% reduction in homeostasis model assessment of insulin resistance (HOMA-IR).[64]

A study by Ernst and colleagues of 36 morbidly obese women (6 of whom were postmenopausal), who, post bariatric surgery, had an average weight loss of 43.1 kg, showed a marked reduction in all testosterone-related androgen markers and dehydroepiandrosterone (DHEA) levels, while SHBG levels markedly increased.[66]

A meta-analysis published in 2017 indicated surgically induced weight loss in women with severe obesity and PCOS resulted in marked decreases in serum levels of total and free testosterone and resolution of hirsutism and menstrual dysfunction in as many as 53% and 96% of the patients, respectively, leading to a PCOS resolution of 96%.[23, 67]

Eid and colleagues,[68] in a retrospective study, have demonstrated a reduction in weight and comorbid hirsutism and diabetes in women with PCOS following Roux-en-Y gastric bypass. [68] Data from 14 women showed a BMI reduction from 44.8 to 29.2 at 12 months. Significant improvements were seen in testosterone, fasting glucose, insulin, cholesterol and triglyceride at 12 months. Ten patients had irregular menses at baseline and all had regular menses at 6 and 12 months. Hirsutism was present in 11 patients at baseline and only 7 patients at 12 months. Most interesting was the fact that most biomarkers, menstrual cycling and hirsutism were not correlated with degrees of weight loss.[68]

Similar results are seen in a systematic review and meta-analysis by Skubleny and colleagues of 2130 women in 13 studies. Participants had a mean age of 30.8 years and a preoperative mean BMI of 46.3, which improved postoperatively to 34.2 at a mean follow-up period of 23.8 months. EWL ranged from 33% to 75%, with a mean of 57.2%.[69] The different bariatric procedures included LAGB, Roux-en-Y gastric bypass, LSG, DJB and VBG; 45.6% of women had PCOS, which decreased to 6.8% postoperatively at 12 months and 7.1% at study endpoint; 56.2% had menstrual irregularity, which decreased to 7.7% at 12 months. The incidence of hirsutism preoperatively was 67% and down to 38.6% at 12 months and 32% at study end.[69] Preoperative infertility was 18.2% and significantly reduced to 4.3% at study end.

So, it can be seen that weight loss in PCOS patients can cause marked improvement in symptoms and fertility and reductions in hyperinsulinemia, insulin resistance, testosterone and hirsutism (Figure 16.2).[70] However, it may not be weight loss alone in relation to bariatric surgery, as the hormonal consequences of certain bariatric procedures, for example Roux-en-Y gastric bypass, could account for some of these

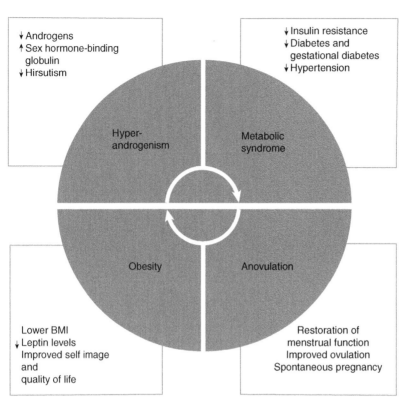

Hyper-
androgenism

↓Androgens
↑Sex hormone-binding
globulin
↓Hirsutism

Metabolic
syndrome

↓Insulin resistance
↓Diabetes and
gestational diabetes
↓Hypertension

Obesity

Anovulation

Lower BMI
↓Leptin levels
Improved self image
and
quality of life

Restoration of
menstrual function
Improved ovulation
Spontaneous pregnancy

Figure 16.2 Key features of polycystic ovarian syndrome and improvements seen after bariatric surgery
Source. Reprinted with permission from S. M. Malik and M. L. Traub. Defining the role of bariatric surgery in polycystic ovarian syndrome patients. World J Diabetes 2012; 3(4): 70, 72–77, 84–85.

changes. An increase in GLP-1 levels certainly leads to a reduction in insulin resistance, improves pancreatic beta-cell function and has an anorectic influence centrally. Reduction in leptin and adiponectin levels decreases HOMA-IR and normalizes lipid parameters.[57, 60, 71]

Bariatric Surgery and Reproduction

Bariatric surgery in reproductive-aged women has been shown to reduce menstrual irregularities,[65, 72, 73] as well as improve hyperandrogenism in PCOS women.[62, 74] Furthermore, there is an increase in SHBG,[74, 75] luteinizing hormone (LH) and follicle-stimulating hormone (FSH) levels after bariatric surgery.[74, 76] Ovulatory function increases with luteal LH and progesterone level improvement.[77] This suggests improved reproductive function and fertility.

As a result of surgery, patients with PCOS who had previously suffered from infertility may become pregnant. The pregnant mother will require closer observation during her pregnancy, as both mother and child will require adequate nutrition for fetal growth and will benefit from

regular assessments of vitamin and nutrients, particularly iron, calcium and vitamin B12 levels and the need for supplementation. It has been recommended that there be a minimum of 12 months post bariatric surgery before attempts at pregnancy be considered, in order to attain stable and normal nutritional status, especially following the malabsorptive and bypass bariatric procedures.[78, 79] Most data show that pregnancy after bariatric surgery is safe.[80–83] A study comparing post–bariatric surgery women to the general population showed a marked decrease in gestational diabetes and caesarean sections, and additionally bariatric surgery did not increase rates of postpartum hemorrhage, infection, shoulder dystocia or fetal demise.[9]

Bariatric Surgery in Adolescents

With the rapid increase of obese adolescents, bariatric surgery has become a consideration with guidelines becoming similar to adults, that is, BMI of > 40 or 35 with significant comorbidities.[84] In considering bariatric surgery in adolescents, procedures must take into account their age and future growth, and therefore procedures considered should have low morbidity and low metabolic side effects.

Bariatric Case Histories with PCOS

The following two presentations illustrate the post-operative course in patients with PCOS.

EM, a 39-year-old, weight 106 kg, BMI 39. Pre-op PCOS diagnosed at 19 with ultrasound ovaries, insulin resistance (IR) high, serum insulin on blood tests, periods light, irregular with hot flushes and anxiety. Laparoscopy showed polycystic ovarian morphology (PCOM), hormonal changes, hair on chin and nipples. On metformin pre-op. Underwent laparoscopic sleeve gastrectomy. At 26 months post-op, weight 70 kg, BMI 26, periods regular, no hirsutism, serum insulin 6.5, blood sugar normal, off metformin. Has been diagnosed with endometriosis and cystic ovaries but anxiety gone.

KK a 40-year-old, weight 133 kg, BMI 48. Pre-op, irregular periods every 18 days, ultrasound cysts on ovaries, normal serum insulin, hair on chin. Underwent laparoscopic sleeve gastrectomy. At 22 months post-op, weight 116 kg, BMI 42.1, painful heavy period every 16 days, some hirsutism and acne. Diagnosed with endometriosis and cystic ovaries; insulin normal.

In summary, two patients approximately the same age and diagnosed with PCOS pre-op, with one returning to normal post-op with good weight loss of 30 kg plus (post-op BMI) and the second still with symptoms and signs having lost only 17 kg (post-op BMI); ironically, both diagnosed with endometriosis post-op.

The question arises that, as the first patient had very good weight loss and the second did not, is it weight loss alone that creates the beneficial effect of bariatric surgery? On this topic, a 2020 article and editorial in the *New England Journal of Medicine* [85, 86] concludes that "in this study involving patients with obesity and Type 2 diabetes, the metabolic benefits of Gastric Bypass Surgery and diet were similar and were apparently related to weight loss itself, with no evident clinically important effects independent of weight loss." This does call into question my discussion of gut hormones and the metabolic effects of Roux-en-Y gastric bypass and the improvement in obese patients with PCOS.

Conclusion

PCOS is a very common condition in reproductive-aged women, with sequelae affecting their metabolic health and fertility, especially in obese and overweight women. Weight loss has been shown to reduce the effects of PCOS and to reverse its characteristics of insulin resistance, hormonal imbalance, hyperandrogenism and fertility. The treatment of obesity, as outlined, is diverse, ranging from lifestyle and diet changes to pharmacotherapy and bariatric surgery, with very good improvements and reproductive outcomes. Bariatric surgery provides effective and sustained weight loss with improvements in all aspects of the metabolic syndrome and is an added modality in the treatment of obese women with PCOS.

References

1 Ehrmann, D. A. Polycystic ovary syndrome. *N Engl J Med* 2005; 352(12): 1223–1236.

2 Flegal, K., Carroll, M., Kuczmarski, R. and Johnson, C. Overweight and obesity in the United States: Prevalence and trends, 1960–1994. *Int J Obes Relat Metab Disord* 1998; 22: 39–47.

3 Kim, S. and Popkin, B. M. Commentary: Understanding the epidemiology of overweight and obesity – a real global public health concern. *Int J Epidemiol* 2005; 35(1): 60–67.

4 Popkin, B. M. The nutrition transition and its health implications in lower-income countries. *Public Health Nutr* 1998; 1(1): 5–21.

5 Wiklund, P., Toss, F., Weinehall, L. et al. Abdominal and gynoid fat mass are associated with cardiovascular risk factors in men and women. *J Clin Endocrinol Metab* 2008; 93: 4360–4366.

6 Wexler, M. ALK gene could be key for obesity treatment, study suggests. *Genetic Obesity News.* May 28, 2020.

7 Harris, M. I., Flegal, K. M., Cowie, C. C. et al. Prevalence of diabetes, impaired fasting glucose, and impaired glucose tolerance in U.S. adults: The Third National Health and Nutrition Examination Survey, 1988–1994. *Diabetes Care* 1998; 21(4): 518–524.

8 Stroh, C., Hohmann, U., Lehnert, H. and Manger, T. PCO syndrome: Is it an indication for bariatric surgery? [Article in German]. *Zentralbl Chir* 2008; 133(6): 608–610.

9 McCullough, A. J. Epidemiology of the metabolic syndrome in the USA. *J Dig Dis* 2011; 12(5): 333–340.

10 Wren, A. M., Seal, L. J., Cohen, M. A. et al. Ghrelin enhances appetite and increases food intake in

humans. *J Clin Endocrinol Metab* 2001; 86(12): 5992.

11 Ballinger, A., McLoughlin, L., Medbak, S. and Clark, M. Cholecystokinin is a satiety hormone in humans at physiological post-prandial plasma concentrations. *Clin Sci (Lond)* 1995; 89(4): 375–381.

12 Kissileff, H. R., Carretta, J. C., Geliebter, A. and Pi-Sunyer, F. X. Cholecystokinin and stomach distension combine to reduce food intake in humans. *Am J Physiol Regul Integr Comp Physiol* 2003; 285(5): R992–R998.

13 Batterham, R. L., Cowley, M. A., Small, C. J. et al. Gut hormone PYY3-36 physiologically inhibits food intake. *Nature* 2002; 418(6898): 650–654.

14 Dakin, C. L., Gunn, I., Small, C. J. et al. Oxyntomodulin inhibits food intake in the rat. *Endocrinology* 2001;142(10):4244–50.

15 Kreymann, B., Ghatei, M. A., Williams, G. and Bloom, S. R. Glucagon-like peptide-1 7–36: A physiological incretin in man. *Lancet* 1987; 330 (8571): 1300–1304.

16 Waterson Michael, J. and Horvath Tamas, L. Neuronal regulation of energy homeostasis: Beyond the hypothalamus and feeding. *Cell Metab* 2015; 22(6): 962–970.

17 Hotta, K., Funahashi, T., Bodkin, N. L. et al. Circulating concentrations of the adipocyte protein adiponectin are decreased in parallel with reduced insulin sensitivity during the progression to type 2 diabetes in rhesus monkeys. *Diabetes* 2001; 50(5): 1126–1133.

18 Ueno, N., Inui, A., Iwamoto, M. et al. Decreased food intake and body weight in pancreatic polypeptide-overexpressing mice. *Gastroenterology* 1999;117(6):1427–32.

19 Malaisse-Lagae, F., Carpentier, J. L., Patel, Y. C., Malaisse, W. J. and Orci, L. Pancreatic polypeptide: A possible role in the regulation of food intake in the mouse. Hypothesis. *Experientia* 1977; 33(7): 915–917.

20 McLaughlin, C. L. and Baile, C. A. Obese mice and the satiety effects of cholecystokinin, bombesin and pancreatic polypeptide. *Physiol Behav* 1981; 26(3): 433–437.

21 Sun, Y. S., Brunicardi, F. C., Druck, P. et al. Reversal of abnormal glucose metabolism in chronic pancreatitis by administration of pancreatic polypeptide. *Am J Surg* 1986; 151(1): 130–140.

22 Batterham, R., Le Roux, C., Cohen, M. A. et al. Pancreatic polypeptide reduces appetite and food intake in humans. *J Clin Endocrinol Metab* 2003; 88: 3989–3992.

23 Escobar-Morreale, H. F. Polycystic ovary syndrome: Definition, aetiology, diagnosis and treatment. *Nat Rev Endocrinol* 2018; 14(5): 270–284.

24 Hart, R., Hickey, M. and Franks, S. Definitions, prevalence and symptoms of polycystic ovaries and polycystic ovary syndrome. *Best Pract Res Clin Obstet Gynaecol* 2004; 18(5): 671–683.

25 Asunción, M., Calvo, R. M., San Millán, J. L., Sancho, J., Avila, S. and Escobar-Morreale, H. F. A prospective study of the prevalence of the polycystic ovary syndrome in unselected Caucasian women from Spain. *J Clin Endocrinol Metab* 2000; 85(7): 2434–2438.

26 Alvarez-Blasco, F., Botella-Carretero, J. I., San Millán, J. L. and Escobar-Morreale, H. F. Prevalence and characteristics of the polycystic ovary syndrome in overweight and obese women. *Arch Intern Med* 2006; 166(19): 2081–2086.

27 Gabriella Garruti R. D., Vita, M. G., Lorusso, F., Giampetruzzi, F., Damato, A. B. and Giorgino, F. Adipose tissue, metabolic syndrome and polycystic ovary syndrome: From pathophysiology to treatment. *Reprod Biomed Online* 2009; 19(4): 552–563.

28 Cussons, A. J., Stuckey, B. G. A. and Watts, G. F. Metabolic syndrome and cardiometabolic risk in PCOS. *Curr Diab Rep* 2007; 7(1): 66.

29 Traub, M. Assessing and treating insulin resistance in women with polycystic ovarian syndrome. *World J Diabetes* 2011; 2: 33–40.

30 Moran, L. J., Misso, M. L., Wild, R. A. and Norman, R. J. Impaired glucose tolerance, type 2 diabetes and metabolic syndrome in polycystic ovary syndrome: A systematic review and meta-analysis. *Hum Reprod Update* 2010; 16(4): 347–363.

31 McGowan, M. P. Polycystic ovary syndrome: A common endocrine disorder and risk factor for vascular disease. *Curr Treat Options Cardiovasc Med* 2011; 13(4): 289–301.

32 Coviello, A. D., Legro, R. S. and Dunaif, A. Adolescent girls with polycystic ovary syndrome have an increased risk of the metabolic syndrome associated with increasing androgen levels independent of obesity and insulin resistance. *J Clin Endocrinol Metab* 2006; 91(2): 492–497.

33 Pfeifer, S. M. and Kives, S. Polycystic ovary syndrome in the adolescent. *Obstet Gynecol Clin North Am* 2009; 36(1): 129–152.

34 Azziz, R. PCOS in 2015: New insights into the genetics of polycystic ovary syndrome. *Nat Rev Endocrinol* 2016; 12(2): 74–75.

35 Escobar-Morreale, H. F. and San Millán, J. L. Abdominal adiposity and the polycystic ovary

syndrome. *Trends Endocrinol Metab* 2007; 18(7): 266–272.

36 Gambineri, A., Pelusi, C., Vicennati, V., Pagotto, U. and Pasquali, R. Obesity and the polycystic ovary syndrome. *Int J Obes Relat Metab Disord* 2002; 26: 883–896.

37 National Task Force on the Prevention and Treatment of Obesity. Overweight, obesity, and health risk. *Arch Intern Med* 2000; 160(7): 898–904.

38 Dunaif, A., Segal, K. R., Futterweit, W. and Dobrjansky, A. Profound peripheral insulin resistance, independent of obesity, in polycystic ovary syndrome. *Diabetes* 1989; 38(9): 1165.

39 Dunaif, A., Segal, K. R., Shelley, D. R., Green, G., Dobrjansky, A. and Licholai, T. Evidence for distinctive and intrinsic defects in insulin action in polycystic ovary syndrome. *Diabetes* 1992; 41(10): 1257.

40 Pantasri, T., Norman, R., Pantasri, T. and Norman, R. J. The effects of being overweight and obese on female reproduction: A review. *Gynecol Endocrinol* 2013; 30: 90–94.

41 Kiddy, D. S., Hamilton-Fairley, D., Bush, A. et al. Improvement in endocrine and ovarian function during dietary treatment of obese women with polycystic ovary syndrome. *Clin Endocrinol (Oxf)* 1992; 36(1): 105–111.

42 Hollmann, M., Runnebaum, B. and Gerhard, I. Infertility: Effects of weight loss on the hormonal profile in obese, infertile women. *Hum Reprod* 1996; 11(9): 1884–1891.

43 Rasmussen, C. B. and Lindenberg, S. The effect of liraglutide on weight loss in women with polycystic ovary syndrome: An observational study. *Front Endocrinol* 2014; 5(140).

44 Suliman, M., Buckley, A., Al Tikriti, A. et al. Routine clinical use of liraglutide 3 mg for the treatment of obesity: Outcomes in non-surgical and bariatric surgery patients. *Diabetes Obes Metab* 2019; 21(6): 1498–1501.

45 Sherman, M. M., Ungureanu, S. and Rey, J. A. Naltrexone/bupropion ER (Contrave): Newly approved treatment option for chronic weight management in obese adults. *Pharm Ther* 2016; 41(3): 164–172.

46 Billes, S. and Greenway, F. Combination therapy with naltrexone and bupropion for obesity. *Expert Opin Pharmacother* 2011; 12: 1813–1826.

47 Greenway, F. L., Whitehouse, M. J., Guttadauria, M. et al. Rational design of a combination medication for the treatment of obesity. *Obesity (Silver Spring)* 2009; 17(1): 30–39.

48 Wadden, T. A., Foreyt, J. P., Foster, G. D. et al. Weight loss with naltrexone SR/bupropion SR combination therapy as an adjunct to behavior modification: The COR-BMOD trial. *Obesity (Silver Spring)* 2011; 19(1): 110–120.

49 Colquitt, J. L., Picot, J., Loveman, E. and Clegg, A. J. Surgery for obesity. *Cochrane Database Syst Rev* 2009; 2: Cd003641.

50 Padwal, R., Klarenbach, S., Wiebe, N. et al. Bariatric surgery: A systematic review of the clinical and economic evidence. *J Gen Intern Med* 2011; 26(10): 1183–1194.

51 Buchwald, H., Avidor, Y., Braunwald, E. et al. Bariatric surgery: A systematic review and meta-analysis. *JAMA* 2004; 292(14): 1724–1737.

52 Dixon, J. B. Obesity surgery and the polycystic ovary syndrome. In G. Kovacs, ed. *Polycystic Ovary Syndrome*. Cambridge: Cambridge University Press, 2007.

53 De Castro, M. L., Morales, M. J., Del Campo, V. et al. Efficacy, safety, and tolerance of two types of intragastric balloons placed in obese subjects: A double-blind comparative study. *Obes Surg* 2010; 20(12): 1642–1646.

54 Giardiello, C., Borrelli, A., Silvestri, E., Antognozzi, V., Iodice, G. and Lorenzo, M. Air-filled vs water-filled intragastric balloon: A prospective randomized study. *Obes Surg* 2012; 22(12): 1916–1919.

55 Tate, C. M. and Geliebter, A. Intragastric balloon treatment for obesity: Review of recent studies. *Adv Ther* 2017; 34(8): 1859–1875.

56 Jankiewicz-Wika, J., Kołomecki, K., Cywiński, J. et al. Impact of vertical banded gastroplasty on body weight, insulin resistance, adipocytokine, inflammation and metabolic syndrome markers in morbidly obese patients. *Endokrynol Pol* 2011; 62(2): 109–119.

57 Mingrone, G. and Castagneto-Gissey, L. Mechanisms of early improvement/resolution of type 2 diabetes after bariatric surgery. *Diabetes Metab* 2009; 35(6 Pt 2): 518–523.

58 Rubino, F., Gagner, M., Gentileschi, P. et al. The early effect of the Roux-en-Y gastric bypass on hormones involved in body weight regulation and glucose metabolism. *Ann Surg* 2004; 240(2): 236–242.

59 Rubino, F. Is type 2 diabetes an operable intestinal disease? A provocative yet reasonable hypothesis. *Diabetes Care* 2008; 31 (Suppl 2): S290–S296.

60 Woelnerhanssen, B., Peterli, R., Steinert, R. E., Peters, T., Borbély, Y. and Beglinger, C. Effects of postbariatric surgery weight loss on adipokines and metabolic parameters: Comparison of laparoscopic Roux-en-Y gastric bypass and laparoscopic sleeve gastrectomy – a prospective randomized trial. *Surg Obes Relat Dis* 2011; 7(5): 561–568.

61 Marantos, G., Daskalakis, M., Karkavitsas, N., Matalliotakis, I., Papadakis, J. A. and Melissas, J. Changes in metabolic profile and adipoinsular axis in morbidly obese premenopausal females treated with restrictive bariatric surgery. *World J Surg* 2011; 35(9): 2022–2030.

62 Mustafa, A., Rizkallah, N. N. H., Samuel, N. and Balupuri, S. Laparoscopic Roux-en-Y gastric bypass versus one anastomosis (loop) gastric bypass for obesity: A prospective comparative study of weight loss and complications. *Ann Med Surg* 2020; 55: 143–147.

63 Lee, W.-J., Ser, K.-H., Lee, Y.-C., Tsou, J.-J., Chen, S.-C. and Chen, J.-C. Laparoscopic Roux-en-Y vs. mini-gastric bypass for the treatment of morbid obesity: A 10-year experience. *Obes Surg* 2012; 22(12): 1827–1834.

64 Escobar-Morreale, H., Botella-Carretero, J., Alvarez-Blasco, F., Sancho, J. and Millán, J. The polycystic ovary syndrome associated with morbid obesity may resolve after weight loss induced by bariatric surgery. *J Clin Endocrinol Metab* 2005; 90: 6364–6369.

65 Eid, G. M., Cottam, D. R., Velcu, L. M. et al. Effective treatment of polycystic ovarian syndrome with Roux-en-Y gastric bypass. *Surg Obes Relat Dis* 2005; 1(2): 77–80.

66 Ernst, B., Wilms, B., Thurnheer, M. and Schultes, B. Reduced circulating androgen levels after gastric bypass surgery in severely obese women. *Obes Surg* 2013; 23(5): 602–607.

67 Escobar-Morreale, H. F., Santacruz, E., Luque-Ramírez, M. and Botella Carretero, J. I. Prevalence of "obesity-associated gonadal dysfunction" in severely obese men and women and its resolution after bariatric surgery: A systematic review and meta-analysis. *Hum Reprod Update* 2017; 23(4): 390–408.

68 Eid, G. M., McCloskey, C., Titchner, R. et al. Changes in hormones and biomarkers in polycystic ovarian syndrome treated with gastric bypass. *Surg Obes Relat Dis* 2014; 10(5): 787–791.

69 Skubleny, D., Switzer, N. J., Gill, R. S. et al. The impact of bariatric surgery on polycystic ovary syndrome: A systematic review and meta-analysis. *Obes Surg* 2016; 26(1): 169–176.

70 Malik, S. M. and Traub, M. L. Defining the role of bariatric surgery in polycystic ovarian syndrome patients. *World J Diabetes* 2012; 3(4): 71–79.

71 Lima, M. M. O., Pareja, J. C., Alegre, S. M. et al. Acute effect of Roux-en-Y gastric bypass on whole-body insulin sensitivity: A study with the euglycemic-hyperinsulinemic clamp. *J Clin Endocrinol Metab* 2010; 95(8): 3871–3875.

72 Deitel, M., Stone, E., Kassam, H. A., Wilk, E. J. and Sutherland, D. J. Gynecologic-obstetric changes after loss of massive excess weight following bariatric surgery. *J Am Coll Nutr* 1988; 7(2): 147–153.

73 Jamal, M., Gunay, Y., Capper, A., Eid, A., Heitshusen, D. and Samuel, I. Roux-en-Y gastric bypass ameliorates polycystic ovary syndrome and dramatically improves conception rates: A 9-year analysis. *Surg Obes Relat Dis* 2012; 8(4): 440–444.

74 Gerrits, E. G., Ceulemans, R., van Hee, R., Hendrickx, L. and Totté, E. Contraceptive treatment after biliopancreatic diversion needs consensus. *Obes Surg* 2003; 13(3): 378–382.

75 Victor, A., Odlind, V. and Kral, J. G. Oral contraceptive absorption and sex hormone binding globulins in obese women: Effects of jejunoileal bypass. *Gastroenterol Clin North Am* 1987; 16(3): 483–491.

76 Bastounis, E. A., Karayiannakis, A. J., Syrigos, K., Zbar, A., Makri, G. G. and Alexiou, D. Sex hormone changes in morbidly obese patients after vertical banded gastroplasty. *Eur Surg Res* 1998; 30(1): 43–47.

77 Rochester, D., Jain, A., Polotsky, A. J. et al. Partial recovery of luteal function after bariatric surgery in obese women. *Fertil Steril* 2009; 92 (4): 1410–1415.

78 American College of Obstetricians and Gynecologists. ACOG Committee Opinion number 315, September 2005: Obesity in pregnancy. *Obstet Gynecol* 2005; 106(3): 671–675.

79 Poitou Bernert, C., Ciangura, C., Coupaye, M. et al. Nutritional deficiency after gastric bypass: Diagnosis, prevention and treatment. *Diabetes Metab* 2007; 33(1): 13–24.

80 Aricha-Tamir, B., Weintraub, A. Y., Levi, I. and Sheiner, E. Downsizing pregnancy complications: A study of paired pregnancy outcomes before and after bariatric surgery. *Surg Obes Relat Dis* 2012; 8(4): 434–439.

81 Burke, A. E., Bennett, W. L., Jamshidi, R. M. et al. Reduced incidence of gestational diabetes with bariatric surgery. *J Am Coll Surg* 2010; 211(2): 169–175.

82 Lesko, J. and Peaceman, A. Pregnancy outcomes in women after bariatric surgery compared with obese and morbidly obese controls. *Obstet Gynecol* 2012; 119(3): 547–554.

83 Sheiner, E., Levy, A., Silverberg, D. et al. Pregnancy after bariatric surgery is not associated with adverse perinatal outcome. *Am J Obstet Gynecol* 2004; 190(5): 1335–1340.

84 Pratt, J. S., Lenders, C. M., Dionne, E. A. et al. Best
    practice updates for pediatric/adolescent weight
    loss surgery. *Obesity (Silver Spring)* 2009; 17(5):
    901–910.

85 Yoshino, M., Kayser, B. D., Yoshino, J. et al.
    Effects of diet versus gastric bypass on

    metabolic function in diabetes. *N Engl J Med*
    2020; 383(8): 721–732.

86 Rosen, C. J. and Ingelfinger, J. R. Bariatric
    surgery and restoration of insulin sensitivity: It's
    weight loss. *N Engl J Med* 2020; 383(8):
    777–778.

Mood Disorders in Polycystic Ovary Syndrome

Anuja Dokras

Introduction

Polycystic ovary syndrome (PCOS), the commonest endocrine disorder in reproductive-aged women, is associated with significant non-endocrine morbidities, namely type 2 diabetes, obesity, dyslipidemia, sleep apnea and hepatic steatosis.[1] Over the past decade, it has become well recognized that PCOS is also associated with significant mental health disorders, including depression and anxiety, with more recent evidence for increased risk of eating disorders (ED). The significant burden of disease associated with both PCOS and mental illness resulted in the Androgen Excess and Polycystic Ovary Syndrome (AE-PCOS) Society's position statement in 2018 recommending routine screening for depression and anxiety and consideration of screening for ED in all women with PCOS.[2] In the general population, it is well recognized that obesity and insulin resistance increase the risk of depression,[3, 4] and depression itself is a known risk factor for cardiovascular disease.[5] Recognizing the importance of timely identification of mood disorders in PCOS, the international PCOS guidelines also endorsed the abovementioned recommendations of the AE-PCOS Society to screen at the time of initial diagnosis. [6] In this chapter, we will review the prevalence of mood disorders in PCOS, underlying etiologies and the impact of current PCOS-related therapies. There are several gaps in the literature, and these will be highlighted as potential research opportunities.

What Is the Risk of Depression in PCOS?

Women with PCOS are at an increased risk of both depressive symptoms and major depressive disorders (MDD). We conducted a survey at a tertiary academic center and reported an increased risk for depression (new cases) in women with PCOS compared to controls (21% vs. 3%; OR 5.11; 95% CI 1.26 to 20.69; $p < 0.03$). [7] The overall OR of depression in women with PCOS was 4.23 (95% CI 1.49 to 11.98; $p < 0.01$) independent of obesity and infertility. We also found a higher prevalence of MDD in the PCOS group (13.6%, $n = 103$), compared to 1.9% in the control group ($n = 103$, $p < 0.002$), with a fivefold increased risk after adjusting for body mass index (BMI) and family history of depression ($p < 0.03$). In the USA, the prevalence of MDD in women in the general population is high (approximately 5%) and significantly affects the lifetime burden of disease.[8] We subsequently surveyed the same cohort of women and reported a 40% prevalence of depression, with 19% new cases of MDD over 22 months.[9] These initial findings have been supported by a large number of cross-sectional studies both in clinic and in population-based settings across the globe. In a large national registry from Sweden, women with PCOS ($n = 24385$) were found to be at a higher risk of depressive disorders (OR 1.25; 95% CI 1.19 to 1.25) compared to 243850 controls after adjusting for other psychiatric comorbidities and matching for age, county of residence, and year of birth.[10] In a meta-analysis, we subsequently reported a median prevalence of depression of 36.6% (IQR 22.3, 50.0%) in the PCOS group and 14.2% (IQR 10.7, 22.2%) in the control group. Women with PCOS had increased odds of any depressive symptoms (OR 3.78; 95% CI 3.03 to 4.72; 18 studies) and of moderate/severe depressive symptoms (OR 4.18; 95% CI 2.68 to 6.52; 11 studies).[11]

In addition to examining data obtained from cross-sectional studies, it is important to understand the risk of depression over time in this population. Several longitudinal studies demonstrate the persistent of depressive symptoms over time. In both an Australian study of hospital records (median follow-up: 8 years)[12] and a Taiwanese study using a national health insurance database (median follow-up: 5 years) [13] women with PCOS, who did not have a psychiatric disorder at baseline, had a significantly higher risk of developing depression during the follow-up period. In the Northern Finland birth cohort population-based study, depressive symptoms were increased at ages 31 and 46 in women with PCOS compared with controls.[14] In a US population, where depression scores were measured every 5 years over a 25-year period, Center for Epidemiologic Studies Depression Scale (CES-D) scores were higher among women with PCOS (2.51; 95% CI 1.49 to 3.54; $p < 0.01$) across the lifespan.[15] Interestingly, depression scores decreased across the lifespan in both women with and women without PCOS (coef −0.1 point per year; $p < 0.001$).

There are limited data on depression during pregnancy, with one population-based study showing PCOS is associated with antenatal but not postpartum depression after controlling for preexisting depression and anxiety.[16] Using a large insurance claims dataset, we have recently shown that the odds of perinatal depression (adjusted odds ratio (aOR) 1.32; 95% CI 1.26 to 1.39) and postpartum depression (OR 1.50; 95% CI 1.39 to 1.62) are higher in women with PCOS than in controls.[17]

Although the above-discussed studies collectively demonstrate an increased burden of depressive symptoms in young reproductive-aged women with PCOS in various parts of the globe, there are limited data on the prevalence of depression in the different PCOS phenotypes.

Why Are Women with PCOS at an Increased Risk of Depressive Symptoms?

Women with PCOS have several recognized risk factors for depression, including insulin resistance, obesity, body image distress and genetic associations. Given the high prevalence of obesity in the PCOS population, several studies have evaluated the independent association between PCOS and depression. In the above-described meta-analysis, when studies with participants matched on BMI were included, women with PCOS had higher odds of depression than controls OR 3.25 (1.73 to 6.09).[11] To identify factors that might increase the risk of depression in this population, we also performed a meta-regression and found a significant though weak correlation between depressive symptoms and BMI and insulin sensitivity (measured by homeostasis model assessment of insulin resistance, HOMA-IR).[11] In a US cohort study of 163 women with PCOS followed over 5.5 years, obesity significantly increased the odds of persistent depression,[18] such that a 1 kg/m^2 increase in BMI increased the odds of converting from a negative to positive depression screen by 10%. In contrast, in a population-based study including 85 women with PCOS followed for 15 years in Finland, BMI did not have an association with depressive symptoms.[14] These studies indicate that obesity may be a significant contributor to the risk of depression; however, the directionality of this association maybe difficult to ascertain, as women with depression may lead a lifestyle that predisposes them to obesity.

Another risk factor unique to PCOS that has been extensively investigated is hyperandrogenism; however, the data is mixed.[7, 19, 20] In the meta-analysis described in the section "What Is the Risk of Depression in PCOS?" we performed a meta-regression and reported a weak correlation between depressive symptoms and Ferriman–Gallwey score for hirsutism but not with serum androgens.[11] This supports the notion that dermatological manifestations of hyperandrogenism, such as acne, hirsutism and alopecia, may mediate depressive symptoms,[21] likely through an impact on body image. Alternatively, it has been suggested that direct and indirect effects of testosterone on neurotransmitters or oversensitivity to the stress hormone adrenocorticotropic hormone, with subsequent production of adrenal androgens, may be associated with depression in PCOS.[22]

Negative body image in women with PCOS, independent of BMI, has also been associated with depression.[23, 24] We have shown that women with PCOS have significantly worse body image distress scores on all five Body-Self Relations Questionnaire–Appearance Scales (MBSRQ-AS) subscales and on the Stunkard Figure Rating Scale compared with the control women.[25] Specifically, the body image domains associated with higher depression scores were appearance evaluation, body areas satisfaction, overweight preoccupation and higher self-classified weight. Interestingly, in this study we found that body image distress significantly mediates much of the relationship between PCOS and depression.

Another known risk factor for depression is adverse childhood experiences (ACEs). A population-based survey conducted in Australia found a high prevalence of ACEs in women with PCOS compared to controls (19.3% vs. 9.2%), and this was the strongest factor associated with psychiatric disorders (ACEs ≥ 4: aOR 2.9; 95 % CI 2.4 to 3.5).[26] Finally, there is genetic evidence for shared biologic pathways between PCOS and depression as indicated in a meta-analysis of genome-wide association studies (GWAS).[27] As BMI and depression are also genetically linked, the independent association of PCOS and depression needs to be further evaluated. It appears that several factors may predispose women with PCOS to an increased risk of depressive symptoms, and based on the above-discussed findings the impact of interventions such as weight loss and improvement of hyperandrogenism on depressive symptoms should be explored.

Impact of PCOS Treatment on Depressive Symptoms

Lifestyle management (LSM) including dietary modifications and increased physical activity is the first-line treatment for overweight/obese women with PCOS and has been reinforced by the international PCOS guidelines (see also Chapter 10).[6] Although few studies have examined the impact of LSM on depressive symptoms, the overall data suggest an improvement in symptoms. In an Australian study, women with PCOS showed improvement in depressive symptoms after 20 weeks in all three groups, namely dietary intervention alone ($n = 14$), diet and aerobic exercise $n = 15$) and a combination of diet and aerobic and resistance exercise ($n = 20$).[28] More recently, a randomized control trial (RCT) conducted in Sweden showed improvements in depressive symptoms and general health in women with PCOS randomized to lifestyle intervention ($n = 23$) compared to women undergoing self-treatment ($n = 26$) for four months.[29] A systematic review has examined the impact of

dietary composition on mood and suggested that a high-protein diet may improve depressive symptoms and self-esteem.[30]

In the general population, cognitive behavioral therapy (CBT) is the first-line treatment for depression and may also aid weight-loss efforts.[31, 32] We conducted a pilot study in overweight/obese women with PCOS who screened positive for depression and randomized them to CBT (8 weeks) and LSM or LSM alone. [33] After 16 weeks' intervention, the group receiving CBT and LSM lost twice as much weight compared to the LSM alone group (3.2 kg vs. 1.8 kg; $p < 0.03$), were more likely to meet their weekly exercise goal (59% vs. 38% of sessions; $p = 0.002$) and were more likely to exercise a higher median number of minutes per week (102 min vs. 90 min; $p = 0.003$). Both groups had similar improvements in depressive symptoms based on CES-D 0.31 points/week (95% CI −0.55 to −0.07; $p = 0.01$). More recently, a RCT from the Netherlands showed that women undergoing LSM and CBT had significant improvement in depression scores compared to women receiving care as usual over 12 months. Collectively, these studies indicate improvement in depression scores with LSM over short study periods and possibly sustained up to one year. It is not clear if these benefits are recognized independent of weight loss.

Oral combined hormonal contraceptive therapy is also used as first-line therapy for management of PCOS in women not seeking fertility treatment. As oral contraceptive pills (OCPs) improve clinical hyperandrogenism by effectively decreasing serum androgens, it can be hypothesized that their use will also improve depressive symptoms. Few studies have examined the effects of OCPs on mood in the PCOS population. In the OWL-PCOS study, overweight/obese women with PCOS were randomized to OCP versus intensive LSM versus combination (OCP + LSM), and we found that the prevalence of depression decreased (13.3% to 4.4%, $p < 0.05$) in the OCP group after 16 weeks compared to baseline.[34] In another study including lean women with PCOS, OCP use for four months did not change depressive symptoms.[35] Metformin is another medication commonly used for management of PCOS; however, there is limited and mixed data on the effects of insulin-sensitizing medications on depressive symptoms in PCOS.[36, 37] The impact of long-term use of OCPs and metformin on mood disorders needs to be evaluated in order to better counsel this high-risk population.

What Is the Risk of Anxiety in PCOS?

Anxiety, or generalized anxiety disorder (GAD), is a common psychiatric disorder. In a meta-analysis by Cooney and colleagues, the prevalence of anxiety was 41.9% in PCOS and 8.5% among controls (OR 5.62; 95% CI 3.22 to 9.80; $n = 9$ studies).[11] In addition, women with PCOS were more likely to have moderate and severe anxiety symptoms (OR 6.55; 95% CI 2.87 to 14.93). In the Swedish national registry study that reported an increased risk of depressive disorders, women with PCOS were also more likely to have anxiety disorders (aOR 1.37; 95% CI 1.32 to 1.43).[10] Furthermore, hospital admissions records of 2566 women with PCOS compared to 25 660 controls also showed a higher prevalence of anxiety in patients with a history of PCOS (14.0% vs. 5.9%).[12]

Few studies have examined the longitudinal prevalence of anxiety in the PCOS population. In a cohort study from Taiwan, the incidence of anxiety increased significantly over a five-year follow-up period after an initial diagnosis of PCOS ($n = 5$ 431) compared to controls.[13] In the 15-year Finnish birth cohort study, the likelihood of an abnormal anxiety score persisted between ages 31 years (16.1% in PCOS vs. 8.2% in controls) and 46 years (12.8% in PCOS vs. 8.3% in controls).[14] Overall, there is evidence for increased risk of anxiety symptoms in women with PCOS residing in different regions of the world; however, similar to depressive symptoms, it is not clear if the prevalence of anxiety differs in PCOS phenotypes.

Why Are Women with PCOS at an Increased Risk of Anxiety Symptoms?

It is likely that similar factors that mediate depression such as obesity, insulin resistance and hyperandrogenism may also play a role in anxiety symptoms. In the meta-regression by Cooney and colleagues, we found a positive association between BMI, hirsutism score and free testosterone levels with anxiety symptoms,

though the effect size was small.[11] In women presenting to dermatologists, self-assessed hirsutism has also been associated with anxiety, indicating a strong association with clinical hyperandrogenism.[38] Interestingly, there is evidence to suggest that prenatal androgen exposure as seen in the rodent model may result in increased anxiety-like symptoms in the next generation.[39] In addition, infertility and alopecia have also been identified as risk factors for anxiety in PCOS.[40] Physical manifestations of PCOS such as acne, hirsutism and obesity also impact body image and low body image impacts anxiety.[41] In fact, we have shown that body image distress significantly mediates anxiety symptoms in women with PCOS.[25] Therapies targeted at improving some of these risk factors may decrease the anxiety symptoms in PCOS.

Impact of PCOS Treatments on Anxiety Symptoms

Few studies targeted at improving weight, insulin resistance and hyperandrogenism specifically examine the impact of these interventions on anxiety symptoms. In the OWL-PCOS trial described in the section "Impact of PCOS Treatment on Depressive Symptoms," overweight/obese women with PCOS randomized to LSM ($n = 44$) showed a significant decrease in prevalence of anxiety from 15.9% to 4.7%, with no significant change in the OCP ($n = 45$) and OCP + LSM ($n = 43$) groups.[34] Of note, subjects in the LSM and combined groups lost significantly more weight over 16 weeks compared to the OCP group (6.4 kg each for LSM and combined; 1.2 kg for OCP). In contrast, in another study where participants underwent LSM not associated with weight loss, there were no differences in anxiety scores over 32 weeks. [42] In the Swedish study by Oberg and colleagues, LSM for four months resulted in improvement in anxiety scores compared to self-treatment.[29] Moreover, women who lost > 5% body weight during the study period had lower normalized anxiety scores, indicating less anxiety, at baseline. These findings indicate that women with increased anxiety may have difficulty achieving weight loss but those who lose weight might show improvement in anxiety scores.

What Is the risk of Eating Disorders and Disordered Eating in PCOS?

As LSM is the mainstay of treatment for all women with PCOS, it is critical to identify factors that influence the ability to engage effectively in weight management programs. Underlying disordered eating and ED can both influence the effectiveness of weight management programs. In a recent meta-analysis, we reported an increased odds of an abnormal ED score (OR 3.05; 95% CI 1.33 to 6.99) and any ED diagnosis (OR 3.87; 95% CI 1.43 to 10.49) in women with PCOS compared to controls.[43] Disordered eating global and subscale scores, as measured by the Eating Disorder Examination Questionnaire (EDE-Q) survey, were significantly higher in women with PCOS, with a higher prevalence of disordered eating in PCOS (12.2%) compared to controls (2.8%, $p = 0.01$).[44] An Australian study reported disordered eating was more prevalent in women with PCOS ($n = 501$) compared to controls ($n = 398$, $p = 0.012$).[45] In this study, increased BMI (OR 1.03; 95% CI 1.01 to 1.05; $p = 0.012$) and older age (OR 1.05; 95% CI 1.02 to 1.08; $p = 0.002$) but not PCOS diagnosis (OR 1.43; 95% CI 0.96 to 2.13; $p = 0.078$) increased the odds of disordered eating. Although there are fewer studies on the prevalence of ED in PCOS, a meta-analysis reported that women with PCOS were more likely to have bulimia nervosa (OR 1.37; 95% CI 1.17 to 1.60), binge eating (OR 2.95; 95% CI 1.61 to 5.42) or any eating disorder (OR 1.96; 95% CI 1.18 to 3.24) but not anorexia nervosa (OR 0.92; 95% CI 0.78 to 1.10).[46] Binge eating disorder is especially relevant in the PCOS population, as it is independently associated with diabetes, obesity and hypertension – all of which are more common in women with PCOS.[47, 48]

Why Are Women with PCOS at Increased Risk for Disordered Eating and ED?

Women with PCOS have several known risk factors for disordered eating behaviors, such as high BMI, early onset of overweight or obesity and frequent dieting.[49, 50] In addition, the high prevalence of moderate to severe depression and anxiety symptoms in this population also predisposes them to ED.[51] After controlling for age

and BMI, Lee and colleagues reported that PCOS subjects with elevated anxiety scores had an increased risk of an abnormal EDE-Q global score compared to those without anxiety (aOR, 5.91; 95% CI 0.61 to 56.9).[44] Another study has shown that obesity at baseline conferred a 6.9-fold increased odds of an elevated EDE-Q score (aOR 6.89; 95% CI 2.70 to 17.62), while a positive depression screen conferred a 3.6-fold increased odds (aOR 3.58; 95% CI 1.74 to 7.35) in women with PCOS ($n = 164$).[52]

Impact of PCOS Treatments on Disordered Eating and ED

LSM, the first-line treatment for PCOS, has the potential for harm in patients with comorbid disordered eating.[53] For example, in the general population, binge eating disorder is associated with less weight loss, more rapid weight regain and more attrition from weight loss treatments, [54, 55] and dietary restriction is associated with an increased risk of bulimia.[56] Although there are no studies specifically in women with PCOS, CBT has been used as an approach for management of ED.[57, 58] On the other hand, as reviewed in this chapter LSM, CBT and OCPs may improve both anxiety and depressive symptoms in this population, thereby decreasing the risk of disordered eating. The high prevalence of disordered eating in PCOS and negative impact of ED on the efficacy of weight-loss interventions necessitates identification of this psychiatric comorbidity in order to identify effective weight-loss strategies. The international PCOS guidelines suggest screening all women with PCOS for disordered eating at their initial evaluation.[6]

Conclusion

In addition to cardiometabolic comorbidities, there is ample evidence to support the claim that women with PCOS also have an increased risk of psychiatric comorbidities. These mental health disorders can further aggravate the long-term risk for cardiovascular disease. Early identification of depression, anxiety and disordered eating followed by appropriate management, including referral for specialized treatment, is critical. Care for women with PCOS is often fragmented, and the development of multidisciplinary models of care will be beneficial in order to effectively manage the multitude of symptoms. All intervention studies should examine the impact on depressive and anxiety symptoms to allow better counseling of the population. Currently, it appears that LSM and CBT will likely improve both weight management and mood symptoms. Also, the few studies that have examined the impact of OCPs on depressive and anxiety symptoms do not indicate worsening of symptoms. Future research should focus on the impact of body image distress and ED in the overall management of this young population.

References

1 Cooney, L. G. and Dokras, A. Beyond fertility: Polycystic ovary syndrome and long-term health. *Fertil Steril* 2018; 110: 794–809.

2 Dokras, A., Stener-Victorin, E., Yildiz, B. O. et al. Androgen excess– Polycystic Ovary Syndrome Society: Position statement on depression, anxiety, quality of life, and eating disorders in polycystic ovary syndrome. *Fertil Steril* 2018; 109: 888–899.

3 Kan, C., Silva, N., Golden, S. H. et al. A systematic review and meta-analysis of the association between depression and insulin resistance. *Diabetes Care* 2013; 36: 480–489.

4 Luppino, F. S., de Wit, L. M., Bouvy, P. F. et al. Overweight, obesity, and depression: A systematic review and meta-analysis of longitudinal studies. *Arch Gen Psychiatry* 2010; 67: 220–229.

5 Van der Kooy, K., van Hout, H., Marwijk, H. et al. Depression and the risk for cardiovascular diseases: Systematic review and meta analysis. *Int J Geriatr Psychiatry* 2007; 22: 613–626.

6 Teede, H. J., Misso, M. L., Costello, M. F. et al. Recommendations from the international evidence-based guideline for the assessment and management of polycystic ovary syndrome. *Fertil Steril* 2018; 110: 364–379.

7 Hollinrake, E., Abreu, A., Maifeld, M., Van Voorhis, B. J. and Dokras, A. Increased risk of depressive disorders in women with polycystic ovary syndrome. *Fertil Steril* 2007; 87: 1369–1376.

8 Guo, N., Robakis, T., Miller, C. and Butwick, A. Prevalence of depression among women of reproductive age in the United States. *Obstet Gynecol* 2018; 131: 671–679.

9 Kerchner, A., Lester, W., Stuart, S. P. and Dokras, A. Risk of depression and other mental health disorders in women with polycystic ovary syndrome: A longitudinal study. *Fertil Steril* 2009; 91: 207–212.

10 Cesta, C. E., Månsson, M., Palm, C. et al. Polycystic ovary syndrome and psychiatric disorders: Co-morbidity and heritability in a nationwide Swedish cohort. *Psychoneuroendocrinology* 2016; 73: 196–203.

11 Cooney, L. G., Lee, I., Sammel, M .D. and Dokras, A. High prevalence of moderate and severe depressive and anxiety symptoms in polycystic ovary syndrome: A systematic review and meta-analysis. *Hum Reprod* 2017; 32: 1075–1091.

12 Hart, R. and Doherty, D. A. The potential implications of a PCOS diagnosis on a woman's long-term health using data linkage. *J Clin Endocrinol Metab* 2015; 100: 911–919.

13 Hung, J. H., Hu, L. Y., Tsai, S. J. et al. Risk of psychiatric disorders following polycystic ovary syndrome: A nationwide population-based cohort study. *PLoS ONE* 2014; 9: e97041.

14 Karjula, S., Morin-Papunen, L., Auvinen, J. et al. Psychological distress is more prevalent in fertile age and premenopausal women with PCOS symptoms: 15-year follow-up. *J Clin Endocrinol Metab* 2017: 102: 1861–1869.

15 Greenwood, E. A., Yaffe, K., Wellons, M. F., Cedars, M. I. and Huddleston, H. G. Depression over the lifespan in a population-based cohort of women with polycystic ovary syndrome: Longitudinal analysis. *J Clin Endocrinol Metab* 2019; 104: 2809–2819.

16 Tay, C. T., Teede, H. J., Boyle, J. A., Kulkarni, J., Loxton, D. and Joham, A. E. Perinatal mental health in women with polycystic ovary syndrome: A cross-sectional analysis of an Australian population-based cohort. *J Clin Med* 2019; 8: 2070.

17 Alur-Gupta, S., Boland, M. R., Barnhart, K. T., Sammel, M. D. and Dokras, A. Postpartum complications increased in women with polycystic ovary syndrome. *Am J Obstet Gynecol* 2020; 224(3): 280.e1–280.e13.

18 Greenwood, E. A., Pasch, L. A., Shinkai, K., Cedars, M. I. and Huddleston, H. G. Clinical course of depression symptoms and predictors of enduring depression risk in women with polycystic ovary syndrome: Results of a longitudinal study. *Fertil Steril* 2019; 111: 147–156.

19 Jedel, E., Gustafson, D., Waern, M. et al. Sex steroids, insulin sensitivity and sympathetic nerve activity in relation to affective symptoms in women with polycystic ovary syndrome. *Psychoneuroendocrinology* 2011; 36: 1470–1479.

20 Weiner, C. L., Primeau, M. and Ehrmann, D. A. Androgens and mood dysfunction in women: Comparison of women with polycystic ovarian syndrome to healthy controls. *Psychosom Med* 2004; 66: 356–362.

21 Ekbäck, M. P., Lindberg, M., Benzein, E. and Årestedt, K. Health-related quality of life, depression and anxiety correlate with the degree of hirsutism. *Dermatology* 2013; 227: 278–284.

22 Barry, J. A., Qu, F. and Hardiman, P. J. An exploration of the hypothesis that testosterone is implicated in the psychological functioning of women with polycystic ovary syndrome (PCOS). *Med Hypotheses* 2018; 110: 42–45.

23 Deeks, A. A., Gibson-Helm, M. E., Paul, E. and Teede, H. J. Is having polycystic ovary syndrome a predictor of poor psychological function including anxiety and depression? *Hum Reprod* 2011; 26: 1399–1407.

24 Himelein, M. J. and Thatcher, S. S. Depression and body image among women with polycystic ovary syndrome. *J Health Psychol* 2006; 11: 613–625.

25 Alur-Gupta, S., Chemerinski, A., Liu, C. et al. Body-image distress is increased in women with polycystic ovary syndrome and mediates depression and anxiety. *Fertil Steril* 2019; 112: 930–938.e1.

26 Tay, C. T., Teede, H. J., Loxton, D., Kulkarni, J. and Joham, A. E. Psychiatric comorbidities and adverse childhood experiences in women with self-reported polycystic ovary syndrome: An Australian population-based study. *Psychoneuroendocrinology* 2020; 116: 104678.

27 Day, F., Karaderi, T., Jones, M. R. et al. Large-scale genome-wide meta-analysis of polycystic ovary syndrome suggests shared genetic architecture for different diagnosis criteria. *PLoS Genet* 2018; 19 (14): e1007813.

28 Thomson, R. L., Buckley, J. D., Lim, S. S. et al. Lifestyle management improves quality of life and depression in overweight and obese women with polycystic ovary syndrome. *Fertil Steril* 2010: 94: 1812–1816.

29 Oberg, E., Lundell, C., Blomberg, L. et al. Psychological well-being and personality in relation to weight loss following behavioral modification intervention in obese women with polycystic ovary syndrome: A randomized controlled trial. *Eur J Endocrinol* 2020; 183: 1–11.

30 Moran, L. J., Ko, H., Misso, M. et al. Dietary composition in the treatment of polycystic ovary syndrome: A systematic review to inform evidence-based guidelines. *J Acad Nutr Diet* 2013; 113: 520–545.

31 Qaseem, A., Barry, M. J., Kansagara, D. and Clinical Guidelines Committee of the American College of Physicians. Nonpharmacologic versus pharmacologic treatment of adult patients with major depressive disorder: A clinical practice guideline from the American College of Physicians. *Ann Intern Med* 2016; 164: 350–359.

32 Abilés, V., Rodríguez-Ruiz, S., Abilés, J. et al. Effectiveness of cognitive-behavioral therapy in morbidity obese candidates for bariatric surgery with and without binge eating disorder. *Nutr Hosp* 2013; 28: 1523–1529.

33 Cooney, L.G., Milman, L. W., Hantsoo, L. et al. Cognitive-behavioral therapy improves weight loss and quality of life in women with polycystic ovary syndrome: A pilot randomized clinical trial. *Fertil Steril* 2018; 110: 161–171.e1.

34 Dokras, A., Sarwer, D. B., Allison, K. C. et al. Weight loss and lowering androgens predict improvements in health-related quality of life in women with PCOS. *J Clin Endocrinol Metab* 2016; 101: 2966–2974.

35 Cinar, N., Harmanci, A., Demir, B. and Yildiz, B. O. Effect of an oral contraceptive on emotional distress, anxiety and depression of women with polycystic ovary syndrome: A prospective study. *Hum Reprod* 2012; 27: 1840–1845.

36 AlHussain, F., AlRuthia, Y., Al-Mandeel, H. et al. Metformin improves the depression symptoms of women with polycystic ovary syndrome in a lifestyle modification program. *Patient Prefer Adherence* 2020; 14: 737–746.

37 Kashani, L., Omidvar, T., Farazmand, B. et al. Does pioglitazone improve depression through insulin-sensitization? Results of a randomized double-blind metformin-controlled trial in patients with polycystic ovarian syndrome and comorbid depression. *Psychoneuroendocrinology* 2013; 38: 767–776.

38 Ekbäck, M. P., Lindberg, M., Benzein, E. and Årestedt, K. Health-related quality of life, depression and anxiety correlate with the degree of hirsutism. *Dermatology* 2013; 227: 278–284.

39 Stener-Victorin, E., Manti, M., Fornes, R., Risal, S., Lu, H. and Benrick, A. Origins and impact of psychological traits in polycystic ovary syndrome. *Med Sci (Basel)* 2019; 7: 86.

40 Chaudhari, A. P., Mazumdar, K. and Mehta, P. D. Anxiety, depression, and quality of life in women with polycystic ovarian syndrome. *Indian J Psychol Med* 2018; 40: 239–246.

41 Kogure, G. S., Ribeiro, V. B., Lopes, I. P. et al. Body image and its relationships with sexual functioning, anxiety, and depression in women with polycystic ovary syndrome. *J Affect Disord* 2019; 253: 385–393.

42 Stener-Victorin, E., Holm, G., Janson, P. O., Gustafson, D. and Waern, M. Acupuncture and physical exercise for affective symptoms and health-related quality of life in polycystic ovary syndrome: Secondary analysis from a randomized

controlled trial. *BMC Complement Altern Med* 2013; 13: 131.

43 Lee, I., Cooney, L. G., Saini, S. et al. Increased odds of disordered eating in polycystic ovary syndrome: A systematic review and meta-analysis. *Eat Weight Disord* 2019; 24: 787–797.

44 Lee, I., Cooney, L. G., Saini, S. et al. Increased risk of disordered eating in polycystic ovary syndrome. *Fertil Steril* 2017; 107: 796–802.

45 Pirotta, S., Barillaro, M., Brennan, L. et al. Disordered eating behaviours and eating disorders in women in Australia with and without polycystic ovary syndrome: A cross-sectional study. *J Clin Med* 2019; 8: 1682.

46 Thannickal, A., Brutocao, C., Alsawas, M. et al. Eating, sleeping and sexual function disorders in women with polycystic ovary syndrome (PCOS): A systematic review and meta-analysis. *Clin Endocrinol (Oxf)* 2020; 92: 338–349.

47 Paganini, C., Peterson, G., Stavropoulos, V. and Krug, I. The overlap between binge eating behaviors and polycystic ovarian syndrome: An etiological integrative model. *Curr Pharm Des* 2018; 24: 999–1006.

48 Kessler, R. C., Berglund, P. A., Chiu, W. T. et al. The prevalence and correlates of binge eating disorder in the World Health Organization World Mental Health Surveys. *Bio Psychiatry* 2013; 73: 904–914.

49 Striegel-Moore, R. H. and Bulik, C. M. Risk factors for eating disorders. *Am Psychol* 2007; 62: 181–198.

50 Moran, L. J., Brown, W. J., McNaughton, S. A., Joham, A. E. and Teede, H. J. Weight management practices associated with PCOS and their relationships with diet and physical activity. *Hum Reprod* 2017; 32: 669–678.

51 Hudson, J. I., Hiripi, E., Pope, H. G., Jr., Kessler, R. C. The prevalence and correlates of eating disorders in the National Comorbidity Survey Replication. *Biol Psychiatry* 2007; 61: 348–358.

52 Greenwood, E. A., Pasch, L. A., Cedars, M. I. and Huddleston, H. G. Obesity and depression are risk factors for future eating disorder-related attitudes and behaviors in women with polycystic ovary syndrome. *Fertil Steril* 2020; 113: 1039–1049.

53 Lim, S. S., Hutchison, S. K., Van Ryswyk, E., Norman, R. J., Teede, H. J. and Moran, L. J. Lifestyle changes in women with polycystic ovary syndrome. *Cochrane Database Syst Rev* 2019; 3: CD007506.

54 Sherwood, N. E., Jeffery, R. W. and Wing, R. R. Binge status as a predictor of weight loss treatment outcome. *Int J Obes Relat Metab Disord* 1999; 23: 485–493.

55 Yanovski, S. Z., Gormally, J. F., Leser, M. S., Gwirtsman, H. E. and Yanovski, J. A. Binge eating disorder affects outcome of comprehensive very-low-calorie diet treatment. *Obes Res* 1994; 2: 205–212.

56 Killen, J. D., Taylor, C. B., Hayward, C. et al. Weight concerns influence the development of eating disorders: A 4-year prospective study. *J Consult Clin Psychol* 1996; 64: 936–940.

57 Grilo, C. M., Masheb, R. M., Wilson, G. T., Gueorguieva, R. and White, M. A. Cognitive-behavioral therapy, behavioral weight loss, and sequential treatment for obese patients with binge-eating disorder: A randomized controlled trial. *J Consult Clin Psychol* 2011; 79: 675–685.

58 Linardon, J., Wade, T. D., de la Piedad Garcia, X. and Brennan, L. The efficacy of cognitive-behavioral therapy for eating disorders: A systematic review and meta-analysis. *J Consult Clin Psychol* 2017; 85: 1080–1094.

Chapter 18

The Long-Term Health Consequences of Polycystic Ovary Syndrome

Lisa Owens and Stephen Franks

Introduction

Polycystic ovary syndrome (PCOS) is one of the most common conditions in women, affecting up to 13% of reproductive-aged women, with up to 70% of affected women remaining undiagnosed. [1–3] There has been a paradigm shift from recognizing PCOS as a predominantly reproductive and metabolic condition toward its recognition as a complex multisystem disorder with comorbidities and long-term health implications (summarized in Figure 18.1). International guidelines now recognize that PCOS is associated with not just reproductive (anovulation, infertility and hyperandrogenism) and metabolic (hyperinsulinemia, diabetes, hyperlipidemia) features but also cardiovascular complications (hypertension and cardiovascular events), psychological illness and reduced quality of life, as well as endometrial cancer. This shift has been aided by some recent longitudinal population-based studies, which have highlighted the increased prevalence of psychiatric and cardiovascular morbidity and will be discussed in detail in this chapter. In particular, the Northern Finland Birth Cohort 1966 (NFBC1966) study, which included 5889 women born in 1966 and followed so far up to the age of 46, is the largest general population-based prospective study that includes longitudinal assessment of women with PCOS from adolescence to late reproductive age.

While there have been studies that highlight the long-term impact of PCOS on women's health, there remains a dearth of evidence around the timing and nature of intervention to prevent health complications in this cohort. PCOS remains a poorly understood, neglected, yet

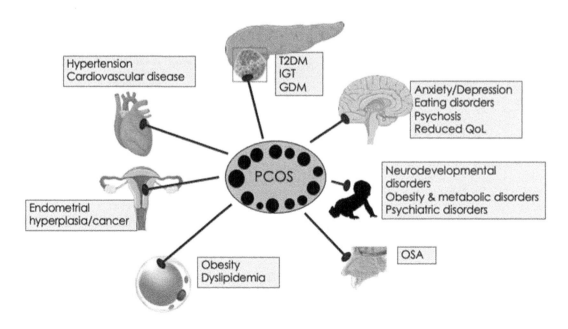

Figure 18.1 The long-term health consequences of PCOS

common condition. Many of the recommendations discussed in this chapter with respect to monitoring and intervention are based on the expert comprehensive reviews published in the 2018 international evidence-based guideline for the assessment and monitoring of women with PCOS.[4]

There are also long-term health consequences for the offspring of women with PCOS. Their children are more likely to be obese with metabolic disorders and are more likely to develop neurodevelopmental or psychiatric disorders. These issues will also be discussed.

Hyperinsulinemia, Insulin Resistance and Diabetes

Hyperinsulinemia and Insulin Resistance

Insulin resistance is a metabolic state in which physiological concentrations of insulin produce subnormal effects on glucose homeostasis and utilization,[5] so that higher than normal concentrations of circulating insulin are required to maintain normal blood glucose levels. Resistance to insulin-mediated glucose disposal leads to compensatory hyperinsulinemia. Up to 75% of lean women and 95% of overweight women with PCOS have been reported to have insulin resistance, as diagnosed by clamp studies.[6] Although these figures are likely to have been inflated by selection of the patient population for study, women with PCOS nevertheless have a greater frequency and degree of both hyperinsulinemia and insulin resistance than age- and weight-matched controls.[2, 7, 8] Hyperinsulinemia, rather than insulin resistance itself, may contribute to the mechanism of anovulation and the pathogenesis of PCOS.[9]

Insulin resistance is independently exacerbated by excess weight in women with PCOS.[8] There are also ethnic variations, with prevalence higher among certain ethnic groups, such as Southeast Asians and Indigenous Australians. Insulin resistance is involved in both the etiology and the clinical features of PCOS.[2] Hyperinsulinemia drives ovarian androgen biosynthesis and increased bioavailability of free androgens, and insulin resistance increases the prevalence and severity of metabolic, reproductive and psychological features of PCOS.[10, 11] Although insulin resistance is not in itself

a disease (and has no specific symptoms), its presence is independently associated with increased risk of cardiovascular morbidity and mortality and type 2 diabetes. Insulin resistance in PCOS is also associated with metabolic inflexibility, or inefficient energy oxidation, a marker of impaired metabolism.[12]

The clinical phenotype of PCOS influences the risk of insulin resistance. There are significant differences in insulin sensitivity between ovulatory and anovulatory women with PCOS. Anovulatory women with PCOS display insulin resistance, whereas the majority of those with a regular menstrual cycle do not.[13] Although there is impaired insulin-mediated glucose metabolism in ovarian granulosa cells, there is no resistance to the steroidogenic action of the higher than normal levels of insulin in the ovaries.[14] Insulin is known to act synergistically with luteinizing hormone (LH) in the ovary to stimulate steroidogenesis and contributes to premature arrest of the follicle development (and hence anovulation).[15]

The clinical implication of these observations is that women with PCOS are very likely to have insulin resistance and hyperinsulinemia, especially if they have irregular cycles and are obese. Insulin resistance is a risk factor for cardiovascular disease (CVD) and type 2 diabetes (T2DM), independent of obesity. Accurate assessment of insulin sensitivity requires time-consuming "clamp" studies, which are not appropriate for routine testing. However, it is not a diagnostic criterion of PCOS and its measurement is not necessary in a routine clinical setting. Insulin resistance can be inferred in obese women with PCOS and the focus should be on its clinical consequences (e.g. impaired glucose tolerance and T2DM). Moderate aerobic exercise improves insulin sensitivity in the short term in PCOS.[16] Weight loss reduces abdominal fat and insulin resistance and improves clinical features of PCOS.[17] Lifestyle interventions are therefore recommended for all with PCOS who are overweight or obese.

Impaired Glucose Tolerance and Type 2 Diabetes

Dysglycemia and type 2 diabetes (T2DM) are more prevalent among women with PCOS, independent of obesity. Meta-analyses show that women with PCOS have increased prevalence of impaired glucose tolerance (IGT) (OR 2.48; 95% CI 1.63 to 3.77) and T2DM (OR 4.43; 95% CI 4.06 to 4.82).[18] A population-based study in Denmark found that T2DM was four times more prevalent and diagnosed four years earlier among women with PCOS.[19] Women with PCOS who are obese and are of high-risk ethnic backgrounds (such as Southeast Asians) have an even higher risk of T2DM.[19]

Fasting blood glucose (together with HbA1c) or a two-hour glucose level during an oral glucose tolerance test (OGTT) are the best indicators of T2DM or IGT, and triglyceride levels, sex hormone-binding globulin (SHBG) and body mass index (BMI) are also predictors for development of T2DM.[19] After correction for age and BMI, fasting glucose, two-hour glucose and triglycerides are the most reliable predictors.[19] It is recommended by the 2018 international evidence-based guideline for the assessment and monitoring of PCOS that glycemic status should be assessed at baseline in all women with PCOS. [4] Subsequent screening for diabetes should be every one to three years, depending on the presence of other risk factors for T2DM.

Gestational Diabetes Mellitus

Gestational diabetes mellitus (GDM), similarly to T2DM, is also more prevalent among women with PCOS, independent of obesity. The risk is estimated to be five-fold that of the general population in Asia, four-fold in America and threefold in European populations. There is no current consensus about optimal screening for GDM in women with PCOS. GDM itself has a high prevalence in the general population and is associated with significant morbidity in pregnancy.[20] International guidelines recommend offering a 75 g OGTT to all women with PCOS when they are planning pregnancy or seeking fertility treatment. If an OGTT is not performed preconception, it should be offered before 20 weeks' gestation and at 24–28 weeks' gestation.[4]

Metabolic Syndrome

Metabolic syndrome in women is defined as having three or more of the following abnormalities: abdominal obesity, high triglyceride level, low HDL cholesterol level, hypertension and an elevated fasting glucose level. It is associated with a heightened risk for developing T2DM and cardiovascular morbidity and mortality. Insulin resistance also appears to play a pathogenic role in the metabolic syndrome. One study showed that the prevalence of the metabolic syndrome among women with PCOS was 43%, nearly two-fold that reported for age-matched women in the general population.[21] The increased prevalence in women with PCOS was observed in age- and BMI-matched groups. Acanthosis nigricans was more frequent in women with PCOS and metabolic syndrome. Women with PCOS and metabolic syndrome had significantly higher levels of serum free testosterone and lower levels of serum SHBG than women with PCOS without it.

Insulin Resistance, Metabolic Syndrome and Diabetes in the Offspring of Women with PCOS

The risk of diabetes and / or metabolic syndrome in the offspring of mothers with PCOS has not been extensively studied to date but the current literature points to the probability of significant transgenerational effects. It is known that maternal GDM is associated with an increased prevalence of diabetes in offspring, and GDM is more prevalent among women with PCOS. One study showed that, during adulthood, sons of women with PCOS exhibited significantly higher fasting insulin, homeostasis model assessment of insulin resistance (HOMA-IR) and two-hour insulin on OGTT and insulin sensitivity index composite significantly lower than in control sons.[22] After adjusting for BMI, two-hour insulin and insulin sensitivity index composite remained significantly different. A 2015 Australian retrospective cohort study found that offspring of PCOS mothers had increased hospitalizations, including for metabolic disorders (7.9% vs. 5.3%; HR 1.43; 95% CI 1.26 to 1.65).[23]

Obesity

The prevalence of obesity is increasing worldwide and is a major public health issue. Obesity is a known independent risk factor for the development of type 2 diabetes and cardiovascular disease. In women with obesity, cardiovascular morbidity and mortality are increased, independent of other risk factors. Obesity is more prevalent in women with PCOS compared to the general population, and the rate of weight gain is accelerated. There is a complex, incompletely understood interplay between PCOS, obesity and fat distribution. Obesity exacerbates the symptoms of PCOS, increasing insulin resistance and hyperandrogenism. However, the risk of PCOS and the severity of PCOS symptoms are not linearly related to increasing BMI.

The prevalence of obesity in women with PCOS varies depending on the population studied and the criteria used to define PCOS. In some reported series, more than 50% of women with PCOS were obese.[24] There are also temporal trends; one study showed an increase in prevalence of obesity from 51% in the 1990s to 74% in the following decades.[25] Women with PCOS also tend to have a central distribution of adiposity.[26, 27] Central obesity is associated with more severe metabolic disturbance in PCOS.[28]

Rates of weight gain also appear higher in women with PCOS. A longitudinal study demonstrated that, for each increase of 1 kg/m^2 in BMI, there is a 9% higher prevalence of PCOS.[29] Obesity and greater weight gain between the ages of 20 and 30 were associated with PCOS status at ages 27–30. The NFBC1966 study found that women with a diagnosis of PCOS by age 46 had a higher BMI at all ages compared with controls. Increase in BMI between the ages of 14 and 31, but not between 31 and 46, was greater in women with PCOS compared to controls. PCOS was associated with higher BMI at all ages. Women with PCOS in the study had a progressive increase in waist-to-hip ratio, even in the absence of weight gain, between the ages of 20–25 and 40–45 years. The observations from these two longitudinal studies highlight a time in a woman's life when she is more vulnerable to the development of PCOS. Earlier age of adiposity rebound (the second BMI rise in childhood at around the age of 6 years) is also associated with PCOS independent of BMI.[30] These studies also emphasize the importance of weight management in early life in order to potentially avoid developing PCOS or attenuating the severity of symptoms.

While it is accepted that obesity is common in PCOS, and exacerbates the symptoms and complications of the condition, it is unclear whether there are specific causal factors that contribute to increased tendency to obesity among women with PCOS or whether it is simply an association. An abnormality in energy expenditure in women

with PCOS, notably in postprandial thermogenesis, has been implicated in increased propensity to weight gain. Postprandial thermogenesis was significantly reduced in women with PCOS and there was a direct correlation of postprandial thermogenesis with insulin resistance.[31] It was calculated by Robinson and colleagues that, if the difference in energy balance demonstrated in the study was maintained long term over a year, women with PCOS would have an excess of 1.9 kg of fat.[31] Reduced postprandial energy expenditure has recently been reported in prenatally androgenized sheep, a reliable animal model of PCOS, suggesting the important role of early androgen exposure in the development of metabolic effects in PCOS.[32]

Obesity has a significant impact on clinical and biochemical manifestations in women with PCOS. Adiposity is associated with insulin resistance and hyperinsulinemia and results in reduced SHBG synthesis and excess ovarian androgen production, further worsening hyperandrogenism.[24] Visceral adiposity increases the risk of type 2 diabetes, especially in high-risk ethnic groups,[33] as well as metabolic syndrome and possibly cardiovascular disease in women with PCOS.[34–36] Obesity has an impact on the reproductive complications of PCOS. It affects ovulation, menstrual cycle regularity, time to conception, fertility and response to ovulation induction agents.[37, 38] It is also associated with a higher prevalence of pregnancy complications, including miscarriage, gestational diabetes, preeclampsia and fetal macrosomia.[25, 39, 40] Obesity also worsens the psychological comorbidities associated with PCOS, including psychological distress, anxiety, depression, low self-esteem and negative body image. Psychological health should be addressed when managing women with obesity and PCOS.[24, 39]

While obesity clearly adversely affects the symptoms and long-term consequences of PCOS, weight loss has been shown to improve symptoms and the biochemical picture. Studies have shown that interventions that reduce total body weight by as little as 5–10% improve the metabolic, reproductive and psychological features of PCOS.[17, 37, 38, 41–43] Pharmacological obesity agents and bariatric surgery (see Chapter 16) are used in women with PCOS, with some evidence of benefit. Bariatric surgery, while still experimental, has been shown to promote successful pregnancy and is considered second-line after lifestyle intervention to improve fertility outcomes in obese women (BMI ≥ 35 kg/m^2) with anovulatory PCOS.[44]

A healthy lifestyle is recommended in women with PCOS, in order to limit weight gain and maintain a healthy weight, particularly in those who are overweight or obese. The international evidence-based guideline for the assessment and management of PCOS recommends monitoring weight at each visit or at a minimum of 6 to 12 months, with frequency planned and agreed between the health professional and the individual. BMI and waist circumference should be measured, and the World Health Organization (WHO) guidelines should be used to categorize them.

Risk of Obesity in Offspring of Women with PCOS

There appears to be some transgenerational transmission of obesity and adverse metabolic features in the offspring of women with PCOS. A 2015 Australian retrospective cohort study found that offspring of PCOS mothers had an increased prevalence of metabolic syndrome, obesity and hospitalization later in life,[23] compared to offspring of age-matched non-PCOS mothers. During adulthood, sons of women with PCOS exhibited higher weight, BMI and waist circumference; however, this was not significant after adjusting for BMI.[22]

Cardiovascular Disease and Risk Factors

Cardiovascular disease (CVD) remains one of the leading causes of death in women. CVD primarily affects women in the later decades of life; however, risk factors for the development of CVD can be detected earlier in life. Women with PCOS clearly display risk factors for CVD and have a higher incidence of metabolic syndrome, a strong risk factor for CVD; however, longitudinal data recording cardiovascular events in older, well-defined cohorts with and without PCOS are lacking. Consequently, the choice of optimal screening for risk factors and indications for intervention remain unclear and controversial. Obesity and diabetes, well-defined risk factors for CVD, have already been discussed in the

chapter. Here, we discuss other CVD risk factors, as well as the existing evidence around cardiovascular events in women with PCOS.

Dyslipidemia

It is well known that lipid abnormalities are associated with risk for CVD. High-density lipoprotein cholesterol (HDL-C)[45, 46] and triglyceride levels are strong independent predictors of cardiovascular death in women and low-density lipoprotein cholesterol (LDL-C) and total cholesterol levels are poorer predictors of cardiovascular mortality.[46]

Lipid abnormalities are more common in women with PCOS than in reference populations. Studies have reported higher total cholesterol, LDL-C,[26, 47–49] very low-density lipoprotein (VLDL) cholesterol,[50, 51] triglycerides[26, 48, 51, 52] and lower HDL-C levels[26, 48, 50] among women with PCOS compared with control women. The NFBC1966 study performed nuclear magnetic resonance metabolomics on 31-year-old women and found that those with PCOS displayed more adverse metabolite profiles than controls. Four lipid fractions in different subclasses of VLDL were associated with PCOS. Those women with PCOS and large waist circumference had significantly lower HDL, Apolipoprotein A1 and albumin compared with controls. In these women with large waist circumference, testosterone levels were also significantly associated with VLDL and serum lipids.[53]

Paradoxically, a large study of young white women with PCOS found that HDL-C levels were significantly higher even among obese subjects; however, this difference was not significant after adjusting for age, BMI, insulin and other variables.[47] Nevertheless, it is possible that increased HDL-C levels could confer some protection against CVD in young women with PCOS. This same study demonstrated that the predominant lipid abnormality in young white women with PCOS was increased LDL-C levels, independent of obesity.[47] Furthermore, women with PCOS have raised concentrations of small dense LDL (LDL III) subfractions,[54] considered to be more atherogenic, and increased hepatic lipase activity compared to weight-matched control women.[51]

These lipid abnormalities in women with PCOS are independent of, but exacerbated by, excess weight.[25, 28, 39] Central obesity and insulin resistance have been shown to be associated with more severe metabolic disturbance.[28] These lipid abnormalities occur not just in later life; studies have shown that lipid abnormalities, particularly elevated triglyceride levels, in women with PCOS are apparent even at a young age, independent of obesity.[36, 55] In the NFBC1966 study, LDL, total cholesterol and triglyceride levels measured in women at the age of 31 were significantly associated with diagnosis of PCOS by age 46. Multivariate analysis showed that triglyceride levels at age 31 were significantly associated with a diagnosis of PCOS independent of obesity (OR = 1.48; 95% CI 1.08 to 2.03).[52]

Apart from obesity, individual symptoms of PCOS may predict dyslipidemia. Women with oligomenorrhea and hirsutism are more likely to have higher triglyceride levels (mean 1.17 mmol/liter; 95% CI 1 to 1.33) and lower HDL-C (mean 1.47 mmol/liter; 95% CI 1.4 to 1.55) than those with hirsutism and regular cycles (mean triglyceride levels 0.91 mmol/liter; 95% CI 0.85 to 0.96; mean HDL-C 1.62 mmol/liter; 95% CI 1.57 to 1.66), suggesting an association between oligomenorrhea and dyslipidemia in hyperandrogenemic women with PCOS.

The 2018 international guideline recommends that overweight and obese women with PCOS of any age should have a fasting lipid profile (including total cholesterol, LDL-C, HDL-C and triglyceride level) at diagnosis. Thereafter, frequency of measurement should be based on the presence of hyperlipidemia and global CVD risk.[4]

Hypertension

Hypertension is a strong independent risk factor for CVD. The NFBC1966 study examined hypertension in women with self-reported PCOS (srPCOS) based on the use of antihypertensive medication, diagnosis of hypertension set by a physician and clinically measured blood pressure.[56] This study found that the use of antihypertensive medication was significantly more common in women with PCOS compared to controls. At age 31, 3.9% of women with srPCOS reported taking antihypertensives compared to 1.9% of control women ($p = 0.022$) and, by age 46, 21.5% of women with srPCOS reported taking antihypertensives compared to 15.5% of control women ($p < 0.001$). At age 31 years, women with

PCOS had significantly higher systolic and diastolic BP than control women. At age 46 years, PCOS was significantly associated with hypertension (adjusted odds ratio (aOR) = 1.56; 95% CI 1.14 to 2.13) independent of BMI, consumption of alcohol, smoking, education and use of combined contraceptive pills.

The 2018 international evidence-based guideline for the assessment and management of PCOS recommends that all women with PCOS should have their blood pressure measured annually, or more frequently based on global CVD risk.[4]

Cardiac Echocardiographic Parameters and Autonomic Function

In the NFBC1966 hypertension study, the hypertensive women with srPCOS also displayed consistent, unfavorable echocardiographic changes at the age of 46 compared with normotensive controls. These changes included higher values for measured interventricular septal thickness at diastole, left ventricular mass index, and left atrial systolic volume, estimated left ventricular filling pressure (suggesting modest alterations in diastolic function) and mildly decreased left ventricular systolic function.

The study also examined cardiac autonomic function in these late reproductive-aged women with PCOS.[57] The authors discovered decreased vagal/parasympathetic activity, manifested as heart rate variability parameters and baroreflex sensitivity. In their multivariate regression analysis, they found that metabolic status was the strongest contributing factor. PCOS, BMI and the free androgen index did not significantly associate with heart rate variability parameters, whereas blood pressure, insulin resistance and triglycerides did.

Cardiovascular Events

The risk of cardiovascular events among women with PCOS remains unclear. Data are limited, because, as mentioned, studies to date have mainly been on small numbers of subjects, have been mostly retrospective and were conducted in younger women.

In the NFBC1966 hypertension study, the women with PCOS exhibited significantly increased cardiovascular morbidity; however, these results need to be interpreted with a degree of caution as the number of affected cases is small. The prevalence of CVD was twice as high in women aged 46 with srPCOS than in controls (6.8% vs. 3.4%), and the prevalence of myocardial infarction was significantly higher in women with PCOS (1.8% vs. 0.5%). By age 46 years, two women with PCOS, but no women in the control group, had died as a result of ischemic heart disease. These figures emphasize the need for large, longitudinal studies beyond the fifth decade of life.

Pierpoint and colleagues, however, undertook a retrospective analysis of a long-term follow-up study of 786 women diagnosed with polycystic ovary syndrome in the UK between 1930 and 1979 to test whether cardiovascular mortality was increased.[58] Hospital records were used and women were followed for an average of 30 years. Standardized mortality ratios (SMRs) were calculated to compare the death rates of women with PCOS with national rates. The SMR for all causes was 0.90 (95% CI 0.69 to 1.17). There were 15 deaths from circulatory disease, (SMR 0.83; 95% CI 0.46 to 1.37). Of these, 13 were from ischemic heart disease (SMR 1.40; 95% CI 0.75 to 2.40) and 2 were from other circulatory disease (SMR 0.23; 95% CI 0.03 to 0.85). There were 6 deaths from diabetes mellitus as underlying/contributory cause, compared with 1.7 expected (OR 3.6; 95% CI 1.5 to 8.4). The authors concluded that, despite having cardiovascular risk factors, women with PCOS do not have markedly higher than average mortality from circulatory disease.

A meta-analysis was completed for the 2018 international evidence-based guideline for the assessment and management of PCOS;[4] however, the authors comment that findings should be interpreted with caution, given the methodological and reporting limitations and small sample sizes of these observational studies, which were mostly completed in young women. The analysis found that there was no statistical difference in prevalence of myocardial infarction (3 studies, $n = 1633$), stroke (4 studies, $n = 3012$), CVD-related death (2 studies, $n = 779$) and coronary artery disease (2 studies, $n = 2152$) between women with and without PCOS. One study suggested that, when a group of women with PCOS are compared to a UK-wide population, the risk of myocardial infarction, but not angina, was increased in women with PCOS over the age of

45 years. When they compared the same women with PCOS to a local population, the risk of MI and angina was increased in women with PCOS. However, when all age groups were combined, there was no difference in risk of myocardial infarction or angina between women with and without PCOS, regardless of whether the control group were local or UK-wide. A more detailed subsequent study by the same research group showed that cardiovascular morbidity and mortality in women with PCOS were similar to those in the general population.[49] Although the history of coronary heart disease was not more common among women with PCOS, the history of cerebrovascular disease was increased. Women with PCOS had higher levels of several cardiovascular and metabolic risk factors such as diabetes, hypertension, hypercholesterolemia, hypertriglyceridemia and increased waist-to-hip ratio. After adjusting for BMI, the differences in prevalence of diabetes, family history of diabetes, hypertension and hypercholesterolemia remained significant.

Overall, it remains unclear whether PCOS is an independent risk factor for CVD. Nor is there sufficient evidence to advise on which is the most effect screening tool or methodology to assess the risk of CVD in women with PCOS. An international position statement on CVD risk assessment in PCOS recommends that assessment of CVD risk in PCOS should include screening for well-established CVD risk factors, including those already known to be important in PCOS, such as weight, BMI, waist circumference, lipid profiles, blood pressure, glucose and physical activity.[59] Management of these risk factors should be as recommended by existing guidelines for the general population.

Obstructive Sleep Apnea

Obstructive sleep apnea (OSA) is a disorder in which a person frequently stops breathing during sleep. It results from an obstruction of the upper airway during sleep that occurs because of inadequate motor tone of the tongue and/or airway dilator muscles.[60] It is associated with oxygen desaturation, sleep arousal and the resumption of ventilation, fragmenting sleep and causing daytime sleepiness. OSA prevalence in the general adult population varies between 2% and 8%.[60] In PCOS, studies demonstrate a high prevalence of OSA.[61, 62] OSA is associated with obesity but the high prevalence of OSA in PCOS is not completely explained by obesity as rates are higher when compared with matched controls.[61] Hyperandrogenism and metabolic syndrome may contribute to OSA.[63, 64]

Randomized controlled trials in the general population demonstrate benefits of treatment of OSA for symptoms, quality of life, mood and productivity with,[65] and improvement in, surrogate markers of CVD.[66] Studies of the effects of treatment of OSA in PCOS are very limited;[64] however, OSA screening is currently warranted in those with symptoms, because of the benefits of treatment that have been demonstrated in the general population.[67]

Psychological Morbidity and Quality of Life

While often the treatment of women with PCOS focuses on the reproductive and metabolic consequences, the psychological impact of the condition can remain overlooked. Several studies have found that women with PCOS have a higher prevalence of psychological distress and psychiatric disorders, as well as a lower health-related quality of life (HRQoL). The prevalence of anxiety and depression is up to eight times higher in women with PCOS compared with controls. In addition to anxiety and depression, women with PCOS also present with increased body dissatisfaction, low self-esteem [68] and disordered eating. Despite these data, and despite the fact that PCOS is common, current recommendations on screening for psychiatric symptoms do not recognize or list PCOS as a high-risk group and, consequently, their symptoms are often underrecognized.

Small studies have suggested that individual features of PCOS promote psychological distress in women, such as subfertility, obesity, metabolic disease and hyperandrogenism,[69, 70] although some studies have found an independent effect of PCOS.[71] Hirsutism either alone or in association with PCOS is associated with psychological distress.[72] The perceived lack of effective treatment is associated with a further psychological burden.[73]

Negative body image is also higher in PCOS and this negative body image predicts both depression and anxiety.[68, 74] Women with PCOS feel less physically attractive, healthy or physically fit and are less satisfied with their body size and appearance.

Depressive Symptoms and Anxiety

The prevalence of depressive symptoms and depression in women with PCOS is two- to eight times higher than in controls. This increased prevalence of depressive symptoms is independent of BMI. A meta-analysis of 10 studies from eight countries reported increased depression scores in women with PCOS compared with controls (OR 4.03; 95% CI 2.96 to 5.5; $p < 0.01$).[75] The Androgen Excess and Polycystic Ovary Syndrome Society (AE-PCOS) undertook a meta-analysis that found that the overall prevalence of abnormal depression scores was 36.6% (IQR, 22.3%, 50.0%) in the PCOS group and 14.2% (IQR, 10.7%, 22.2%) in the control group.[69] The odds of moderate and severe depressive symptoms in women with PCOS were increased compared with controls (OR 4.18; 95% CI 2.68 to 6.52) and were independent of obesity.

Most of the individual studies have been small but a large population-based study carried out in Sweden also reported a significantly increased adjusted risk of depressive disorders in women with PCOS (AOR 1.25; 95% CI 1.1.9 to 1.31).[76] Most of the individual studies have lacked a population-based approach and longitudinal follow-up but the NFBC1966 study, which has the longest follow-up data, found that women with PCOS experienced increased anxiety and/or depression symptoms up until premenopausal age.[72] They found that coexistence of anxiety and depression was more prevalent in PCOS compared with controls and that PCOS had an independent effect on psychological distress. They also found that women who were aware of their diagnosis had a higher anxiety score compared with the ones who were not aware (42.3% vs. 20%, $p = 0.032$), and a similar trend was shown in depression (38.5% vs. 21.7%, NS).

Meta-analyses of available studies have consistently reported higher anxiety scores in PCOS compared to controls. One recent meta-analysis of 10 studies showed increased moderate/severe anxiety symptoms in PCOS (OR 5.38; 95% CI 2.28 to 12.67), with a prevalence of 41.9% in PCOS, compared to 8.5% in controls.[69] The abovementioned large population-based Swedish study showed increased diagnosis of an anxiety disorder in women with PCOS matched for sex, age and country of birth (OR 1.37; 95% CI 1.32 to 1.43).[76]

Overall, these studies indicate increased anxiety and depressive symptoms and disorders in women with PCOS, across varied ethnic groups. Therefore, it is recommended, in the AE-PCOS Society position statement on depression, anxiety, quality of life, and eating disorders in PCOS that women with PCOS "should be routinely screened for depressive symptoms at the time of diagnosis, using simple screening tools validated in the region of practice. If the screening test is positive, practitioners should further assess, refer appropriately, or offer treatment."[77]

Health-Related Quality of Life and Life Satisfaction

The NFBC1966 study is also the largest longitudinal study thus far of HRQoL in women with PCOS. They found that women with PCOS or hirsutism have a lower HRQoL than controls at ages 31 and 46.[78] This low HRQoL in PCOS was significant even after adjusting for BMI, hyperandrogenism and socioeconomic status. Mental distress was found to be the strongest contributing factor to HRQoL. Moreover, women with PCOS were more likely to report decreased life satisfaction and four times more likely to report poor health status at ages 31 and 46 compared to women without PCOS symptoms. The reduction in HrQoL was similar to that of women with other chronic health conditions such as asthma, depression and rheumatoid arthritis that are well recognized to be associated with reduced QoL.

Psychosis

The NFBC1966 study has also examined the incidence of psychosis in women with PCOS (unpublished data). They showed an increased hazard ratio for any psychosis up to the age of 50 of 2.99 (95% CI 1.52 to 5.82), even after adjustment for parental history of psychosis. The risk for schizophrenia was not increased. They used scales of psychopathology as a measure of psychological disturbance, which were higher in PCOS than in controls. BMI, socioeconomic status, isolated hyperandrogenism and oligo/amenorrhoea were not individually associated with an increased risk of psychosis.

Eating Disorders and Disordered Eating

There is a lack of good evidence regarding the prevalence of eating disorders and disordered eating in women with PCOS.[77] Available data suggest that the prevalence of any eating disorder is higher in PCOS than in the general community (21% vs. 4%).[79] A large population-based Swedish study of women with PCOS (n = 24385) and matched controls reported increased bulimia nervosa but not anorexia nervosa.[76] Risk factors for disordered eating are more prevalent in women with PCOS, including obesity, depression, anxiety, low self-esteem and poor body image.[71, 80]

Many women with eating disorders are undiagnosed and unaware that they have an eating disorder. The National Institute for Health and Care Excellence (NICE) guidance for eating disorders suggests considering an eating disorder in individuals with a range of symptoms relevant to PCOS. The 2018 international evidence-based guideline for the assessment and management of polycystic ovary syndrome states that increased awareness of these conditions, and effective assessment when clinically suspected, is important. Increasing recognition and management of eating disorders and disordered eating are important in improving the psychological functioning and overall quality of life in women with PCOS and reducing the associated health risks.[4]

Psychosexual Dysfunction

Psychosexual dysfunction refers to sexual problems or difficulties that have a psychological origin such as depression, low self-esteem and negative body image. The prevalence of psychosexual dysfunction varies from 13.3% to 62.5% in PCOS;[81, 82] and, while studies are limited in this area, prevalence appears to be greater than the general population,[83–85] although some studies suggest it is not.[86] Sexual satisfaction, arousal, lubrication and orgasm appear to be impaired in PCOS, and sexual self-worth is lower.[87] PCOS symptoms such as hirsutism, infertility and obesity are likely to impact on feelings of sexuality and feelings of being unattractive.[85, 88] Therapies such as the combined oral contraceptive pill can also affect psychosexual function, although data pertaining to this in women with PCOS are limited.

Mental Health Disorders in Offspring of Women with PCOS

Researchers in Karolinska Institutet, Sweden, carried out a population-based cohort study in Finland including all live births between 1996 and 2014. They examined a wide range of neuropsychiatric disorders in offspring exposed to maternal PCOS.[89] They compared data from 24682 (2.2%) children born to Finnish mothers with PCOS or anovulatory infertility with 1073071 children born to mothers without PCOS. A total of 105409 (9.8%) children were diagnosed with a neurodevelopmental or psychiatric disorder during the follow-up period. Children born to mothers who had PCOS had an increased risk of neurodevelopmental and psychiatric disorders. This included a number of psychiatric diagnoses, including mood, anxiety, eating and sleeping disorders, intellectual disabilities, specific developmental, autism spectrum disorders, attention-deficit/hyperactivity disorder, conduct and tic disorders, as well as other behavioral and emotional disorders. The risk was increased independent of the babies' gender and maternal obesity.

The observational nature of the study shows only an association between maternal PCOS and psychiatric and neurodevelopment problems and does not prove causality. Other familial factors may affect the association between PCOS in mothers and problems in offspring, for example there was no information about weight gain in pregnancy. In addition, the prevalence of PCOS in the Finnish registries was lower than that reported in other studies and therefore may have captured only the most severe cases.

Endometrial Cancer

An association between PCOS and endometrial carcinoma was first suggested in 1949, 14 years after the original description of the syndrome.[90] Since then, several studies have been published that support this association. Women with PCOS have been thought to be at increased risk for endometrial cancer through chronic anovulation with unopposed estrogen exposure to the endometrium. However, the risk of developing endometrial cancer is likely a complex interplay between estrogen exposure, obesity, nulliparity and infertility.[91] Overall, the risk to women with PCOS appears to be two to six times that of the general population.[92] However, the evidence for such an association in epidemiological studies is incomplete and inconsistent,[93] either because sample sizes were too small or because there was no measure of relative risk compared to the general population. In addition the meta-analyses that report increased risk of endometrial cancer in PCOS all include estimates from analyses that did not take BMI into account.[94, 95]

Women with anovulatory infertility are at risk of developing endometrial hyperplasia, which can be atypical and therefore premalignant.[91, 96] However, in one of these studies, the risk for endometrial carcinoma was increased only among the obese subgroup of anovulatory women.[96] Not all women with chronic anovulation have PCOS, and not all women with PCOS have anovulation, so these data cannot be directly applied to all women with PCOS.

Obese women in the general population are at increased risk of endometrial cancer compared to normal weight women, and hypertension and relative hyperglycemia were found to be significant markers of risk.[97, 98] Women with diabetes mellitus have also been shown to be at increased risk for endometrial cancer.[98] Therefore, the apparent association between PCOS and endometrial carcinoma may be related to metabolic abnormalities arising as a result of the syndrome.

There are no prospective studies demonstrating increased risk for endometrial carcinoma among women with PCOS. It is also unclear whether the mortality from endometrial cancer among women with PCOS is increased. It has been suggested that metformin may have a role in prevention or treatment of endometrial cancer, particularly in obese women. However, the conclusion from recent meta-analyses of available studies is that there is not yet any clear evidence of a beneficial effect.[99, 100] A small non-significant increased risk of endometrial cancer has been shown with clomiphene,[101] and letrozole has not been studied in this context. Oral contraceptives reduce risk for endometrial cancer in the general population.

Owing to limited data, universal screening or preventative strategies for these women cannot be applied at present, although endometrial surveillance by transvaginal ultrasound or endometrial biopsy is recommended for women with PCOS who have thickened endometrium, prolonged amenorrhea, unopposed estrogen exposure or abnormal vaginal bleeding, based on clinical suspicion.[4] A pragmatic approach taken by clinicians and recommended by international guidelines is to induce a withdrawal bleed with a progestogen at least every three months among women with PCOS with infrequent cycles.[4]

Summary

Polycystic ovary syndrome is a common, chronic multisystem disorder associated with long-term health consequences. Women with PCOS are at risk of metabolic, cardiovascular and psychological morbidities as well as cancer. While there have been several comprehensive longitudinal studies identifying these long-term consequences, there are, thus far, few long-term interventional studies that evaluate the treatment of these comorbidities in women with PCOS. It is important to recognize and monitor these conditions, along with pragmatic approaches to treatment based on available evidence in PCOS and evidence from the general population. International guidelines highlight the importance of diagnosis and surveillance of these comorbidities, as well as providing sensible approaches to treatment, based on both evidence (where it exists) and expert opinion (where there is little or no conclusive evidence).[4]

Women with PCOS are therefore at significantly increased risk of developing prediabetes, type 2 diabetes and GDM during their lifetime compared to the general population. The risk of developing T2DM is estimated to be four times higher than controls and the risk is not dependent on obesity.[5, 18, 19, 58, 102, 103] Women with PCOS are predisposed to obesity. In some series, more than 50% of women with PCOS were obese,[24] with central adiposity,[26, 27] and higher rates of weight gain throughout adulthood. Obesity has a significant clinical impact on women with PCOS, worsening hyperandrogenism[24] and affecting fertility[37, 38] and pregnancy.[25, 39, 40] Obesity worsens the psychological comorbidities associated with PCOS.[24, 39] Thus weight management in early life is important in order to potentially avoid developing PCOS or attenuating the severity of symptoms. Studies have shown that interventions that reduce body weight by as little as 5–10% improve the metabolic, reproductive and psychological features of PCOS.[17, 37, 38, 41–43]

Hypertension is more prevalent in women with PCOS.[56] Women with PCOS should have their blood pressure measured annually, or more frequently in the presence of other cardiovascular risk factors.[4] Lipid abnormalities are more common in women with PCOS than in the general population, even at a young age.[36, 55] Studies have reported higher total cholesterol, LDL-C,[26, 47–49] VLDL-cholesterol,[50, 51] triglycerides [26, 48, 51, 52] and lower HDL-C levels.[26, 48, 50, 104] These lipid abnormalities in women with PCOS are independent of, but exacerbated by, excess weight.[25, 28, 39] Overweight or obese women with PCOS should have a fasting lipid profile at diagnosis. Thereafter, frequency of measurement should be based on the presence of hyperlipidemia and cardiovascular risk.[4]

Women with PCOS clearly display risk factors for CVD and have a higher incidence of insulin resistance, obesity and metabolic syndrome, all independently associated with CVD; however, longitudinal data of cardiovascular events are lacking. The limited longitudinal studies to date have shown conflicting results, with some showing that women with PCOS have no increased mortality from CVD,[58] whereas others show an increased risk of myocardial infarction[56] and cerebrovascular disease.[49] Assessment and management of CV risk factors are recommended for women with PCOS. Studies have shown an increased prevalence of OSA in women with PCOS, independent of obesity.[61, 62] Studies of treatment of OSA in PCOS are very limited.[64]

In addition to the physical complications of PCOS, it also has psychological complications. Several studies have found that women with PCOS have a higher prevalence of psychological distress and psychiatric disorders, as well as a lower HRQoL. Women with PCOS have a higher prevalence of anxiety and depression, as well as negative body image and low self-esteem.[72] The incidence of psychosis is also higher in women with PCOS. Eating disorders appear to be more prevalent in PCOS,[79] especially among obese women with psychological issues. Psychosexual dysfunction, although, again, poorly studied, appears to be more common in women with PCOS than in the general population, including difficulties with sexual self-worth and satisfaction.[83, 87]

Women with PCOS have been thought to be at increased risk for endometrial cancer through a complex interplay between estrogen exposure, obesity, nulliparity and infertility.[91] A pragmatic approach to prevent this is to induce a withdrawal bleed at least every three months among women with PCOS with infrequent cycles.[4]

PCOS also appears to affect the next generation. A large population-based cohort study in Finland found that children born to mothers who had PCOS had an increased risk of neurodevelopmental and psychiatric disorders.[89] These included mood, anxiety, eating and sleeping disorders, intellectual disabilities, autism spectrum disorders, attention-deficit/hyperactivity disorder and other behavioral disorders. A study showed that, during adulthood, sons of women with PCOS exhibited significantly higher insulin resistance and hyperinsulinemia, as well as higher BMI and waist circumference; however, this was not significant after adjusting for BMI.[22] Another study found that offspring of PCOS mothers had an increased prevalence of metabolic syndrome, obesity and hospitalization later in life compared to offspring of age-matched mothers.[23]

Longitudinal studies have highlighted the long-term health consequences of PCOS, although data with regards to certain complications are lacking. Future studies are essential to target and determine the timing, nature and impact of medical interventions to reduce the effect of these health consequences on the lives of women with PCOS.

In conclusion, PCOS is a complex endocrine disorder with comorbidities and long-term health implications. It is associated with an increased prevalence of abnormal glucose tolerance, including IGT, T2DM and GDM, as well as psychological sequalae, including anxiety, depression, disordered eating, psychotic disorders and reduced quality of life. Other long-term consequences associated with PCOS include obesity, hypertension, dyslipidemia and possible CVD, as well as endometrial cancer and OSA. Offspring of mothers with PCOS are predisposed to neurodevelopmental and psychiatric disorders, obesity and metabolic disease. (Some of the individual images have been obtained, and amended, from Servier Art: https://smart.servier.com)

References

1 Azziz, R. et al., Positions statement: Criteria for defining polycystic ovary syndrome as a predominantly hyperandrogenic syndrome: an Androgen Excess Society guideline. *J Clin Endocrinol Metab* 2006; 91(11): 4237–4245.

2 Diamanti-Kandarakis, E. and Dunaif, A. Insulin resistance and the polycystic ovary syndrome revisited: an update on mechanisms and implications. *Endocr Rev* 2012; 33(6): 981–1030.

3 March, W. A., et al., The prevalence of polycystic ovary syndrome in a community sample assessed under contrasting diagnostic criteria. *Hum Reprod* 2010; 25(2): 544–551.

4 Teede, H. J., et al., Recommendations from the international evidence-based guideline for the assessment and management of polycystic ovary syndrome. *Hum Reprod* 2018; 33(9): 1602–1618.

5 Reaven, G. M., Banting Lecture 1988:. Role of insulin resistance in human disease. *Diabetes*, 1988; 37(12): 1595–1607.

6 Stepto, N. K., et al., Women with polycystic ovary syndrome have intrinsic insulin resistance on euglycaemic-hyperinsulaemic clamp. *Hum Reprod* 2013; 28(3): 777–784.

7 Robinson, S., et al., Postprandial thermogenesis is reduced in polycystic ovary syndrome and is associated with increased insulin resistance. *Clin Endocrinol (Oxf)* 1992; 36(6): 537–543.

8 Cassar, S., et al., Insulin resistance in polycystic ovary syndrome: A systematic review and meta-analysis of euglycaemic-hyperinsulinaemic clamp studies. *Hum Reprod* 2016; 31(11): 2619–2631.

9 Abbott, D. H., Dumesic, D. A. and Franks, S. Developmental origin of polycystic ovary syndrome: A hypothesis. *J Endocrinol* 2002; 174(1): 1–5.

10 Diamanti-Kandarakis, E. and Papavassiliou, A. G. Molecular mechanisms of insulin resistance in polycystic ovary syndrome. *Trends Mol Med* 2006; 12(7): 324–332.

11 Teede, H. J., et al., Insulin resistance, the metabolic syndrome, diabetes, and cardiovascular disease risk in women with PCOS. *Endocrine* 2006; 30(1): 45–53.

12 Rimmer, M., et al., Metabolic inflexibility in women with polycystic ovary syndrome: A systematic review. *Gynecol Endocrinol* 2020; 36(6): 501–507.

13 Robinson, S., et al., The relationship of insulin insensitivity to menstrual pattern in women with hyperandrogenism and polycystic ovaries. *Clin Endocrinol (Oxf)*, 1993; 39(3): 351–355.

14 Rice, S., et al., Impaired insulin-dependent glucose metabolism in granulosa-lutein cells from anovulatory women with polycystic ovaries. *Hum Reprod* 2005; 20(2): 373–381.

15 Willis, D., et al., Modulation by insulin of follicle-stimulating hormone and luteinizing

hormone actions in human granulosa cells of normal and polycystic ovaries. *J Clin Endocrinol Metab* 1996; 81(1): 302–309.

16 Richter, E. A., et al., Effect of exercise on insulin action in human skeletal muscle. *J Appl Physiol* 1989; 66(2): 876–885.

17 Holte, J., et al., Restored insulin sensitivity but persistently increased early insulin secretion after weight loss in obese women with polycystic ovary syndrome. *J Clin Endocrinol Metab* 1995; 80(9): 2586–2593.

18 Moran, L. J., et al., Impaired glucose tolerance, type 2 diabetes and metabolic syndrome in polycystic ovary syndrome: A systematic review and meta-analysis. *Hum Reprod Update* 2010; 16(4): 347–363.

19 Rubin, K. H., et al., Development and risk factors of type 2 diabetes in a nationwide population of women with polycystic ovary syndrome. *J Clin Endocrinol Metab* 2017; 102(10): 3848–3857.

20 Bodmer-Roy, S., et al., Pregnancy outcomes in women with and without gestational diabetes mellitus according to the International Association of the Diabetes and Pregnancy Study Groups criteria. *Obstet Gynecol* 2012; 120(4): 746–752.

21 Apridonidze, T., et al., Prevalence and characteristics of the metabolic syndrome in women with polycystic ovary syndrome. *J Clin Endocrinol Metab* 2005; 90(4): 1929–1935.

22 Recabarren, S .E., et al., Metabolic profile in sons of women with polycystic ovary syndrome. *J Clin Endocrinol Metab* 2008; 93(5): 1820–1826.

23 Doherty, D. A., et al., Implications of polycystic ovary syndrome for pregnancy and for the health of offspring. *Obstet Gynecol* 2015; 125(6): 1397–1406.

24 Gambineri, A., et al., Obesity and the polycystic ovary syndrome. *Int J Obes Relat Metab Disord* 2002; 26(7): 883–896.

25 Yildiz, B. O., Knochenhauer, E. S. and Azziz, R. Impact of obesity on the risk for polycystic ovary syndrome. *J Clin Endocrinol Metab* 2008; 93(1): 162–168.

26 Talbott, E., et al., Coronary heart disease risk factors in women with polycystic ovary syndrome. *Arterioscler Thromb Vasc Biol* 1995; 15(7): 821–826.

27 Taponen, S., et al., Hormonal profile of women with self-reported symptoms of oligomenorrhea and/or hirsutism: Northern Finland birth cohort 1966 study. *J Clin Endocrinol Metab* 2003; 88(1): 141–147.

28 Pasquali, R., Obesity and androgens: Facts and perspectives. *Fertil Steril* 2006; 85(5): 1319–1340.

29 Teede, H. J., et al., Longitudinal weight gain in women identified with polycystic ovary syndrome: Results of an observational study in young women. *Obesity (Silver Spring)*, 2013; 21(8): 1526–1532.

30 Koivuaho, E., et al., Age at adiposity rebound in childhood is associated with PCOS diagnosis and obesity in adulthood-longitudinal analysis of BMI data from birth to age 46 in cases of PCOS. *Int J Obes (Lond)* 2019; 43(7): 1370–1379.

31 Robinson S, Chan SP, Spacey S, Anyaoku V, Johnston DG, Franks S. Postprandial thermogenesis is reduced in polycystic ovary syndrome and is associated with increased insulin resistance. *Clin Endocrinol (Oxf)*. 1992 Jun;36(6):537–43.

32 Siemienowicz, K., et al., Insights into manipulating postprandial energy expenditure to manage weight gain in polycystic ovary syndrome. *iScience* 2020; 23(6): 101164.

33 Diamanti-Kandarakis, E., Role of obesity and adiposity in polycystic ovary syndrome. *Int J Obes (Lond)* 2007; 31 (Suppl 2): S8–13.

34 Dunaif, A., et al., Defects in insulin receptor signaling in vivo in the polycystic ovary syndrome (PCOS). *Am J Physiol Endocrinol Metab* 2001; 281 (2): E392–E399.

35 Hudecova, M., et al., Prevalence of the metabolic syndrome in women with a previous diagnosis of polycystic ovary syndrome: Long-term follow-up. *Fertil Steril* 2011; 96(5): 1271–1274.

36 Schmidt, J., et al., Cardiovascular disease and risk factors in PCOS women of postmenopausal age: A 21-year controlled follow-up study. *J Clin Endocrinol Metab* 2011; 96(12): 3794–3803.

37 Clark, A. M., et al., Weight loss in obese infertile women results in improvement in reproductive outcome for all forms of fertility treatment. *Hum Reprod* 1998; 13(6): 1502–1505.

38 Clark, A. M., et al., Weight loss results in significant improvement in pregnancy and ovulation rates in anovulatory obese women. *Hum Reprod* 1995; 10 (10): 2705–2712.

39 Lim, S. S., et al., The effect of obesity on polycystic ovary syndrome: A systematic review and meta-analysis. *Obes Rev*, 2013 14(2): 95–109.

40 Legro, R. S., Obesity and PCOS: Implications for diagnosis and treatment. *Semin Reprod Med* 2012; 30(6): 496–506.

41 Moran, L. J., et al., Dietary composition in restoring reproductive and metabolic physiology in overweight women with polycystic ovary syndrome. *J Clin Endocrinol Metab* 2003; 88(2): 812–819.

42 Crosignani,G., et al., Overweight and obese anovulatory patients with polycystic ovaries:

Parallel improvements in anthropometric indices, ovarian physiology and fertility rate induced by diet. *Hum Reprod* 2003; 18(9): 1928–1932.

43 Jakubowicz, D. J. and Nestler, J. E. 17 alpha-Hydroxyprogesterone responses to leuprolide and serum androgens in obese women with and without polycystic ovary syndrome offer dietary weight loss. *J Clin Endocrinol Metab* 1997; 82(2): 556–560.

44 Benito, E., et al., Fertility and pregnancy outcomes in women with polycystic ovary syndrome following bariatric surgery. *J Clin Endocrinol Metab* 2020; 105(9): 1–8.

45 Wilson, W., Abbott, R. D. and Castelli, W. P. High density lipoprotein cholesterol and mortality: The Framingham Heart Study. *Arteriosclerosis* 1988; 8 (6): 737–741.

46 Bass, K. M., et al., Plasma lipoprotein levels as predictors of cardiovascular death in women. *Arch Intern Med* 1993; 153(19): 2209–2216.

47 Legro, R. S., Kunselman, A. R. and Dunaif, A. Prevalence and predictors of dyslipidemia in women with polycystic ovary syndrome. *Am J Med* 2001; 111(8): 607–613.

48 Talbott, E., et al., Adverse lipid and coronary heart disease risk profiles in young women with polycystic ovary syndrome: Results of a case-control study. *J Clin Epidemiol* 1998; 51(5): 415–422.

49 Wild, S., et al., Cardiovascular disease in women with polycystic ovary syndrome at long-term follow-up: A retrospective cohort study. *Clin Endocrinol (Oxf)* 2000; 52(5): 595–600.

50 Wild, R. A., et al., Lipoprotein lipid concentrations and cardiovascular risk in women with polycystic ovary syndrome. *J Clin Endocrinol Metab* 1985; 61 (5): 946–951.

51 Pirwany, I. R., et al., Lipids and lipoprotein subfractions in women with PCOS: Relationship to metabolic and endocrine parameters. *Clin Endocrinol (Oxf)* 2001; 54(4): 447–453.

52 Ollila, M. M., et al., Weight gain and dyslipidemia in early adulthood associate with polycystic ovary syndrome: Prospective cohort study. *J Clin Endocrinol Metab* 2016; 101(2): 739–747.

53 Couto Alves, A., et al., Metabolic profiling of polycystic ovary syndrome reveals interactions with abdominal obesity. *Int J Obes (Lond)* 2017; 41 (9): 1331–1340.

54 Clements, M. K., et al., FMRFamide-related neuropeptides are agonists of the orphan G-protein-coupled receptor GPR54. *Biochem Biophys Res Commun* 2001; 284(5): 1189–1193.

55 Diamanti-Kandarakis, E., et al., Pathophysiology and types of dyslipidemia in PCOS. *Trends Endocrinol Metab* 2007; 18(7): 280–285.

56 Ollila, M. E., et al., Self-reported polycystic ovary syndrome is associated with hypertension: A Northern Finland birth cohort 1966 study. *J Clin Endocrinol Metab* 2019; 104(4): 1221–1231.

57 Ollila, M. M., et al., Effect of polycystic ovary syndrome on cardiac autonomic function at a late fertile age: A prospective Northern Finland Birth Cohort 1966 study. *BMJ Open* 2019; 9(12): e033780.

58 Pierpoint, T., et al., Mortality of women with polycystic ovary syndrome at long-term follow-up. *J Clin Epidemiol* 1998; 51(7): 581–586.

59 Wild, R. A., et al., Assessment of cardiovascular risk and prevention of cardiovascular disease in women with the polycystic ovary syndrome: A consensus statement by the Androgen Excess and Polycystic Ovary Syndrome (AE-PCOS) Society. *J Clin Endocrinol Metab* 2010; 95(5): 2038–2049.

60 Park, J. G., K. Ramar, and E. J. Olson, Updates on definition, consequences, and management of obstructive sleep apnea. *Mayo Clin Proc* 2011; 86 (6): 549–554.

61 Fogel, R. B., et al., Increased prevalence of obstructive sleep apnea syndrome in obese women with polycystic ovary syndrome. *J Clin Endocrinol Metab* 2001; 86(3): 1175–1180.

62 Vgontzas, A. N., et al., Polycystic ovary syndrome is associated with obstructive sleep apnea and daytime sleepiness: Role of insulin resistance. *J Clin Endocrinol Metab* 2001; 86(2): 517–520.

63 Andersen, M. L. and Tufik, S. The effects of testosterone on sleep and sleep-disordered breathing in men: Its bidirectional interaction with erectile function. *Sleep Med Rev* 2008; 12(5): 365–379.

64 Tasali, E., et al., Treatment of obstructive sleep apnea improves cardiometabolic function in young obese women with polycystic ovary syndrome. *J Clin Endocrinol Metab* 2011; 96(2): 365–374.

65 McEvoy, R. D., et al., CPAP for prevention of cardiovascular events in obstructive sleep apnea. *N Engl J Med* 2016; 375(10): 919–931.

66 Hu, X., et al., The role of continuous positive airway pressure in blood pressure control for patients with obstructive sleep apnea and hypertension: A meta-analysis of randomized controlled trials. *J Clin Hypertens (Greenwich)* 2015; 17(3): 215–222.

67 Jonas, D. E., et al., Screening for obstructive sleep apnea in adults: Evidence report and systematic

review for the US Preventive Services Task Force. *JAMA* 2017; 317(4): 415–433.

68 Himelen M. J. and Thatcher, S. S. Depression and body image among women with polycystic ovary syndrome. *J Health Psychol* 2006; 11(4): 613–615.

69 Cooney, L. G., et al., High prevalence of moderate and severe depressive and anxiety symptoms in polycystic ovary syndrome: A systematic review and meta-analysis. *Hum Reprod* 2017; 32(5): 1075–1091.

70 Shi, X., et al., Co-involvement of psychological and neurological abnormalities in infertility with polycystic ovarian syndrome. *Arch Gynecol Obstet* 2011; 284(3): 773–778.

71 Hollinrake, E., et al., Increased risk of depressive disorders in women with polycystic ovary syndrome. *Fertil Steril* 2007; 87(6): 1369–1376.

72 Karjula, S., et al., Psychological distress is more prevalent in fertile age and premenopausal women with PCOS symptoms: 15-Year follow-up. *J Clin Endocrinol Metab* 2017; 102(6): 1861–1869.

73 Drosdzol, A., Skrzypulec, V. and Plinta, R. Quality of life, mental health and self-esteem in hirsute adolescent females. *J Psychosom Obstet Gynaecol* 2010; 31(3): 168–175.

74 Bazarganipour, F., et al., Body image satisfaction and self-esteem status among the patients with polycystic ovary syndrome. *Iran J Reprod Med* 2013; 11(10): 829–836.

75 Dokras, A., et al., Increased prevalence of anxiety symptoms in women with polycystic ovary syndrome: Systematic review and meta-analysis. *Fertil Steril* 2012; 97(1): 225–30.e2.

76 Cesta, C. E., et al., Polycystic ovary syndrome and psychiatric disorders: Co-morbidity and heritability in a nationwide Swedish cohort. *Psychoneuroendocrinology* 2016; 73: 196–203.

77 Dokras, A., et al., Androgen Excess- Polycystic Ovary Syndrome Society: Position statement on depression, anxiety, quality of life, and eating disorders in polycystic ovary syndrome. *Fertil Steril* 2018; 109(5): 888–899.

78 Karjula, S., et al., Population-based data at ages 31 and 46 show decreased HRQoL and life satisfaction in women with PCOS symptoms. *J Clin Endocrinol Metab* 2020; 105(6).

79 Månsson, M., et al., Women with polycystic ovary syndrome are often depressed or anxious: A case control study. *Psychoneuroendocrinology* 2008; 33 (8): 1132–1138.

80 Karacan, E., et al., Body satisfaction and eating attitudes among girls and young women with and without polycystic ovary syndrome. *J Pediatr Adolesc Gynecol* 2014; 27(2): 72–77.

81 Dashti, S., et al., Sexual dysfunction in patients with polycystic ovary syndrome in Malaysia. *Asian Pac J Cancer Prev* 2016; 17(8): 3747–3751.

82 Eftekhar, T., et al., Sexual dysfunction in patients with polycystic ovary syndrome and its affected domains. *Iran J Reprod Med* 2014; 12(8): 539–546.

83 Pastoor, H., et al., Sexual function in women with polycystic ovary syndrome: A systematic review and meta-analysis. *Reprod Biomed Online* 2018; 37 (6): 750–760.

84 Janssen, O. E., et al., Mood and sexual function in polycystic ovary syndrome. *Semin Reprod Med* 2008; 26(1): 45–52.

85 Elsenbruch, S., et al., Quality of life, psychosocial well-being, and sexual satisfaction in women with polycystic ovary syndrome. *J Clin Endocrinol Metab* 2003; 88(12): 5801–5807.

86 Ercan, C.M., et al., Sexual dysfunction assessment and hormonal correlations in patients with polycystic ovary syndrome. *Int J Impot Res* 2013; 25 (4): 127–132.

87 Drosdzol, A., et al., Quality of life and marital sexual satisfaction in women with polycystic ovary syndrome. *Folia Histochem Cytobiol* 2007; 45 (Suppl 1): S93–S97.

88 Hahn, S., et al., Clinical and psychological correlates of quality-of-life in polycystic ovary syndrome. *Eur J Endocrinol* 2005; 153(6): 853–860.

89 Chen, X., et al., Association of polycystic ovary syndrome or anovulatory infertility with offspring psychiatric and mild neurodevelopmental disorders: A Finnish population-based cohort study. *Hum Reprod* 2020; 35(10): 2336–2347.

90 Speert, H., Carcinoma of the endometrium in young women. *Surg Gynaecol Obstet* 1949; 88(3): 332–336.

91 Dahlgren, E., et al., Endometrial carcinoma; ovarian dysfunction: A risk factor in young women. *Eur J Obstet Gynecol Reprod Biol* 1991; 41 (2): 143–150.

92 Charalampakis, V., et al., Polycystic ovary syndrome and endometrial hyperplasia: An overview of the role of bariatric surgery in female fertility. *Eur J Obstet Gynecol Reprod Biol* 2016; 207: 220–226.

93 Hardiman, P. Pillay, O. C., and Atiomo, W. Polycystic ovary syndrome and endometrial carcinoma. *Lancet*, 2003; 361(9371): 1810–1812.

94 Chittenden, B. G., et al., Polycystic ovary syndrome and the risk of gynaecological cancer: A systematic review. *Reprod Biomed Online* 2009; 19(3): 398–405.

95 Barry, J. A., Azizia, M. M. and Hardiman, J. Risk of endometrial, ovarian and breast cancer in women

with polycystic ovary syndrome: A systematic review and meta-analysis. *Hum Reprod Update* 2014; 20(5): 748–758.

96 Coulam, C. B., Annegers, J. F. and Kranz, J. S. Chronic anovulation syndrome and associated neoplasia. *Obstet Gynecol* 1983; 61(4): 403–407.

97 Furberg, A. S. and Thune, I. Metabolic abnormalities (hypertension, hyperglycemia and overweight), lifestyle (high energy intake and physical inactivity) and endometrial cancer risk in a Norwegian cohort. *Int J Cancer* 2003; 104(6): 669–676.

98 Weiderpass, E., et al., Body size in different periods of life, diabetes mellitus, hypertension, and risk of postmenopausal endometrial cancer (Sweden). *Cancer Causes Control* 2000; 11(2): 185–192.

99 Harris, H. R. and Terry, K. L. Polycystic ovary syndrome and risk of endometrial, ovarian, and breast cancer: A systematic review. *Fertil Res Pract* 2016; 2: 14.

100 Chu, D., et al., Effect of metformin use on the risk and prognosis of endometrial cancer: A systematic review and meta-analysis. *BMC Cancer* 2018; 18(1): 438.

101 Brinton, L. A., et al., Fertility drugs and endometrial cancer risk: Results from an extended follow-up of a large infertility cohort. *Hum Reprod* 2013. 28(10): 2813–2821.

102 Azziz, R., et al., Polycystic ovary syndrome. *Nat Rev Dis Primers* 2016; 2: 16057.

103 Teede, H., A. Deeks, and L. Moran, Polycystic ovary syndrome: A complex condition with psychological, reproductive and metabolic manifestations that impacts on health across the lifespan. *BMC Med* 2010; 8: 41.

104 Cortón, M., et al., Differential gene expression profile in omental adipose tissue in women with polycystic ovary syndrome. *J Clin Endocrinol Metab* 2007; 92(1): 328–337.

Polycystic Ovary Syndrome
The Patient's Perspective

Chapter 19

Sabra Lane

As a young journalist I was told "You should never be the story." However, in this case, I think my story is a good example of what some PCOS women endure throughout their lives.

Imagine being told as a 16-year-old teenage girl "You'll never have children." It was shocking. I also clearly remember being told "You have polycystic ovary syndrome" and being utterly confused about what it was, as I'd never heard of it before. Mum says I cried for about 24 hours. Then I boldly declared, "If I can't have children, I'll have a career instead." I don't remember saying that at all, but Mum says I did. I do remember signing paperwork, acknowledging the risks of taking anti-androgen medication. This medication was rarely prescribed then, and I was told there were only about 75 women in Australia at the time who had been diagnosed with the condition.

The diagnosis had been a long time coming. At age 15, I'd visited the family doctor with some puzzling symptoms. I'd only experienced menstruation twice during my life, with a long 18-month gap in between. I was also particularly hairy. It was sprouting everywhere it shouldn't be for a young woman; it was a mortifying thing for a teenager. That first family doctor told me I was worrying too much about things that didn't really matter, that young girls and women shouldn't worry about things "they'd grow out of." Really? Thick, dark hair on my arms, legs, and my face. I had begged my parents to allow me to shave my legs, because I was so embarrassed. An elderly aunt had asked my Mum, "What are you going to do about her mustache?" Thank goodness for that intervention; it eventually led to me being allowed to see a beautician for waxing and electrolysis. During my 30s, a twin combination of anti-androgen medication and intense pulsed light treatment delivered huge relief in reducing my hair growth.

Let us jump back, however, to that very first diagnosis, which essentially was "nothing to see here." My mum wasn't convinced, and we sought a second opinion from a female GP. This doctor had an inkling that my condition might be the very thing she'd just read about in her regular medical journal. The doctor kept her suspicion about PCOS to herself and referred me to a specialist in a capital city, more than 500 kilometers from my hometown; and he was the one who delivered the dreaded declaration about "no children." He advised it was congenital and hopefully the prescribed drugs, including the Pill, would regulate my period and would lead to less hair growth.

Weight wasn't an issue then, but it became a big one by the age of 21. I went from a size 10 to 18 within 6 months. I'd moved to a capital city by then and was seeing a new endocrinologist who welcomed my rapid weight gain with the greeting, "My, how matronly we've become."

I think I've tried every diet and exercise known to womankind. It's only in the past two years (I'm now 53) that I have found the 5:2 "Fast Diet" has helped me lose kilos. Combined with my passion for hiking in the great outdoors, these two things have finally helped keep my weight in check. It is a daily dilemma deciding what to eat and drink. If I lust after cake, I know I'll have to make sure I walk it off over an entire week.

Exercise has been part of my life and I know my symptoms are improved when I am very active. This should be made crystal clear to every PCOS woman; and it should be made really clear that it is substantial exercise that is required, including weight resistance exercise. This has helped me stave off insulin resistance. Many PCOS women become diabetic by their 40s and I am determined to do everything within my power to prevent that. As mentioned, I'm now in my 50s . . . so far, so good.

Yet, let's jump back into the time-warp machine again. Around the age of 32, I was told by a new specialist endocrinologist (I'd moved cities again), "You know the diagnosis about not having children is not correct?" Actually, no I didn't. Slowly, day by day and week by week I wondered, what if? What if it was possible to have kids? I stopped taking the Pill and the anti-androgen medication. I also had to coax my then partner, who hadn't been keen on the idea, that maybe we should try for our own family. After some months, it was finally time to see a specialist.

When I was 36, we consulted a fertility specialist and his first-line treatment recommendation was Clomid tablets. I had three rounds of treatment with it, the third round occurring while I was being made redundant from a much-loved job. These tablets caused massive hormonal swings. Combined with the trauma of losing my beloved job, it was a devastating and lonely time.

This fertility expert wanted to fast-track me for IVF treatment. I wasn't so sure, and I sought a second opinion from a female fertility specialist. She suggested a laparoscopy first, to check my tubes and to carry out ovarian diathermy, if she thought it appropriate. This operation revealed previously undiagnosed endometriosis and it took three hours to cut it out. No wonder the Clomid didn't work – how could it with all this foreign tissue in my womb? Sadly, none of this resulted in a small bundle of joy; and my partner wasn't keen on IVF and I couldn't convince him to change his mind, so that's where it ended.

I grieved over that for a long time, indeed years. In the months that followed, I would exclude myself from social situations where I knew young children would be; it was a self-preservation mechanism. My partner would counsel friends to be cautious in sharing news about their pregnancies or kids.

Some colleagues knew about my situation and some were oblivious to it, but it's not something I wanted to make public. At a morning editorial meeting, one coworker shared their news of an "unexpected" pregnancy. This child was an "inconvenience" as it meant the dream of a foreign posting would have to go on hold for a couple of years. Somehow I held it together to avoid a total meltdown in the office. I snuck away to the women's toilet and bit my bottom lip, hoping my quivering chin wouldn't give me away ... fancy that, the inconvenience of another child? If only I could have just one.

It's important to note three out of four PCOS women will have their own children. Many will need some form of assistance, but exercise and weight loss are the best ways to restore fertility in women. Women shouldn't believe the myth that PCOS women are infertile. In my case, that is true, but many women who've relied on this "fake" advice as their form of contraceptive have found consequence weighs about 2 kilos and sometimes cries and smiles. That might be a welcome result for many, and for some it might not.

It was no surprise to read some years ago about a study that found PCOS women experience the same level of anxiety as breast cancer patients. Many of us live the social taboos of being fat, hairy and infertile in a society that idolizes thin, hair-free, pimple-free, childbearing women.

During the 2000s, I served on the board of the volunteer-run Australian PCOS patient support and advocacy group: PCOS Awareness Association (POSAA). Frustrated by frequent stories about women being misdiagnosed or undiagnosed for years, I thought something needed to change. From 2005, I started a letter-writing campaign, peppering MPs, health experts and medical groups with letters, calls and visits about the need for nationally agreed guidelines on diagnosing and treating PCOS. I argued there was an urgent need among GPs and the broader community to know this syndrome existed, together with agreed guidelines on managing the various symptoms. I was also spurred into action because too many women were using "Dr. Google" for information and clinging to highly questionable sources and websites as their guidance for treatment. I was joined in this effort by Lucy Wicks, who was then a little-known telco executive; she is now an MP in Federal Parliament. We included in our "letter-bombing" campaign Professor Helena Teede, Professor Rob Norman and Professor Gab Kovacs. Lucy and I knew it might be a long campaign, requiring years not months. In 2009, the Federal Government led by a female health minister, Nicola Roxon, announced it would fund a research alliance to consult and craft national PCOS guidelines. These became a reality in September 2011.

At times, having PCOS can seem like you're in a dark and lonely place; but friendships with other

PCOS women have been liberating in escaping that isolation. Knowing you are not alone is a relief. Yoga has also helped restore some balance and calm in my life. PCOS is not me. Yes I have it, but I won't let it define me. I think having the syndrome has made me the determined, stoic and pragmatic journalist I am. If I can endure this, I can endure just about anything and anyone.

I wish more women had access to holistic care, places where they can receive advice on treating their symptoms, along with diet and exercise guidance and counseling all in one place. Sometimes it is no wonder many resort to "Dr. Google" for information. Consultations in 15- and 30-minute blocks are not enough to make clear to patients that behavioral and lifestyle change are absolutely essential in becoming healthy and happy. Women need explicit, lengthy advice, including the caution that it may take many months and some experimentation with medications and exercise to discover what key combination will work for them. Every patient needs a specially tailored plan and that might require some time to discover exactly what the winning combination is. Early on, I was advised to avoid stress, alcohol and shift work to enable a "good balance" in my life to help get symptoms under control. My response was, "I'm a journalist, all those things are part of my life and that's probably not going to happen."

Unfortunately, there is no magic pill. Maybe one day there might be. For now, though, a woman's informed choice on what she eats, how she exercises and what medicines she takes – all together – is the best form of treatment in becoming healthy and happy. And yes, that is possible.

Chapter 20

Cancer and Polycystic Ovary Syndrome

Paul Hardiman

The possibility that women with polycystic ovary syndrome (PCOS) could be at increased risk of cancer was first suggested 14 years after the description of the syndrome by Stein and Leventhal in 1935.[1] This report was related to endometrial cancer, an association that could have some basis, at least in women with anovulatory PCOS, who are exposed to estrogen unopposed by progesterone, which when used as menopausal therapy was shown to increase the risk of endometrial cancer.[2] Based on the same mechanism, there could theoretically be an association between PCOS and cancers of breast and ovary.

However, more than 70 years after the risk of cancer in women with PCOS was first considered, conclusive evidence is still not available. Some of the reasons for the lack of robust evidence (imprecise diagnostic criteria for PCOS and confounding effects of obesity) apply equally to other possible long-term morbidities in women with PCOS. Moreover, many of the studies are case series, case repots or (at best) cohorts reliant on population data to calculate incidence ratios. Most scientific attention has been directed at the risk of endometrial cancer, but we will also review the evidence for breast and ovarian malignancy. The chapter will conclude with a review of the mechanisms that might contribute to neoplastic change in the endometrium of women with PCOS.

Endometrial Cancer

The seminal studies to investigate a potential association between endometrial cancer and PCOS and those that followed are summarized in Table 20.1.

An association between PCOS and endometrial carcinoma was first suggested in a case series by Speert in 1949.[3] Two years later, Dockerty

and colleagues published another case series of 36 women aged less than 40 with endometrial cancer. [4] Fourteen of the subjects had cystic ovaries but histology was not available in eight. Six year later, Dockerty coauthored a study that described 43 patients with Stein-Leventhal syndrome (PCOS). [5] Sixteen of these women were identified by examining surgical specimens removed from a group of several thousand patients with endometrial cancer. The remaining 27 patients were women with a confirmatory ovarian biopsy and symptoms of Stein-Leventhal syndrome. Endometrial tissue was available for examination in only 15 of these cases. Thirteen samples showed "thickening," two were atrophic, but there were no reported cases of endometrial carcinoma. The authors concluded that "our most important observation in Stein-Leventhal syndrome concerns the complication of endometrial carcinoma," despite the fact that the study design did not allow comparison of the risk in PCOS women with that in women who did not have the syndrome or even that in the general population.

In some later studies, polycystic ovarian morphology was used as a surrogate for PCOS. It is likely therefore that around half the subjects in these studies did not have the clinical syndrome. In 1979, Ramzy and Nisker assessed ovarian morphology in 15 patients aged less than 40 with endometrial cancer, 25 from women with PCOS and 21 aged-matched controls.[6] The results showed that the ovaries of patients with endometrial adenocarcinoma were more similar to normal ovaries than to polycystic ovaries (11.1% of ovaries of the endometrial cancer group having features suggestive of polycystic ovarian disease). However, the results only just reached levels of statistical significance. In 1984, Gallup and Stock reported the prevalence of histological features of polycystic ovaries in women treated for endometrial cancer.[8] The prevalence in the patients

Table 20.1 Studies investigating the association between endometrial cancer and PCOS

Authors	Study design	Participants	Findings	Comments
Speert 1949[3]	Case series	14 women under 40 years with endometrial carcinoma	8 with cystic and 1 with sclerotic ovaries	No controls
Dockerty et al. 1951[4]	Case series	36 women under 40 years with endometrial carcinoma	14 with cystic ovaries (no histology in 8)	No controls
Jackson and Dockerty 1957[5]	Case series	"many thousands" of endometrial cancer cases Cross-sectional	16 women with PCOS	No evidence of association
Ramzy and Nisker 1979 [6]		Case-control endometrial cancer, 25 from women with PCOS, 21 from	27 women with PCOS on biopsy	None had endometrial carcinoma
			15 ovaries from cases of cases more similar to the normal than to PCOS	Ovaries from endometrial carcinoma No evidence of association
Coulam et al. 1983[7]	Retrospective cohort	1270 women with chronic anovulation	SMR for endometrial carcinoma 3.1	No data for women with PCOS
Gallup and Stock 1984 [8]	Case series	111 cases of endometrial cancer	PCOS in 31.2% of women under 40, 2.3% over 40	No controls
Dahlgren et al. 1991[9]	Case-control	147 cases of endometrial cancer; 409 controls	Increased hirsutism in cases with endometrial cancer	No data for PCOS
Escobedo et al. 1991 [10]	Case-control	399 cases of endometrial cancer; 3040 controls	OR 4.2 for "ovarian factor" infertility	No data for women with PCOS
Ho et al. 1997[11]	Retrospective cohort	116 cases of endometrial hyperplasia	Prevalence of endometrial carcinoma not increased in cases with PCOS	No evidence of association
Wild et al. 2000[12]	Retrospective cohort	345 surviving women from Pierpoint cohort	OR 5.3	Obesity a possible confounder
Niwa et al. 2000[13]	Case-control	136 cases of endometrial cancer; 376 controls	OR 1.17	
Iatrakis et al. 2006[14]		Case-control	OR 8.96	

Study	Study type	Sample	Results	Comments
Zucchetto et al. 2009 [15]	Case-control	454 cases of endometrial cancer; 908 controls	Increased risk not statistically significant	PCOS self-reported
Fearnley et al. 2010[16]	Case-control	156 cases of endometrial cancer; 398 controls	OR 4.0	OR 2.02 after adjusting for BMI
Holm et al. 2012[17]	Cohort study	963 women with PCOS	Endometrial cancer incidence 0.1%	Incidence less than general in premenopausal population (0.4%)
Hart and Doherty 2015 [18]	Cohort study	2566 cases of PCOS	HR 22.52 (6.94 –73.14)	No significant increased risk Lack of uniform diagnostic criteria for PCOS
Gottschau et al. 2015 [19]		Cohort study	12070 women with PCOS	SIR 3.9 (2.2–6.3)
Ding et al. 2018[20]	Cohort study	8155 women with PCOS; 32620 matched controls	HR 17.7 (4.9–64.2)	No adjustment for confounder Short follow-up Prevalence of PCOS may have been underestimated

Note. HR = hazard ratio, OR= odds ratio, SIR = standardized incidence ratio, SMR= standardized mortality ratio.

aged less than 40 was 31.2% compared to 2.3% in older women. The rate in the younger women is similar to that found using ultrasound, in the general population so the result of this study is not supporting a much higher risk of endometrial cancer. However, this was a small study including only 117 cases and the clinical utility of data obtained on the basis of ovarian histology is very limited. Polycystic ovarian morphology was also used by Wild and colleagues, who followed up 309 women with features of polycystic ovaries (54%), operating records of women who had undergone culdoscopy, wedge resection or ovarian biopsy (22%) or from hospital discharge records (16%). [12] The study was designed to assess mortality from cardiovascular disease but mention was made in the discussion of seven cases of endometrial cancer (standardized mortality ratio (SMR) was 6.1 after adjusting for BMI). In a cohort study of patients aged less than 50 with endometrial cancer,[21] 6 had features of polycystic ovaries. Pillay and colleagues studied the ovarian morphology from 128 women with endometrial cancer and 83 with benign gynecologic conditions. [22] Overall, the prevalence of polycystic ovaries was similar to that in a group of controls with benign gynecologic conditions (e.g. fibroids). However, in a subset of patients aged less than 50 years, polycystic ovary morphology was more prevalent in women with endometrial cancer (62.5% vs. 27.3%, p = 0.033) than in the controls. The authors concluded that any association between the two conditions might be confined to those who are premenopausal.

In some other studies, the risk of endometrial cancer is reported in women with symptoms associated with PCOS. In a cohort of 1260 subjects with chronic anovulation,[7] the relative risk was 3.1 compared to the rate in the local population. Similar concerns apply to studies reported by Dahlgren (subjects with "ovarian factor"), Escobedo and colleagues (subjects with hirsutism) and a study of histology in women with a previous diagnosis of endometrial hyperplasia.[9–11] In this study, repeat histology was obtained after treatment, which was in some cases progestogen administration and in others hysterectomy. Only one of the women with cancer and three who did not have cancer on the repeat biopsy had "PCOS"; the difference in proportion with the syndrome was not significant. However, this study almost certainly underreported PCOS, as the prevalence

in the 116 women with hyperplasia on the first biopsy was less than 4% (below that found using even very strict modern diagnostic criteria). [11] Thirty-nine percent of the young women with endometrial cancer reported by Soliman and colleagues had a history of irregular periods but only 7% had a recorded diagnosis of PCOS (diagnostic criteria unspecified), which is at the lower end of prevalence found in the general population.[21] Brinton and colleagues reported a twofold increase in a cohort of 2560 infertile women with menstrual irregularity or androgen excess.[23] The result was not statistically significant in those with only androgen excess. A significantly increased risk of endometrial cancer was reported in another case control study. [16] PCOS was diagnosed in those women with hirsutism, severe acne as an adult or irregular periods and those who self-reported the condition. The results showed a significant positive association between PCOS and endometrial cancer, although this was reduced after adjusting for BMI. Significant positive associations were also observed with hirsutism and irregular periods.

Even in those studies that report increased risk in women with PCOS, the syndrome is often self-reported with no defined diagnostic criteria. In a case control, the proportion with self-reported PCOS was not significantly increased in 454 women with endometrial cancer compared to 908 hospital controls; the risk in premenopausal women was not significantly increased.[15] Similarly, there were no strict diagnostic criteria in the Danish cohort study reported by Holm and colleagues.[17] The subjects were 963 women with a "referral diagnosis" of PCOS or hirsutism. One case of endometrial cancer was identified, so the prevalence was lower than in the general population. A very different result was reported by Hart and Doherty.[18] The subjects were 2566 women with a diagnosis of PCOS on a database of hospital admissions in Western Australia. The hazard ratio was 22.5 compared to 25660 randomly selected age-matched women without a PCOS diagnosis. The authors acknowledge that the diagnosis of PCOS was not standardized until halfway through the recruitment period so that some women labeled as having a PCOS diagnosis would not have met the revised definition.

In another Danish cohort study, Gottschau and colleagues identified patients with an International Disease Code of PCOS from the

National Patient Register, but the criteria used to make that diagnosis were not stated. The SIR (incidence of endometrial cancer in the cohort compared with that in the general population) was 3.9.[19] A sub-analysis was presented with significantly increased SIR in those diagnosed with PCOS between the ages of 9 and 29 years but this raises some concerns about the diagnostic criteria as most clinicians would be reluctant to diagnose the syndrome in young girls or adolescents. The subjects in a cohort from Taiwan were diagnosed using nonstandard criteria of hormone levels (including luteinizing hormone, LH), ultrasound or both.[20] The results showed a 17-fold increase in endometrial cancer

Robust (Rotterdam) criteria were used to diagnose PCOS in 412 of the subjects with chronic anovulation reported by Brinton and colleagues.[23] In this subset, the SIR was increased to a similar level seen in those with androgen excess or menstrual disorders but this increase was not statistically significant.

Breast Cancer

Table 20.2 lists studies of the association between breast cancer and PCOS.

No significant increased risk was found (before or after adjusting for BMI) in the 31-year follow-up of the Pierpoint cohort (of women with histological features of polycystic ovaries).[25] The risk was also not increased in the study of women with chronic anovulation.[7] No significant increased risk was found in the women with PCOS reported by Brinton and colleagues, although the risk was increased in those with androgen excess or menstrual disorder.[23] In the studies from Denmark and Australia, the incidence was similar to the general population.[19, 18] Yin and colleagues similarly found no increased risk in a cohort of 14764 women with diagnosed PCOS from a Swedish register, but as discussed in relation to endometrial cancer studies, the prevalence of PCOS was far below accepted levels in the general population, which casts doubt on the validity of the hazard ratios obtained.[24]

Meta analyses by Chittenden and colleagues, Barry and colleagues and Shobeiri and Jenabi did not find significant increased risks of breast cancer in women with PCOS.[26–28]

Ovarian Cancer

The available evidence does not suggest an association between PCOS and ovarian cancer (Table 20.3).

The risk of ovarian cancer was not increased women with PCOS or the larger group with menstrual irregularity or androgen excess.[23] The results of a study designed to investigate the risk of ovarian cancer found no increased risk of ovarian cancer in women with a self-reported diagnosis of PCOS, hirsutism or acne.[29] In a study designed to assess the effect of metformin on the risk of ovarian cancer, Bodmer and colleagues reported the odds ratio for women with a recorded diagnosis of PCOS.[30] The subjects and controls were identified from the UK General Practice Research Database. Although the authors interpreted the results as showing a tendency toward an increased risk of ovarian cancer in the women with PCOS, the 95% confidence interval ranged from less than one to more than four so this cannot be accepted as a positive finding. The study of Danish women reported a similar nonsignificant result.[19] Both cohort studies from Taiwan by Shen and colleagues and Ding and colleagues also found no increased risk.[31, 20] Subjects in the study by Harris and colleagues consisted mainly of women with irregular or long menstrual cycles but included a small number with self-reported PCOS.[32] The risk of ovarian cancer was not increased overall, or in these three subgroups. No increased risk was found on sub-analysis by histological subtype. Women with BMI < 25 and irregular cycles had reduced risk while those with BMI > 25 had no altered risk except in those who had never used the oral contraceptive pill, who had increased risk for borderline tumors. The number of cases on which the latter finding was based is not stated so this might be a type I error resulting from small size.

Potential Mechanisms for Increased Endometrial Cancer Risk

PCOS is associated with multiple risk factors for endometrial cancer. Many of these risk factors are interrelated and exacerbated by obesity, so that it is difficult to assess their individual contribution to the increased risk observed in women with the syndrome.

193

Table 20.2 Studies investigating the association between breast cancer and PCOS

Author	Study design	Participants	Findings	Comments
Coulam et al. 1983[7]	Cohort	1270 women with chronic anovulation	RR 1.5 (0.75–2.55)	No data for women with PCOS
Wild et al. 2000[12]	Cohort	345 cases of PCOS	OR 1.5 (0.7–2.9) 1.3 (0.6–2.80) after adjusting for BMI	No significant increased risk 31-year follow-up of Pierpoint cohort
Brinton et al. 2010[23]	Cohort study	2560 infertile women with androgen excess or menstrual disorders including 412 with PCOS	SIR 0.90 (0.4–1.7)	No increase in women with PCOS or androgen excess alone Significantly increased risk in women with androgen excess or menstrual disorders
Hart and Doherty 2015[18]	Cohort	2566 cases of PCOS	HR 0.91 (0.44 –1.88)	No significant increased risk Lack of uniform diagnostic criteria for PCOS
Gottschau et al. 2015[19]	Cohort study	12070 women with PCOS	SIR 1.1 (0.8–1.4)	No significant increased risk
Yin et al. 2019[24]	Case cohort	14764 cases of PCOS: 3478840 controls	Adjusted HR 0.85 (0.64–1.13)	No significant increased risk No diagnostic criteria for PCOS Prevalence of PCOS 0.4%

Note. HR = hazard ratio, RR = relative risk, SIR = standardized incidence ratio.

Table 20.3 Studies investigating the association between ovarian cancer and PCOS

Author	Study design	Participants	findings	Comments
Olsen et al. 2008[29]	Cohort study	1276 cases of PCOS and 1508 controls	OR 1.1 (0.6–2.0)	No increased risk observed in women with self-reported PCOS, hirsutism or acne
Brinton et al. 2010[23]	Cohort study	2560 infertile women with androgen excess or menstrual disorders	SIR 1.76 (0.91–3.07)	No increased risk observed. Risk not reported in 412 cases of PCOS (Rotterdam criteria)
Bodmer et al. 2011[30]	Case control study	1611 cases of ovarian cancer; 9170 controls	OR 1.63 (0.65–4.08)	No increased risk observed
Gottschau et al. 2015[19]	Cohort study	12070 women with PCOS	SIR 1.8 (0.8–3.2)	No increased risk observed
Shen et al. 2015[31]	Cohort study	3566 cases of PCOS and 14264 controls	HR 1.33 (0.30–5.870)	No increased risk observed
Harris et al. 2017[32]	Case control study	41 cases of epithelial ovarian cancer; 37 cases of PCOS	OR 0.87(0.69–1.10)	No increased risk observed in much larger number of women with irregular or long cycles. PCOS self-reported
Ding et al. 2018[20]	Cohort study	8155 women with PCOS; 3260 matched controls	Adjusted HR 1.64 (0.63–4.27)	No increased risk observed

HR = Hazard ratio, OR = Odds ratio, SIR = standardized incidence ratio.

Body Mass Index

The incidence of obesity in PCOS is between 14% and 75% in different ethnic groups.[33] High BMI was also an independent risk factor for endometrial cancer.[34, 35, 12] Studies have shown that about 57% of endometrial cancer in the USA are thought to be caused by being overweight and obesity.[36, 37] A meta-analysis of 26 studies conducted by the American Institute for Cancer Research, showed that the risk of endometrial cancer increased by 50% for every 5 unit increase in BMI (relative risk [RR], 1. 50; 95% CI 1. 42 ~ 1. 59).[38] In addition, the histologic subtypes of endometrial cancer are mainly associated with obesity. Kristensen and colleagues found that the overall survival rate of type 1 endometrial cancer was significantly higher than that of type 2 endometrial cancer, and high BMI was significantly associated with the increased mortality from type 2 endometrial cancer.[39] The incidence of non-endometrioid subtypes, such as serous clear-cell cancer and carcinosarcoma, were also increased with the BMI.[40]

Adipose tissue is a major source of estrogen in obese women. In addition, the level of sex hormone-binding globulin (SHBG) decreases with the increase of obesity, thus increasing the reserves of bioactive estrogen.[41, 42] After binding to the receptor, excessive estrogen, as a mitogen, can directly regulate the transcription of various proliferative genes and stimulate endometrial proliferation by activating the MAPK and AKT signaling pathways.[43, 44] In addition, the genotoxic metabolites of estrogen react with DNA, which can lead to the accumulation of broken double-stranded DNA, resulting in genetic instability and the occurrence of genetic mutations that tend to cause tumors.[45–47]

Insulin

Insulin resistance and/or hyperinsulinemia are present in around 75% of lean PCOS and 95% of overweight PCOS women.[48] Hernandez and colleagues conducted a meta-analysis involving 25 studies, showing that insulin-related indexes in endometrial cancer patients were significantly higher than those in non-endometrial cancer patients, including the fasting insulin level, non-fasting/fasting C-peptide levels and the level of homeostasis model assessment of insulin resistance (HOMA-IR).[49] Insulin levels are correlated with endometrial cancer independent of BMI.[50] Shah and colleagues found that high insulin levels can not only increase the risk of type 1 endometrial cancer (OR = 45.2) but also increase the risk of atypical hyperplasia of the endometrium (OR = 18.7).[51, 52]

Hyperinsulinemia can also increase bioavailability of IGF-1 by reducing the secretion of IGF-binding proteins 1 and 2 in the liver.[53] After insulin is combined with IGF-1, the activation of PI3 K/Akt and MAPK signaling pathways can directly promote the proliferation of endometrial cells and contribute to tumor induction and metastasis.[36, 54] In addition to the proliferation and anti-apoptotic properties of IGF, its angiogenic effect plays an important role in the development of endometrial cancer. Besides, hyperinsulinemia and IGF-1 inhibit the synthesis of SHBG in the liver and increase the bioavailability of sex hormones, which is thought to worsen hormone-dependent cancers such as endometrial cancer and breast cancer.[55, 56] Also, there is extensive mutual interference between the estrogen signaling pathway and the insulin–IGF axis. Insulin upregulates the activity of aromatase in endometrial glands and stroma and increases the production of endogenous estrogen.[57] In vitro, insulin and IGF-1 in PCOS can accelerate the growth of endometrial cancer cells.[58]

Luteinizing Hormone

Hypersecretion of LH, present in around 65% of PCOS women, has also been implicated in the development of endometrial cancer in women with PCOS. Konishi and colleagues demonstrated overexpression of receptors for LH and follicle-stimulating hormone (FSH) in endometrial hyperplasia (with stronger staining in complex or atypical hyperplasia) and endometrial carcinoma.[59] All 24 patients were 49 years old, but only 3 of the 24 noncontrol cases were documented to have features of PCOS. Of these 24 patients, 15 were less than 40 years of age, of whom 13 had serum testosterone measured. Eight of the 13 (62%) women showed elevated levels of testosterone. Three were in the complex hyperplasia group, two were in the atypical hyperplasia group, and all three adenocarcinomas had raised serum testosterone. Thus none of the subjects aged less than 40 years and with raised testosterone were in the simple hyperplasia group. The authors concluded that the overexpression of receptors for LH and human chorionic gonadotropin (hCG) was a feature of complex endometrial hyperplasia and endometrial carcinoma, developing in younger anovulatory women, including those with PCOS. More recently, Dabizzi and colleagues studied the invasive potential of endometrial cancer and primary endometrial cell lines using invasion and adhesion assays with polymerase chain reaction (PCR) and concluded that LH/hCG regulates endometrial cancer cell invasiveness.[60]

Androgens

Human and animal studies show a stimulatory effect of androgens on endometrial cancer cell lines. Well-differentiated endometrial adenocarcinoma cells maintained a full complement of endometrial receptors for estrogen, progesterone and androgens, based on immune-histochemical staining, radioactive binding studies, reverse transcription and Northern blot analysis.[61] Testosterone stimulates DNA synthesis (similar to the greatest response to estradiol) in MCF7, OMC-2, HEC-59 and Ishikawa cell lines.[62] Using in vitro human tissue culture and a 5α-dihydrotestosterone-treated rat model, Li and colleagues showed that androgen receptor expression is higher in PCOS patients than non-PCOS patients with hyperplasia while AMPKα activation and that androgen receptor and Ki-67 are colocalized in epithelial cell nuclei in endometrial hyperplasia.[63] The authors suggest that androgen receptor-mediated regulation of AMPKα activation might play a role in the development of endometrial hyperplasia.

Dyslipidemia

Abnormal changes of lipid-generating genes at multiple levels, such as transcription, translation, posttranslational modification and enzyme activity, may affect oncogenes.[64] For example, FAS, ACC and ACLY, as well as SREBP1, a key transcription regulator that regulates their expression and activity, can be used as targets to inhibit tumor growth, and the growth of tumor cells can be effectively reduced through corresponding gene knockdown or chemical inhibitors.[65] There is epidemiological evidence that dyslipidemia, a common finding in women with PCOS, is associated with endometrial cancer.[66] Triglyceride levels are also correlated with endometrial cancer. Swanson and colleagues reported that women with the lowest serum triglycerides had a 25% lower risk of developing endometrial cancer than the healthy controls.[67]

Gene and Protein Expression

Genes involved in carcinogenesis (Disc-large homolog 7, drosophila) (DLG7, a tumor suppressor gene) and osteopontin (a secreted noncollagen, sialic acid-rich protein) appeared to be switched on at a much earlier level in histologically normal endometrium in women who did not cycle regularly.[68, 22] Endometrial Bcl-2 expression was higher in PCOS than both the control proliferative phase and the secretory phase.[69] This inhibits apoptosis in the endometrium and plays an important regulatory role in the abnormal proliferative changes of endometrium in PCOS. Elevated levels of Cyr61 (a unique marker of estrogen action), ER a, Ki67 and cFos were found in the midsecretory endometrium of ovulatory PCOS patients, endometrial cancer patients and patients with endometrial hyperplasia.[70] This raises the possibility that Cyr61 overexpression may be an early biomarker of hyperplasia or adenocarcinoma in the PCOS group of women.

Conclusions

More than 70 years after the first report of increased cancer risk in women with PCOS, we still do not have conclusive evidence. The results from numerous studies suggest an association with endometrial carcinoma but estimates of the risk range from 1.17- to 22.5-fold. Increased risk in these women could be explained by chronic anovulation, insulin resistance or dyslipidemia. However, these results are based on studies of women with some symptoms of the syndrome or a self-reported diagnosis and are subject to confounding by obesity, diabetes, low parity, age at first pregnancy and use/length of use of hormonal contraception. Studies of breast and ovarian cancer do not show an increased risk in women with PCOS. There have been no long-term longitudinal studies with robust diagnostic criteria for PCOS.

This uncertainty will not be resolved by further case control studies, the design of which allows limited scope to controlling for the confounding factors and interactions between them. Priority should be given to an appropriately powered prospective longitudinal cohort study. The results of such a study not only will define the risk more clearly but could facilitate the development of screening of subgroups at greatest risk. This is important because there may be primary interventions, such as lifestyle changes and metformin treatment.[71, 72]

For the present, women who have PCOS should be made aware that there is evidence, albeit imperfect, that they are at increased risk of developing endometrial cancer. While multiple mechanisms might contribute to the increased risk, the evidence that unopposed estrogen can induce hyperplasia and carcinoma has led to recommendations that women with oligomenorrhea receive treatment with a progestogen to induce a withdrawal bleed at least every 3 to 4 months. Based on the current evidence, it would seem unnecessary to cause additional anxiety regarding additional risk of breast or ovarian cancer.

References

1   Azziz, R. and Adashi, E. Y. Stein and Leventhal: 80 years on. *Am J Obstet Gynecol* 2016; 214(2): 247. e241–247.e211.

2   Ziel, H. K. and Finkle, W. D. Increased risk of endometrial carcinoma among users of conjugated estrogens. *N Engl J Med* 1975; 293(23): 1167–1170.

3   Speert, H. Carcinoma of the endometrium in young women. *Surg Gynecol Obstet* 1949; 88(3): 332–336.

4   Dockerty, M. B., Lovelady, S. B. and Foust, G. T., Jr. Carcinoma of the corpus uteri in young women. *Am J Obstet Gynecol* 1951;61(5):966–81.

5   Jackson, R. L. and Dockerty, M. B. The Stein-Leventhal syndrome: Analysis of 43 cases with special reference to association with endometrial carcinoma. *Am J Obstet Gynecol* 1957; 73(1): 161–73.

6   Ramzy, I. and Nisker, J. A. Histologic study of ovaries from young women with endometrial adenocarcinoma. *Am J Clin Pathol* 1979; 71: 253–256.

7   Coulam, C. B., Annegers, J. F. and Kranz, J. S. Chronic anovulation syndrome and associated neoplasia. *Obstet Gynecol* 1983; 61(4): 403–407.

8   Gallup, D. G. and Stock, R. J. Adenocarcinoma of the endometrium in women 40 years of age or younger. *Obstet Gynecol* 1984; 64(3): 417–420.

9   Dahlgren, E., Friberg, L. G., Johansson, S. et al. Endometrial carcinoma; ovarian dysfunction: A risk factor in young women. *Eur J Obstet Gynecol Reprod Biol* 1991; 41(2): 143–150.

10   Escobedo, L. G., Lee, N. C., Peterson, H. B. and Wingo, P. A. Infertility-associated endometrial cancer risk may be limited to specific subgroups of infertile women. *Obstet Gynecol* 1991; 77(1): 124–128.

11   Ho, S. P., Tan, K. T., Pang, M. W. and Ho, T. H. Endometrial hyperplasia and the risk of endometrial carcinoma. *Singapore Med J* 1997; 38 (1): 11–15.

12   Wild, S., Pierpoint, T., Jacobs, H. and McKeigue, P. Long-term consequences of polycystic ovary syndrome: Results of a 31 year follow-up study. *Hum Fertil (Camb)* 2000; 3: 101–105.

13   Niwa, K., Imai, A., Hashimoto, M. et al. A case-control study of uterine endometrial cancer of pre- and post-menopausal women. *Oncol Rep* 2000; 7(1): 89–93.

14   Iatrakis, G., Zervoudis, S., Saviolakis, A. et al. Women younger than 50 years with endometrial cancer. *Eur J Gynaecol Oncol* 2006; 27(4): 399–400.

15   Zucchetto, A., Serraino, D., Polesel, J. et al. Hormone-related factors and gynecological conditions in relation to endometrial cancer risk. *Eur J Cancer Prev* 2009; 18(4): 316–321.

16   Fearnley, E. J., Marquart, L., Spurdle, A. B., Weinstein, P. and Webb, P. M. Polycystic ovary syndrome increases the risk of endometrial cancer in women aged less than 50 years: An Australian case-control study. *Cancer Causes Control* 2010; 21 (12): 2303–2308.

17   Holm, N. S., Glintborg, D., Andersen, M. S., Schledermann, D. and Ravn, P. The prevalence of endometrial hyperplasia and endometrial cancer in women with polycystic ovary syndrome or hyperandrogenism. *Acta Obstet Gynecol Scand* 2012; 91(10): 1173–1176.

18   Hart, R. and Doherty, D. A. The potential implications of a PCOS diagnosis on a woman's long-term health using data linkage. *J Clin Endocrinol Metab* 2015; 100(3): 911–919.

19   Gottschau, M., Kjaer, S. K., Jensen, A., Munk, C. and Mellemkjaer, L. Risk of cancer among women with polycystic ovary syndrome: A Danish cohort study. *Gynecol Oncol* 2015; 136 (1): 99–103.

20   Ding, D. C., Chen, W., Wang, J. H. and Lin, S. Z. Association between polycystic ovarian syndrome and endometrial, ovarian, and breast cancer: A population-based cohort study in Taiwan. *Medicine* 2018; 97(39): e12608.

21   Soliman, P. T., Oh, J. C., Schmeler, K. M. et al. Risk factors for young premenopausal women with endometrial cancer. *Obstet Gynecol* 2005; 105(3): 575–580.

22 Pillay, O. C., Wong Te Fong, L. F. and Crow, J. C. The association between polycystic ovaries and endometrial cancer. *Hum Reprod* 2006; 21(4): 924–929.

23 Brinton, L. A., Moghissi, K. S., Westhoff, C. L., Lamb, E. J. and Scoccia, B. Cancer risk among infertile women with androgen excess or menstrual disorders (including polycystic ovary syndrome). *Fertil Steril* 2010; 94(5): 1787–1792.

24 Yin, W., Falconer, H., Yin, L., Xu, L. and Ye, W. Association between polycystic ovary syndrome and cancer risk. *JAMA Oncol* 2019; 5(1): 106–107.

25 Pierpoint, T., McKeigue, P. M., Isaacs, A. J., Wild, S. H. and Jacobs, H. S. Mortality of women with polycystic ovary syndrome at long-term followup. *J Clin Epidemiol* 1998; 51(7): 581–86.

26 Chittenden, B. G., Fullerton, G., Maheshwari, A. and Bhattacharya, S. Polycystic ovary syndrome and the risk of gynaecological cancer: A systematic review. *Reprod Biomed Online* 2009; 19(3): 398–405.

27 Barry, J. A., Azizia, M. M. and Hardiman, P. J. Risk of endometrial, ovarian and breast cancer in women with polycystic ovary syndrome: A systematic review and meta-analysis. *Hum Reprod Update* 2014; 20(5): 748–758.

28 Shobeiri, F. and Jenabi, E. The association between polycystic ovary syndrome and breast cancer: A meta-analysis. *Obstet Gynecol Sci* 2016; 59(5): 367–372.

29 Olsen, C. M., Green, A. C., Nagle, C. M. et al. Epithelial ovarian cancer: Testing the "androgens hypothesis." *Endocr Relat Cancer* 2008; 15(4): 1061–1068.

30 Bodmer, M., Becker, C., Meier, C, Jick, S. S. and Meier, C. R. Use of metformin and the risk of ovarian cancer: A case-control analysis. *Gynecol Oncol* 2011; 123(2): 200–204.

31 Shen, C. C., Yang, A. C., Hung, J. H., Hu, L. Y. and Tsai, S. J. A nationwide population-based retrospective cohort study of the risk of uterine, ovarian and breast cancer in women with polycystic ovary syndrome. *Oncologist* 2015; 20(1): 45–49.

32 Harris, H. R., Titus, L. J., Cramer, D. W. and Terry, K. L. Long and irregular menstrual cycles, polycystic ovary syndrome, and ovarian cancer risk in a population-based case-control study. *Int J Cancer* 2017; 140(2): 285–291.

33 Ehrmann, D. A. Polycystic ovary syndrome. *New Engl J Med* 2005; 352(12): 1223–1236.

34 Lim, S. S., Davies, M. J., Norman, R. J. and Moran, L. J. Overweight, obesity and central obesity in women with polycystic ovary syndrome: A systematic review and meta-analysis. *Hum Reprod Update* 2012; 18(6): 618–637.

35 Onstad, M. A., Schmandt, R. E. and Lu, K. H. Addressing the role of obesity in endometrial cancer risk, prevention, and treatment. *J Clin Oncol* 2016; 34(35): 4225–4230.

36 Calle, E. E. and Kaaks, R. Overweight, obesity and cancer: Epidemiological evidence and proposed mechanisms. *Nat Rev Cancer* 2004; 4(8): 579–591.

37 Renehan, A. G., Tyson, M., Egger, M., Heller, R. F. and Zwahlen, M. Body-mass index and incidence of cancer: A systematic review and meta-analysis of prospective observational studies. *Lancet* 2008; 371 (9612): 569–578.

38 World Cancer Research Fund and American Institute for Cancer Research. *Food, Nutrition, Physical Activity, and the Prevention of Endometrial Cancer*. Continuous Update Project Report, 2013.

39 Kristensen, A. B., Hare-Bruun, H., Høgdall, C. K. and Rudnicki, M. Influence of body mass index on tumor pathology and survival in uterine cancer: A Danish register study. *Int J Gynecol Cancer* 2017; 27(2): 281–288.

40 McCullough, M. L., Patel, A. V., Patel, R. et al. Body mass and endometrial cancer risk by hormone replacement therapy and cancer subtype. *Cancer Epidemiol Biomarkers Prev* 2008; 17(1): 73–79.

41 Simó, R., Sáez-López, C., Barbosa-Desongles, A., Hernández, C. and Selva, D. M. Novel insights in SHBG regulation and clinical implications. *Trends Endocrinol Metab* 2015; 26(7): 376–383.

42 Simó, R., Saez-Lopez, C., Lecube, A., Hernandez, C., Fort, J. M. and Selva, D. M. Adiponectin upregulates SHBG production: Molecular mechanisms and potential implications. *Endocrinology* 2014; 155(8): 2820–2830.

43 Deng, L., Feng, J. and Broaddus, R. R. The novel estrogen-induced gene EIG121 regulates autophagy and promotes cell survival under stress. *Cell Death Dis* 2010; 1(4): e32.

44 Thomas, C. and Gustafsson, J. The different roles of ER subtypes in cancer biology and therapy. *Nat Rev Cancer* 2011; 11(8): 597–608.

45 Cavalieri, E., Chakravarti, D., Guttenplan, J. et al. Catechol estrogen quinones as initiators of breast and other human cancers: Implications for biomarkers of susceptibility and cancer prevention. *Biochim Biophys Acta* 2006; 1766(1): 63–78.

46 Cavalieri, E. and Rogan, E. The molecular etiology and prevention of estrogen-initiated cancers: Ockham's Razor: Pluralitas non est ponenda sine necessitate. Plurality should not be posited without necessity. *Mol Aspects Med* 2014; 36: 1–55.

47 Cavalieri, E. L. and Rogan, E. G. Depurinating estrogen-DNA adducts, generators of cancer initiation: Their minimization leads to cancer prevention. *Clin Transl Med* 2016; 5(1): 12.

48 Stepto, N. K., Cassar, S., Joham, A. E. et al. Women with polycystic ovary syndrome have intrinsic insulin resistance on euglycaemic-hyperinsulaemic clamp. *Hum Reprod* 2013; 28(3): 777–784.

49 Hernandez, A. V., Pasupuleti, V., Benites-Zapata, V. A., Thota, P., Deshpande, A. and Perez-Lopez, F. R. Insulin resistance and endometrial cancer risk: A systematic review and meta-analysis. *Eur J Cancer* 2015; 51(18): 2747–2758.

50 Burzawa, J. K., Schmeler, K. M., Soliman, P. T. et al. Prospective evaluation of insulin resistance among endometrial cancer patients. *Am J Obstet Gynecol* 2011; 204: 355.e351–357.

51 Shan, W., Ning, C., Luo, X. et al. Hyperinsulinemia is associated with endometrial hyperplasia and disordered proliferative endometrium: A prospective cross-sectional study. *Gynecol Oncol* 2014; 132(3): 606–610.

52 Mu, N., Zhu, Y., Wang, Y., Zhang, H. and Xue, F. Insulin resistance: A significant risk factor of endometrial cancer. *Gynecol Oncol* 2012; 125(3): 751–757.

53 Giovannucci, E. Insulin, insulin-like growth factors and colon cancer: A review of the evidence. *J Nutr* 2001; 131(11): 3109s–3120s.

54 Carlson, M. J., Thiel, K. W., Yang, S. and Leslie, K. K. Catch it before it kills: Progesterone, obesity, and the prevention of endometrial cancer. *Discov Med* 2012; 14(76): 215–222.

55 Hoeben, A., Landuyt, B., Highley, M. S. et al. Vascular endothelial growth factor and angiogenesis. *Pharmacol Rev* 2004; 56(4): 549–580.

56 Ibrahim, Y. H. and Yee, D. Insulin-like growth factor-I and cancer risk. *Growth Horm IGF Res* 2004; 14(4): 261–269.

57 Mihm, M., Gangooly, S. and Muttukrishna, S. The normal menstrual cycle in women. *Anim Reprod Sci* 2011; 124(3–4): 229–236.

58 Davis, S. R., Lambrinoudaki, I., Lumsden, M. et al. Menopause. *Nature Rev Dis Primers* 2015; 23(1): 15004.

59 Konishi, I., Koshiyama, M., Mandai, M. et al. Increased expression of LH/hCG receptors in endometrial hyperplasia and carcinoma in anovulatory women. *Gynecol Oncol* 1997; 65(2): 273–280.

60 Dabizzi, S., Noci, I., Borri, P. et al. Luteinizing hormone increases human endometrial cancer cells invasiveness through activation of protein kinase A. *Cancer Res* 2003; 63(14): 4281–4286.

61 Apparao, K. B., Lovely, L. P., Gui, Y., Lininger, R. A. and Lessey, B. A. Elevated endometrial androgen receptor expression in women with polycystic ovarian syndrome. *Biol Reprod* 2002; 66(2): 297–304.

62 Tada, A., Sasaki, H., Nakamura, J., Yoshihama, M. and Terashima, Y. Aromatase activity and the effect of estradiol and testosterone on DNA synthesis in endometrial carcinoma cell lines. *J Steroid Biochem Mol Biol* 1993; 44(4–6): 661–666.

63 Li, X., Pishdari, B., Cui, P. et al. Regulation of androgen receptor expression alters AMPK phosphorylation in the endometrium: In vivo and in vitro studies in women with polycystic ovary syndrome. *Int J Biol Sci* 2015; 11(12): 1376–1389.

64 Currie, E., Schulze, A., Zechner, R., Walther, T. C. and Farese, R. V., Jr. Cellular fatty acid metabolism and cancer. *Cell Metab* 2013; 18(2): 153–161.

65 Swinnen, J. V., Brusselmans, K. and Verhoeven, G. Increased lipogenesis in cancer cells: New players, novel targets. *Curr Opin Clin Nutr Metabol Care* 2006; 9(4): 358–365.

66 Hirasawa, A., Makita, K., Akahane, T. et al. Hypertriglyceridemia is frequent in endometrial cancer survivors. *Jpn J Clin Oncol* 2013; 43(11): 1087–1092.

67 Swanson, C. A., Potischman, N., Barrett, R. J. et al. Endometrial cancer risk in relation to serum lipids and lipoprotein levels. *Cancer Epidemiol Biomarkers Prev* 1994; 3(7): 575–581.

68 Pillay, O. C., Sharkey, L. A., Catalano, R. and Hardiman, P. Endometrial gene expression in women with PCOS. *Human Reprod* 2005; 20: 20.

69 Chen, Y., Wang, Y. and Li, M. Expression of apoptosis regulatory protein bcl-2 and bax in endometrium of polycystic ovary syndrome [Article in Chinese]. *Zhonghua fu chan ke za zhi* 1999; 34(11): 652–654.

70 MacLaughlan, S. D., Palomino, W. A., Mo, B., Lewis, T. D., Lininger, R. A. and Lessey, B. A. Endometrial expression of Cyr61: A marker of estrogenic activity in normal and abnormal endometrium. *Obstet Gynecol* 2007; 110(1): 146–154.

71 Birks, S., Peeters, A., Backholer, K., O'Brien, P. and Brown, W. A systematic review of the impact of weight loss on cancer incidence and mortality. *Obes Rev* 2012; 13(10): 868–891.

72 Perez-Lopez, F. R., Pasupuleti, V., Gianuzzi, X., Palma-Ardiles, G., Hernandez-Fernandez, W. and Hernandez, A. V. Systematic review and meta-analysis of the effect of metformin treatment on overall mortality rates in women with endometrial cancer and type 2 diabetes mellitus. *Maturitas* 2017; 101: 6–11.

Index